□

Reframing Bodies

□

Reframing Bodies

AIDS,

BEARING WITNESS,

AND THE QUEER

MOVING IMAGE

Roger Hallas

Duke University Press

Durham and London

2009

© 2009 Duke University Press
All rights reserved
Printed in the United States
of America on acid-free
paper ⊗ Designed by
Amy Ruth Buchanan
Typeset in Quadraat by Tseng
Information Systems, Inc.
Library of Congress Cataloging-
in-Publication Data appear
on the last printed page
of this book.

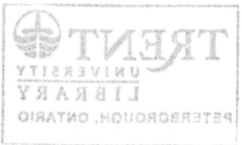

■

To M.B.,

and in memory

of my mother,

Brigitte Hallas

◻

Contents

Illustrations

□

Acknowledgments

In the long process of writing this book, I have benefited from the support, inspiration, and critical input of a large number of people. They have, each in their own way, contributed to my understanding of what it means to bear witness.

The book began as an independent study with Chris Straayer early in my graduate career at New York University. As the project morphed into a dissertation, her deep commitment to my scholarship, coupled with her encouragement to take intellectual risks, has nourished this work all the way to its present form. Furthermore, her dedication to using teaching and scholarship to help sustain queer media from the margins has served as a powerful model for my own practice. Other faculty members at New York University provided vital insight and guidance, particularly those who served on my dissertation committee: Toby Miller was an important early influence on my graduate studies, while Anna McCarthy would consistently ask the right questions, the difficult ones that you dread because you know they need to be addressed. I was also very fortunate to have Ann Cvetkovich and Michael Renov serve as external committee members, given the major influence of their scholarship on this project.

At Syracuse University, Steve Cohan continues to be an invaluable colleague and a wonderful mentor through his cogent feedback, intellectual comradeship, and savvy professional advice. I also received very constructive commentary on several parts of this book from a faculty writing group facilitated by my generous colleague Susan Edmunds. The other members of the group whom I thank include Monika Siebert, Mike Goode, Amy Schrager Lang, Claudia Klaver, Linda Shires, Bob Gates, Gail Hamner, Jolynn Parker, and Sarah Brouillette. My ideas about queer AIDS media have additionally benefited from the students in several courses I have taught at Syracuse University, particularly my undergraduate course, "The Media of Witnessing." Since coming to Syracuse, I have been very fortunate to have met several people—namely, Margaret Himley, Andrew London, and Kendall Phillips—who have proven that intellectual collaborators can quickly become wonderful friends.

Amy Shore, Petra Hammerl-Mistry, Jonathan Kahana, and Frances Guerin all very generously committed considerable time and effort to closely read and comment on various chapter drafts across the years. I am particularly indebted to Frances, with whom I have enjoyed a stimulating intellectual conversation about witnessing and visual culture as we have collaborated as coeditors on *The Image and the Witness* (2007), a book I consider a companion to the present project. Other friends and colleagues in film studies who must be thanked are Patricia Zimmerman, Patricia White, Lynne Joyrich, José Muñoz, Jeff Smith, Alisa Lebow, Bliss Cua Lim, Keith Harris, Denise McKenna, and Ken Rogers. Elsewhere, in the world of AIDS activism, I learned a great deal from Chris Bartlett. One of the great pleasures of working on independent media is the willingness of media makers to discuss their practice with scholars like me. I am thus grateful to the following media makers and activists for our conversations about their work: Gregg Bordowitz, Jim Hubbard, Sarah Schulman, Alex Juhasz, Matthias Müller, John Greyson, Jack Lewis, Robert Semper, Robert Hilferty, and Shanti Avirgan. Numerous other people have helped secure vital research materials, including James Wentzy, Mike Hoolboom, Matt Wolf, Charles Lum, William Yang, Michael Wallin, Ellen Schneider, Basil Tsiokos, Robin Vachal, Dean Otto, Marnie Fleming, Scott Burnham, and Denah Johnston.

The completion of this project has been financially supported by the College of Arts and Sciences at Syracuse University, which provided a semester leave during the revision process, and by the Graduate School of Arts and Sciences at New York University, which provided a Dean's Dissertation Fellowship at an earlier stage in the project's development.

At Duke, I am enormously grateful to Ken Wissoker for his faith in this project. He has sustained its development with his astute judgment and patient generosity. Courtney Berger and Neal McTighe have been wonderful guides in steering me through the production process. Amy Villarejo and Alex Juhasz, the two readers for the press, provided meticulous and highly perceptive commentaries, which have substantially helped me improve the organization and argument of the book.

The long journey that was the writing of this book could not have been completed without the personal encouragement of family and friends, including Ingrid Hallas, Jenny Ward, Mary and Jay Brightman, Lizzie Horn, Shawn Shimpach, Jessica Scarlata, and Nitin Govil. Moreover, I would not have been able to begin my academic career in the United States if it were not for the financial and personal support of my parents, Tony and Brigitte Hallas. It was my mother who first opened my eyes to how cinema could bear witness to historical trauma when we watched together Claude Lanzmann's Shoah over several nights on British television in the late 1980s. Her ethical response to the film engendered a powerful process of coming to terms with the legacy of her childhood in Nazi Germany. She always retained a deep ethical commitment to others throughout her life, a commitment that continues to inspire me in the years since her death. One of my great regrets is that she is not able to witness the publication of this book.

My deepest gratitude must go to Matthew Fee, for all his love, wisdom, and care. We have been together for as many years as it has taken me to complete this project, so he must be credited as its most ardent advocate, especially at those moments at which I have myself felt doubt about it. He has patiently and with infinite grace listened to my fears and frustrations, nurtured my love of cinema with his brilliant analytical eye, and quietly revealed his own profound sagacity to me. Thank you, my cinematic soul mate.

□

Introduction

If I'm dying from anything—I'm dying from the fact that not enough rich, white, heterosexual men have gotten AIDS for anybody to give a shit. You know, living with AIDS in this country is like living in the twilight zone. Living with AIDS is like living through a war which is happening only for those people who happen to be in the trenches. Every time a shell explodes, you look around and you discover that you've lost more of your friends, but nobody else notices.
—VITO RUSSO, "Why We Fight"

I would say, that in this horrible, selfish, dishonest, "private" social moment, the kind of "activism" based on an ethic that people are responsible for how others act and how they are treated is pretty much impossible. . . . I'm glad I witnessed the gorgeousness of ACT UP so that I know that it is right and possible to intervene on behalf of others. But I don't expect to see a moment like that right now. The status quo on AIDS is a consequence of this moment. It will change and this change requires a different counter-culture of personal values. I believe that it will come, and *talking about it is part of making it possible*—even if the timeline of change is a long one.
—SARAH SCHULMAN, "Gentrification of the Mind"

Attending Fever in the Archive, a retrospective of AIDS activist videos from the 1980s and 1990s at the New York Guggenheim in December 2000, I was struck by a bitter irony framing the context in which the work was shown.[1] When I arrived at the museum, a crowd was thronging around the ticket counter. I felt a pang of excitement at the possibility of a substantial audience for the screening, coupled with a twitch of anxiety that it might actually be already sold out. Waiting in line, I soon recognized my initial misconception. Wrapped up in its expensive winter wear and completely ignorant of the screenings, the bourgeois crowd around me was vying to get into the blockbuster show on the designer Giorgio Armani.

In the relatively small audiences of the screenings I attended, I recognized mostly the familiar faces of the downtown independent queer media scene. While this small community of viewers tucked away in the museum's basement worked through our memories of a painfully exigent, but in many ways empowering, historical moment, the oblivious crowds upstairs enjoyed a hugely popular show celebrating a designer whose fashion epitomized the conspicuous consumption of the Reagan-Bush era. The twilight zone that Vito Russo famously invoked in his keynote speech at an ACT UP (AIDS Coalition to Unleash Power) rally in 1988 had returned to haunt the historical moment of the retrospective, a reminder of what Douglas Crimp has called "the incommensurability of experiences" that structures AIDS as a historical trauma.[2] Public indifference to queer people's experience of the AIDS epidemic as a collective trauma was yet again exacerbating the latter's magnitude. Yet in her testimonial to the "gloriousness of ACT UP," Sarah Schulman reminds us that our collective memory is as open to the utopian impulse of hope as it is to the act of mourning. This book takes heed of Schulman's advice.

The conditions under which I rewatched videos from Fever in the Archive in the New York Public Library as I was finishing this book in 2007 intensified the sense of disjuncture that I experienced during the Guggenheim screenings. With over six hundred tapes, the New York Public Library holds the largest collection of AIDS activist videos in the world, a collection initiated by the film archivist Jim Hubbard in the late 1990s.[3] Since the videos are held by the Manuscripts and Archives Division, potential viewers can only see them in the rarefied setting of the division's reading room with its security doors, its pencil-only rule, and wall-to-wall glass cabinets of rare manuscripts. While other scholars silently pored over fragile, yellowed papers from much earlier ages, I sat in the corner next to the room's single video monitor watching images no older than two decades. The necessity to use headphones, so as not to break the silence in the room, engendered a brutal paradox for screening videos made to speak out and act up. Moreover, these urgently produced works of cultural activism created in and for the collective space of a social movement had now become archival objects subject to the individualized scrutiny of my scholarly viewing. The New York Public Library's archiving of these videos has undoubtedly provided valuable institutional recognition of their historical value, but it also admits their historicity as media productions now largely out of use and in need of preservation. Their entry into the archive constituted a process of reframing, but not the first in which they were involved.

Reframing Bodies examines an important group of queer films and videos made between the mid-1980s and the early 2000s in response to the AIDS epidemics in North America, Europe, Australia, and South Africa. This body of what I am calling "queer AIDS media" radically reframed not only the representation of HIV/AIDS but also the mediated spaces in which they circulated.[4] Referring both to the practice of placing a painting or drawing in a new physical frame and to the film technique of moving the camera to alter its spatial perspective, the term *reframing* provides a rich, multifaceted metaphor for the dynamics of discursive appropriation and transformation to be found in these works. Videos such as Stuart Marshall's essayistic *Bright Eyes* (1984) and Gregg Bordowitz's autobiographical *Fast Trip, Long Drop* (1993) and films such as John Greyson's musical feature *Zero Patience* (1993) and Matthias Müller's experimental short film *Pensão Globo* (World Hotel) (1997), were neither mere ideological critiques of the dominant media representation of the epidemic nor corrective attempts to produce "positive images" of people living with HIV/AIDS. Rather, I contend that their significance lies in their ability to bear witness to the simultaneously individual and collective trauma of AIDS. This discursive act required a sustained dialectical tension between directly *attesting* to the medical, psychological, and political imperatives produced by AIDS and *contesting* the enunciative position available to people with HIV/AIDS in dominant media representations, which had consistently subjected their speech to either a shaming abjection or a universalizing humanism. Moreover, the dialectical dynamic of these works reframed not only the bodies of the witnesses seen and heard on the screen but also the relationship of such represented bodies to the diverse viewing bodies in front of the screen. The films and videos that I have chosen to analyze in my book illuminate the specific capacities of these two moving-image media to bear witness to the historical trauma of AIDS. As I shall explain in more detail shortly, to bear witness to such trauma constitutes more than a straightforward representational act, for it must be performed in discursive spaces fraught with the risks of confession, pathology, and depoliticization.

Although some of the films and videos that I discuss in this book have received prior critical attention, it has generally offered only brief considerations of their formal complexity or has situated its analysis in specific generic frameworks that disconnect the individual film or video from other works of queer AIDS media.⁵ Yet for several reasons these works deserve the depth of formal analysis presented in this book, as well as the considerable attention I afford their histories of production and reception. First, it is precisely because of their capacity to hold the complex interplay of political, psychological, and social imperatives in productive tension that queer AIDS media constitute a vital legacy for current and future media practices connected to social movements forged in response to collective trauma. Second, the optic of witnessing also allows me to analyze and connect works usually separated by the critical and institutional distinctions made between film and video, documentary and experimental work, the individual and the collective, the political and the aesthetic. Finally, in bringing the conception of witnessing forged by the interdisciplinary field of trauma studies to bear on this body of documentary and experimental AIDS media, I challenge a number of assumptions in trauma studies that have arisen from the centrality of the Holocaust and the role of psychoanalysis in the development of the field and its theorization of witnessing practices.

The relationship between trauma and time, especially the concept of belatedness, remains a key preoccupation of trauma studies. But the historical trauma of AIDS reveals the limits in directly transposing conceptual frameworks from our understanding of one historical trauma to that of another. Whereas Holocaust studies have stressed the psychic and historical impossibility of bearing witness to the event as it occurred, queer cultural practices of bearing witness to AIDS were widely performed during the traumatic intensity of the gay male epidemics in the global North, affording quite different engagements with traumatic temporality. The psychoanalyst Dori Laub has argued that the Holocaust constituted an event that produced no witnesses *during* its occurrence because "the inherently incomprehensible *and* deceptive psychological structure of the event precluded its own witnessing, even by its very victims."⁶ Cathy Caruth takes such an "inherent latency of the event" to be central to the experience of historical trauma, "a history that can be grasped only in the very inaccessibility of its occurrence."⁷ Within this psychoanalytic understanding of historical trauma established by Holocaust studies, the act of bearing witness thus constitutes the necessarily belated attempt to establish the psychic reality of the event and to thus permit the subject and/or society to work through the trauma. The narrativizing process performed by the act of bearing witness permits the traumatized subject to externalize, and thus psychically realize, the event that her or his psyche, in self-defense, refused to acknowledge during the time it occurred.[8]

A different kind of trauma culture emerged from the AIDS crisis in the 1980s, one fundamentally structured around immediacy and exigency rather than latency and belatedness. As Ann Cvetkovich argues, "Public recognition of traumatic experience has often been achieved only through cultural struggle, and one way to view AIDS activism, particularly in the 1980s, is the demand for such recognition."[9] This trauma culture was not the pervasive late twentieth-century spectacle of helpless, wounded victims criticized by many contemporary thinkers for evacuating a genuine public culture, but "the provocation to create alternate life worlds" (237). Although AIDS activism, like the pandemic itself, was not exclusively queer during the 1980s and early 1990s, gay men and lesbians undoubtedly played the most prominent roles in this emergent trauma culture. Decimating queer lives, the AIDS crisis has constituted a historical trauma for lesbians and gay men, who have suffered illness, death, and loss both on an intensely personal and on a larger collective social level. Individual survival and mutual support demanded an array of immediate responsibilities, including extended periods of caretaking, the negotiation of inadequate healthcare and social services, the distribution of life-saving treatment information, the development of community-based prevention practices, political mobilization against discrimination, and a cultural politics of representation.

By the turn of millennium, the struggle of queer AIDS activism and its cultural production had shifted to the need for its preservation and archiving in the face of the increasing threat of oblivion. Even the queer independent media scene had shown fatigue over AIDS for a number of years by the turn of the millennium. For instance, submissions of new work about HIV/AIDS to lesbian and gay film festivals had been declining since the mid-1990s.[10] In fact, by the late 1990s, it had become a critical commonplace among many gay and lesbian intellectuals in the global North that "no one talks about AIDS anymore."[11] The combination of countless deaths, emotional and political burnout after almost two decades of illness and loss, the growing perception of HIV/AIDS as now a chronic manageable disease under newly developed antiretroviral combination therapies (ARVs), and the less combative political environment of the mid-1990s all appeared to contribute to this waning of interest in AIDS. After almost two decades during which dominant media representation figured the person with HIV/AIDS as the deviant other against which the normative general public could be posited, advertising for the new antiretroviral drugs now invited people with HIV/AIDS to join that general public as a targeted consumer demographic. In their invocation of an affirmative, well-regimented lifestyle, the bodies presented in such advertisements were barely distinguishable from the normative body of contemporary fitness culture.[12] However, the reality of the situation was far more complicated. A number of gay writers, such as Andrew Sullivan and Eric Rofes, called for the recognition of a post-AIDS era. While Sullivan, a gay conservative commentator, understood this to mean the end of the AIDS epidemic (at least for the privileged citizens of the global North like himself who have access to ARVs), the community activist Rofes used the term to advocate for a shift in HIV prevention and in gay men's healthcare, which would take account of the change in gay communities away from perceiving AIDS as an ongoing emergency.[13]

But the normalization of AIDS in the global North has not brought an end to discourses that pathologize gay men and people living with HIV/AIDS. In fact, one of the key divisive strategies of the emergent gay Right in the United States has been to lecture gay men on their need to "grow up" and "be responsible" in the face of AIDS.[14] The implicit message is clear: give up the "infantile" habits of an obsolete sexual permissiveness and embrace the "maturity" of assimilation into the normative. Since the virulent pathologization of gay men's lives that defined the initial media reporting of AIDS in the United States during the early 1980s, several further waves of gay moralism have resuscitated figures from that archive of pathology and abjection. In the mid-1990s, calls by several gay commentators, such as Gabriel Rotello and Michelangelo Signorile, for gay men, especially HIV-positive ones, to take "sexual responsibility" played right into the Rudy Giuliani administration's efforts to clean up Times Square and erase New York City's vibrant culture of public sex.[15] More recently, pathologizing moralism has again resurfaced in the mainstream coverage of rising HIV seroconversion rates and the crisis around crystal methamphetamine addiction among gay men. Found in widely disseminated and discussed publications, such as Rolling Stone, the New York Times Magazine, and the New Yorker, these articles share an ethnographic fascination that recalls the initial reporting of AIDS in the early 1980s, in which journalists reported on their journeys into the "heart of darkness" of a hidden sexual underworld flush with the "deviant" behaviors of crystal meth addiction, barebacking (unprotected anal sex), and bug chasing (intentional HIV seroconversion).[16]

An equally hysterical approach to the complexities of HIV prevention for gay men in the post-AIDS era could be found in The Gift (2003), a widely discussed documentary by the lesbian filmmaker Louise Hogarth that remains woefully oblivious to the representational politics developed by AIDS activist video. Aping the audiovisual design of tabloid television programming, *The Gift* relies heavily on sensationalist digital graphics, sound bites, and an ominous electronic score to communicate its alarmist warning about the alleged suicidal tendencies of contemporary gay male culture. This is nowhere more apparent than in the opening credit sequence that includes a digital graphic of an erect, translucent golden penis with a smoking gun embedded within it. Like much of the moralist discourse on HIV infection rates among gay men, Hogarth's documentary consistently conflates the increasingly prevalent and complexly motivated practice of barebacking among gay men with the much rarer phenomenon of so-called bug chasing, in which HIV-negative gay men are presumed to deliberately seek opportunities for seroconversion (potentially for a number of equally complex reasons that *The Gift* fails to interrogate).[17]

Rather than tackle the consequences for HIV prevention of the widening gaps between gay men separated by generation and serostatus, the documentary relies on highly conventional talking heads that work to bolster those divisions. The two young gay men interviewed as case studies in bug chasing, Kenboy and Doug, are continuously placed in individualizing confessional frameworks that allow their speech to be framed by the authoritative discourse of expert witnesses (clinicians) and a "panel conversation" of older HIV-positive gay men, who berate the ignorance and irresponsibility of young gay men like Doug and Kenboy, but without ever being given the opportunity to speak directly to them. Many gay and lesbian film festivals programmed *The Gift* in the hope of stimulating a critical debate about the state of HIV prevention for gay men. But the sensationalist tenor of the documentary proved far more successful in gaining the attention of dominant media channels and conservative blogs, where the misconceptions, elisions, and pathologizing moralism of *The Gift* were significantly amplified.[18] When the ongoing challenges for gay men in the post-AIDS era are represented by such forms of gay moralism that have internalized the toxic ideology of dominant AIDS representation, it is clearly time to recall and recover the testimonial legacy of queer AIDS media from the 1980s and 1990s.

The very notion of a post-AIDS era continues, however, to be disputed, not only in the context of the mushrooming global AIDS pandemic (where it becomes an obscene notion) but also in the context of the antiretroviral drugs themselves, which have considerable side effects (especially heart disease) and unknown long-term effects and to which there is the growing problem of drug resistance. Yet it is now clear that a specific historical period of the AIDS pandemic ended in the mid-1990s and became part of its history. That era, which encompassed barely a decade, produced not only the radicalization of AIDS activism by groups like ACT UP and AIDS Action Now but also an incredible body of AIDS cultural activism that helped to sustain, inspire, and at times criticize such radicalism.

Crimp coined the term AIDS *cultural activism* to describe forms of cultural production dedicated to the critical rethinking of AIDS in terms "of language and representation, of science and medicine, of health and illness, of sex and death, of the public and private realms."[19] It is the loss of this type of activism that so many lesbians and gay men mourn when they lament the absence of discussion about AIDS—for instance, the empowering mutuality of ACT UP demonstrations, the graphic art of collectives like Gran Fury and General Idea, the conceptual installations of Felix Gonzalez-Torres, or the politicized performance art of Ron Athey and Tim Miller.[20] However, the significance of that historical period in AIDS activism and queer cultural production continues to be felt well beyond the communities and organizations from which it emerged, whether it be in the culture-jamming and queering appropriation of anticorporate activism, the decentered alternative networks of Indymedia, the public address of locative media art, or the proliferating use of moving-image technologies in mediated acts of witnessing, exemplified by the human rights organization WITNESS.[21] AIDS activism and its cultural production also continue, but in a landscape that has undergone significant medical, psychic, political, and cultural transformations.

As major contributors to AIDS cultural activism, queer media makers produced an extraordinary body of films and videos during this key period of the pandemic in North America, Europe, and Australia. Independent, local and often artisanal productions, these works came out of New York, San Francisco, Los Angeles, Toronto, Sydney, and London, the epicenters of the gay epidemic, as well as from a network of long-established lesbian and gay communities that together facilitated a transnational queer counterpublic within which these works could circulate.[22] Within this counterpublic, both the makers themselves and queer critics and scholars rigorously discussed these works.[23] In fact, AIDS cultural activism of the late 1980s and early 1990s engendered a politicized community, at once local and transnational, in which the distinctions between activists, artists, and critics became increasingly fluid. In the present work, I return to this rich period of queer AIDS media from the historical position of afterward not only to assess the productions' historical importance but also to interrogate how time has transformed them.

To what do these works now bear witness in this different historical moment of the AIDS pandemic? How should we understand their relation to the much smaller body of queer AIDS media produced in the global North since the mid 1990s? And what value may they hold for the burgeoning global AIDS activist movement? My discussion of videos from and about South Africa becomes central to this latter question, given that country's recent intersection of highly active social movements around gay rights and the global AIDS crisis.[24]

This book is neither a comprehensive history of the representation of AIDS and homosexuality in independent film and video nor an attempt to analyze the entire media output of the social movement of AIDS activism, what Alexandra Juhasz calls "alternative AIDS media."[25] Rather, I delineate and analyze queer AIDS media as an important strand of both AIDS cultural activism and alternative AIDS media. They are documentary, experimental, and narrative films and videos by and/or about gay men that, in the face of the "crisis of representation" engendered by AIDS, produced transformative means to bear witness to the historical trauma of the epidemic.[26] The AIDS crisis provoked an unprecedented level of alternative media output, with hundreds of films and videos produced by diverse makers with different purposes in a multiplicity of economic and cultural contexts. After viewing over 150 films and videos for the landmark compilation *Video against AIDS* (1989), John Greyson delineated nine different forms of "AIDS tapes": cable-access shows for people with AIDS, the documentation of performances, documentary portraits, experimental critiques of mass media, prevention tapes, promotional tapes for service organizations, safer-sex videos, activist videos, and treatment-information tapes.[27] Moreover, thousands of hours of unused video footage shot at demonstrations, meetings, performances, and other political and cultural events have been stored in archives, warehouses, and apartments.[28] But do all these moving images bear witness to the AIDS epidemic? On a certain level they do, in the sense that all these works and all this footage were driven by an underlying testimonial demand for recognition by those most directly affected by AIDS, articulating a sense of "I'm here, I count."[29] However, in this book I focus my critical attention on queer films and videos that explicitly structure themselves as mediated acts of bearing witness through the development of a testimonial address to the viewer. These works achieve such an address by reframing the intersubjective space between the speaking subject and the listening viewer through a range of formal strategies that include self-reflexive performance, hand-held cinematography, doubled autobiographical subjects, musical spectacle, found footage, and sound design. Queer AIDS media are therefore not merely media of direct address but of direct address reframed. Before examining this process of reframing more closely, we must first consider the discursive complexity of bearing witness as a speech act and precisely how it may be performed through moving-image media.

Bearing Witness

Constructed across several discursive fields including law, psychoanalysis, history, and religion, the act of bearing witness provides a conceptually rich prism through which to examine the complex set of queer responses to the AIDS epidemic. Much of the queer trauma culture of AIDS can be understood through this conceptual framework of witnessing, including such diverse activities as the direct action of ACT UP and its culture of graphic publicity, the collective quilt making of the Names Project, the widespread volunteerism among lesbian and gay communities, and the wealth of queer cultural production within the visual and performing arts, including works in film and video. Such cultural practices have often been framed through explicit reference to a discourse of witnessing. For example, William Yang declares in Sadness (1992), his photographic monologue about AIDS mourning, that "I see myself as a photographic witness to our times."[30] Some projects even made direct titular reference, such as Nan Goldin's group exhibition Witnesses: Against Our Vanishing (1989) at Artists Space in New York City, Thomas McGovern's 1999 photographic monograph Bearing Witness (to AIDS), and André Téchiné's feature film Les témoins (The Witnesses) of 2007.[31]

What binds these various acts of bearing witness together is an ethical imperative at the center of each of these performative acts. Bearing witness involves an address to an other; it occurs only in a framework of relationality, in which the testimonial act is itself witnessed by another. In its address to an other, be that an analyst, a jury, or an audience, bearing witness affirms the reality of the event witnessed; moreover, it produces its "truth."[32] Grounded in this structure of relationality, the act of bearing witness in legal, religious, and psychoanalytic discourses necessitates the bodily copresence of the witness and his or her addressee.[33] Indeed, the witness requires an other as witness to hear the testimony, to be present to the speaking body of the witness. The performativity of the act itself, the power of the truth it produces, relies on the condition of an embodied enunciation. The body of the witness thus commands critical importance; it can even risk imprisonment (of a material witness), torture, and execution (of religious martyrs).[34]

To *witness* requires one's physical presence at the event. To *bear witness* (to testify) to that event also requires the physical presence of the selfsame witness at the moment of enunciation. Such reciprocal presences of the body produce the truth value of this particular speech act. In bearing witness to trauma, the alignment of these two corporeal presences in the singular body of the testifying witness provides the necessary enunciative condition for the listener to sense—both cognitively and affectively—the magnitude of the event. For example, the nineteenth-century abolitionist lecture circuit in the United States privileged the testimonial performance of former slaves over that of white abolitionists or the reading of written slave testimonies. The African American bodies present on stage produced the highest rhetorical degree of authenticity and truth to the testimony presented to the audience. Yet, as Dwight A. McBride points out, the enunciative conditions that facilitate such articulation also restrict it: "Before the slave ever speaks, we know the slave, we know what his or her experience is, and we know how to read that experience."[35] Whether in the context of slavery or of the AIDS crisis, the possibility of public testimony may be just as much a disciplinary trap for the witness as it is a liberating opportunity. Behind the promise of cultural visibility and voice for any marginalized group hovers the potential threat that its publicized bodies merely become a confessional spectacle. In recognizing this trap, queer AIDS media developed a multiplicity of formal techniques to enable and simultaneously transform the discursive space of testimony.

The discursive conditions that enable the act of bearing witness show significant parallels to those facilitating the disciplinary act of confession.[36] Following Michel Foucault, confession is a ritual grounded in the relations of power and knowledge. The presence of the confessor—the one who receives the confession—provides the necessary authority through which the confessant discovers the "truth" of the self and therein achieves personal redemption. Whether a priest, a therapist, or a talk-show host, the confessor does not possess power but merely mediates it. The power dynamic in confession is thus *centripetal* in that it is brought to bear on the body of the confessing subject, pulled in by the subjective cause or origin which is its precondition. The transformative effects of this performative act consequently center around the self. Similar to confession, testimony or bearing witness does not escape the dynamics of power. Rather, it produces a *centrifugal* effect with regard to power. The presence of an addressee for testimony functions not as a mediator directing power onto the subject, as in confession, but as a witness who participates in the horizontal dispersal of power onto other bodies, that is to say, in sharing the responsibility for the historical and social conditions that necessitate testimony. The truth produced by testimony is not the privatized and internalized truth of the subject generated in confession, but rather a truth that locates the subject and his or her experience relationally and historically.[37] This critical distinction between confession and testimony illuminates the risks and limitations of the liberal humanist imperative simply to give a voice and a face to people living with HIV/AIDS. They can end up bearing responsibility for the AIDS crisis, rather than the social order that produced it. For example, the recurrent images of emaciated gay men in hospital beds that circulated in the press during the first decade of AIDS often did more to sustain stigmatizing ideological narratives about homosexuality's "innate pathology" than they did to persuade readers to demand a greater political and medical response to the AIDS crisis.

There is a further distinction in the discourse of witnessing that proves vital for understanding both the cultural politics of AIDS representation and the capacity of moving-image media to bear witness. In his exploration of the Holocaust witness, Giorgio Agamben notes that Latin has two words for witness: "The first word, testis, from which our word 'testimony' derives, etymologically signifies the person who, in trial or lawsuit between two rival parties, is in the position of a third party (*terstis). The second word, superstes, designates a person who has lived through something, who has experienced an event from beginning to end and can therefore bear witness to it."[38] The witness as testis derives enunciative authority from his or her exterior relation to the event witnessed, whereas the witness as superstes relies on his or her interior relation to the event, witnessing it from the inside and surviving it. The witness as superstes is indeed a survivor (superstite). The testis signifies an autonomous, exterior body appropriate for the objectivity demanded by evidentiary discourses such as law and history. These discourses often remain suspicious of the subjective authority claimed by the superstes, whose bodily presence alone can bear witness to surviving the event.[39] The testis responds to an externally generated imperative to bear witness to an event, often received in the form of a summons, whereas the superstes is driven by a subjective impetus to bear witness to the event. The ethical address of the superstes entails a request to listen, to acknowledge, to affirm, and to share the experience of the event, in other words, to bear witness to the witness, to become a secondary witness.[40] Psychoanalysis understands the performative process of bearing witness for the superstes as a form of transference in which the patient/witness and therapist/listener both undergo a transformation.[41] The witness begins to come to terms with the event, to truly experience it for the first time, while the listener shares the burden and, with it, the responsibility to participate in the struggle produced by the experience of the event. This responsibility offers the promise of transforming the psychic recognition of the trauma into praxis, which may entail political engagement, forms of social and psychological support, or the establishment and maintenance of the event's place in collective memory. Since AIDS cultural activism worked to achieve these specific types of praxis, it is tempting to contrast its forms of *superstes* witnessing to the *testis* witnessing of dominant AIDS representation, which persistently took the enunciative position of an observer witnessing the AIDS crisis from the outside. However, such a neat binary not only helps sustain the ideological distinction between the general population and the infected other but also overlooks the complicated relations of difference within AIDS cultural activism itself. Each index of difference became tied up in the interplay between supposedly internal and external enunciative positions: the infected and the uninfected, the dying and the living, gay men and lesbians, older and younger generations of gay men, white queers and queers of color, the insured and the uninsured, members and nonmembers of ACT UP, urban epicenters and elsewhere, North America and Europe, the global North and South. My analysis of queer AIDS media thus illuminates how their witnessing practices necessarily involved multiple and shifting positions of enunciation and address.

Since the conception of witness as *testis* — or external witness — is grounded in a human act of visual perception, it has provided the principal framework for understanding how images may bear witness.[42] To witness in this sense is to register a visual perception, producing a cognitive trace, a memory of the event, which may be accessed at a later date in an evidentiary context. The truth value of such eyewitness testimony relies on the production of a credible witness through the verification of his or her objectivity and competence.[43] Testimonial objectivity arises from the corroboration of the witness's disinterest in and autonomy from the event and its participants; testimonial competence depends on a demonstration of the witness's human ability to perceive and recall accurately. For example, the witness to an assault who testifies in a legal trial will potentially compromise his or her reliability as witness if it is discovered that he or she was earlier involved in an argument that eventually prompted the assault or that he or she was drunk at the time.

In this framework, the camera, with its "instrumentality of a nonliving agent," came to be popularly understood as a type of witness, and this notion continues to shape the professional rationale of photojournalism.[44] The indexical relationship in photography between the event and its representation necessitates the camera's physical presence, as with the human witness, at the scene of the event. The objective credibility of the human and the camera witness relies on the belief that this imprint of the event is a process of passive registration by the human mind and the photosensitive film. The registration of the event is of course mediated in both cases by the interpretative work of the human mind. The human witness relies on his or her mind to make sense of the visual impressions received through the eye, while the camera witness depends on its human operator to decide where, when, and how to register the event photographically.

For a human witness to testify, to bear witness to what he or she has externally witnessed, an act of perception must be transformed into a speech act; mediated by human memory, visual perception thus becomes verbal enunciation. How, then, may we understand the process by which a camera-produced image bears witness? For such an image to bear witness to the event it has "captured," it must rely on an external human agency to name in language the event for which it provides visual evidence.[45] The fate of the Rodney King video in the courtroom demonstrates the problematic significance of this linguistic component. The jury decided to accept the defense attorneys' naming of the event witnessed by the video camera, rather than the one offered by the prosecutors. The verdict thus derived from the belief among jurors that the camera witnessed the pacification of a violent suspect rather than the violent subjugation of a citizen. Similar problems arise with much mainstream documentary media that claim to bear witness to the AIDS pandemic. Disconnected and autonomous from the social and historical world it seeks to represent, the external witness of the camera produces visual evidence of the pandemic that largely depends for its meaning and significance on the framing discourse of its exhibition or dissemination (for example, its voice-over commentary or its title captions) and on its intertextual resonance with prior representation. This question of discursive framing has proven particularly important in the documentary representation of the AIDS pandemic in Africa, given the long-standing ideological construction of the continent in the pathological terms of contagion.[46] Observational approaches that efface the presence of the camera and the relationship of the image-maker to his or her subject risk performing a pathological gaze in which the bodily image of the person with AIDS "confesses" the truth of its subject as victim, carrier, deviant, or criminal.

The relationship between visual media and the witness as *superstes*—or internal witness—constructs a quite different visual mode of bearing witness, one in which the articulation of experience as a form of embodied knowledge supersedes the production of evidence as a form of disinterested knowledge. As this sense of bearing witness does not center on generating objective evidence, its employment of the visual image does not require the indexicality of photographic technologies. In fact, it does not require a documentary image at all, although many visual manifestations of such bearing witness do choose to employ documentary techniques. Moreover, the internal witness may be the maker of the image, its subject, or both.

What defines this mode of bearing witness through visual media is the articulation of magnitude in the sense proposed by Bill Nichols, who uses the term to explore the ethical stakes in the documentary representation of traumatic events.[47] Magnitude involves the incommensurable gap experienced by the viewer between the representation of trauma and its referent in the historical world: "The magnitudes opened up by a text are not merely a matter of naming something of profound importance but, more tellingly, of situating the reader in a position where these magnitudes receive subjective intensity" (232). Generating that position entails a "politics of phenomenology" that recognizes the priority of embodied experience, "not as a structure to bracket and describe but as the social ground or foundation for actual praxis" (232). The encounter between the witness and his or her addressee occurs precisely on this ground of embodied experience that can facilitate the registration of magnitude. Nichols stresses how questions of magnitude necessarily run up against the limits of any given system of representation. Magnitude invokes that which exceeds all our discursive frames. Visual media entail processes of representation in which that remnant or trace of magnitude may be viscerally encountered by the viewer. The image always leaves an excess that remains after signification, that which, as surplus, evades the construction of meaning through discourse. But it would be a mistake to treat the revelation of a nondiscursive surplus or excess as the ultimate aim of visual witnessing practices like queer AIDS media. The exigencies of an ongoing historical trauma, such as the AIDS pandemic, demand a communicative functionality that magnitude's excess cannot alone provide. Whether in relation to domestic melodrama or political modernism, film and media studies have often fetishized nondiscursive excess as a radical form in and of itself. But, as queer AIDS media demonstrate, the value of such excess lies in its potential to sustain the embodied experience necessary for the ethical encounter of bearing witness, a discursive act that is itself always more than a mere articulation of the impossibility to represent the magnitude of historical trauma.[48]

The photographic image of the body, a sign that consistently exceeds the process of signification, leaves the most important trace of magnitude. As

Nichols points out in relation to documentary representation, magnitude wields "a relentless demand for *habeas corpus*" (232). Similarly, in the act of bearing witness through moving-image media, questions of the body become paramount. How can films and videos produce the encounter of bearing witness as an embodied experience for the viewer? When may the deliberate visual inscription of corporeal absence prove more effective in sustaining that embodied experience than the visual inscription of the body? How can representational strategies maintain the act of bearing witness as the viewer's encounter with an other and prevent its reduction to an encounter with the other? Queer AIDS media have had to especially engage with such questions since the politics of AIDS representation have revolved so vociferously around the question of the body and its cultural visibility. As audiovisual media, film and video possess technical qualities that can foster the encounter of bearing witness as much as they can forestall it. In documentary practices, the camera need not be the objectifying apparatus that produces the docile bodies of the other; it may function as an active participant in the social and historical world it seeks to represent. Acknowledging the camera as a technological prosthesis, the maker may employ techniques that illuminate rather than disavow the embodied vision of the camera, the maker's relationship to the body before the camera, and the viewer's relationship to that body. In fictional narrative cinema, the actors need not disavow the gaze of the camera nor of the viewer in the service of sustaining the autonomy of the fictional world for the purposes of the viewer's identificatory pleasure; in their use of direct address, actors may extend their speech and their look across the boundary separating the film's diegesis from the historical world of the viewer. Voice-over techniques need not produce a disembodied "voice of God" narration nor a confessional interiority for the documentary subject; they may address the viewer obliquely through a poetic voice that articulates magnitude through the very gap between the heard voice and the seen body. In fact, the space of the moving image, within its frame and in its relation to a viewer, is endlessly open to the possibilities of reframing.

Analyzing queer AIDS media thus requires us to attend both to the speech act performed by the witness in the film or video and to the visual inscription of the body (or bodies) to which that speech act refers, to which it bears witness. For example, in works such as Tom Joslin's and Peter Friedman's *Silverlake Life: The View from Here* (1993) and Marlon Riggs's *No Regret (Non, je ne regrette rien)* (1992), in which gay men bear witness before the camera to their experience of living with HIV/AIDS, the witness's visualized body corresponds to the body invoked by his speech act. That is to say, the men speak of their own bodies. In a memorializing work such as *Sadness* (Tony Ayres, 1999), the relation between body and speech act becomes more complicated. In *Sadness*, William Yang employs his photographs and accompanying commentary to bear witness to the lives and deaths of several gay friends and former lovers. Yet through his own bodily inscription and verbal commentary in the film, Yang also bears witness to his own experience of loss, grief, and mourning related to those deaths. Simultaneously documentary and autobiographical, *Sadness* encompasses both polarities of witness: the external witness/observer of the *testis* and the internal witness/survivor of the *superstes*. Yang is witness to the other and to the self—physically outside illness and death, but inside psychic pain and loss. But the visual testimony of an other's life and death offered by Yang's photographs is born not from the photographer's position as an objective, detached witness (the typical *testis*), but from Yang's position inside the gay community and from his deeply rooted relationships with his subjects. Moreover, to be outside infection and illness marks an especially contingent position for gay men in the era of AIDS. In their similar movement between bearing witness to one's own and to others' experiences, many of the works that I analyze in the present book incorporate structures of relationality that offer an alternative to the unbridgeable gulf between the normative self and the deviant other that has animated dominant AIDS representation. In extending this intersubjective relationality to the construction of their address, these queer films and videos demonstrate how the camera can relate and connect as much as it can objectify. Proximity is as possible as distance.

Reframing Queer Bodies

During the first decade of the epidemic, the high level of cultural visibility afforded homosexuality in dominant media discourses pathologized gay men more than it empowered them. Yet this visibility, which Simon Watney dubbed "the spectacle of AIDS," paradoxically engendered the invisibility of queer trauma that Russo so eloquently expressed in "Why We Fight."[49] Homosexual bodies were put on display as a traumatizing threat to the general public, while traumatized queer lives were discounted.

The fundamental problems of visibility in AIDS representation were substantially played out in the critical reception to two photographic exhibitions of AIDS portraiture in the late 1980s: Nicholas Nixon's Pictures of People (Museum of Modern Art, New York, 1988) and Rosalind Solomon's Portraits in the Time of AIDS (Grey Art Gallery, New York, 1988). These exhibitions proved that the spectacle of AIDS was as much a problem of the liberal humanism of social documentary photography as it was of the melodramatic hysteria of news coverage. Countering the art establishment's critical acclaim for the shows and the alleged registration of their subjects' "true selves," Crimp and Jan Zita Grover argued that the photographs in fact engendered a loss of identity by their subjects.[50] In their isolation of the suffering human subject, Nixon's and Solomon's photographs erased the political and social context to the epidemic, articulating nothing of the historical battles fought over AIDS and its representation. Such photographs perpetuated the assurance of visibility to the general public: the contamination of sickness and death could remain visibly contained in the vessel of the emaciated, dying body of a person with AIDS. Members of ACT UP/New York picketed the Nixon exhibition at the Museum of Modern Art, challenging the dominant iconography of the PWA (Person With AIDS) and demanding access to representation in the public sphere: "We demand the visibility of PWAs who are vibrant, angry, loving, sexy, beautiful, acting up and fighting back. Stop Looking at Us; Start Listening to Us."[51] But, as Watney warns in relation to these protests, "we should not be tempted simply to duplicate the disavowal of the mass media with our own forms of denial."[52]

Queer media makers consequently demonstrated a distinct suspicion toward the ostensible transparency of realist forms in mainstream media, particularly those of news broadcasts and television documentaries, which arguably played the most important role in shaping the dominant representation of AIDS. As a result, queer media makers constructed a testimonial address to the viewer that interrupted particular media conventions, genres, and dynamics. Yet each of them had to negotiate between the imperative to bear witness as directly as possible and the need to interfere with the discursive structures of the kind of mass-mediated representation that functioned to silence, objectify, or marginalize through its ideology of realist transparency. Juhasz points out that the majority of alternative AIDS media in the 1980s and early 1990s in fact strategically appropriated the conventions of documentary realism such as the talking-head interview, the observational long take, and montage sequences with voice-over.[53] She emphasizes the need to consider the integration of realist and antirealist techniques in alternative AIDS media, rather than to continue to dichotomize them as inherently conservative and progressive forms.[54] However, for queer AIDS media it was less a matter of the integration of realist and antirealist techniques than a dialectical tension kept in play between them. Crucial to this dialectic between "the urgency of the said" and "the self-consciousness of the saying" was the ability of such works to reframe the queer body of the AIDS witness.[55]

The imperative to reframe the body of the AIDS witness stems from the question of how, in attempting to bear witness, one avoids being spoken by the dominant discursive regime. In other words, what kind of discursive strategies reduce the likelihood of an audience reading queer people's testimony as confession, as evidence of homosexuality's supposedly inevitable pathology? Jerry Tartaglia's experimental film A.I.D.S.C.R.E.A.M. (1988) illuminates this very dilemma through the continuous reframing of the discourses and the images he appropriates in his short but compelling film. Although the film's ominous, domineering voice-over is read by a single male voice, its numerously reiterated statements shift between a critical description of how homophobic AIDS discourses function and the blunt citation of them: "A.I.D.S. is the excuse to desexualize gay culture . . . A.I.D.S. proves that homosexuality is contagious." The film's primary images amplify the sense of psychological pressure that these discourses exert on gay men: old gay porn footage that has been reprocessed as a negative image, tinted, and scratched. Reduced to a series of abstracted systematic movements, the once liberating rhythms of gay sex now resonate with the indoctrinating rhythm of erotophobic AIDS propaganda.

In this book, I contend that queer AIDS media have resisted the confessional imperative by explicitly reframing the discursive space within which the queer body may speak and the listening viewer may hear. To reframe in the technical sense refers to the cinematographic practice of moving the camera within the shot to change the perspective or orientation of the image. But it is not merely a matter of new elements entering the frame as others recede. Even in the most subtle instances of reframing spectators experience a dynamic transformation of space not only in the image but also in the space between their world and the one framed by the shot. In this book, I use the term *reframing* in an expansive sense to include the range of formal elements and techniques deployed by queer media makers to forge a discursive space for bearing witness to AIDS amid the confessional pressure of dominant media. As I mentioned earlier, these techniques include self-reflexive performance, hand-held cinematography, doubled autobiographical subjects, musical spectacle, found footage, and sound design. The chapters of the book each examine how these six formal techniques and elements facilitate specific discursive strategies for maintaining the dynamics of testimony.

If to reframe may transform the discursive space of the moving image, then it also has the capacity to reconfigure the phenomenological space in which the moving image is implicated. In other words, the media of film and video involve the production of specific interrelated spaces: the space between the camera and its subject, the space of the frame, the space of address between the film and its viewer, and the space of exhibition. The structure and the dynamics of those spaces are constituted by the relationship between the bodies within them. As Vivian Sobchack and Bill Nichols have extensively argued, these intersubjective relations constitute the "ethical space" of film and video.[56] It is within such ethical space that the act of bearing witness can be performed. The corporeal dimensions to intersubjectivity are particularly significant in the context of HIV/AIDS, where the physical relations between bodies can facilitate desire, care, and political action as much as infection, abjection, and violence. The principal achievement of queer AIDS media is, I argue, to reframe the body of the AIDS witness not just on a representational level on the screen but also in its relation to other bodies—in front of and behind the camera, in front of the screen, off screen, and in the world.

Produced by a generation of media makers steeped in postmodern genre hybridity and caring little about the sanctity of medium specificity that consumed the generation before them, queer AIDS media also reframe discursive space by moving fluidly between documentary, experimental, and narrative modes, as well as between the physical media of film and video. Hence I have organized the book around analyses of poetic and rhetorical techniques rather than around a chronological account. The poetic dimensions of these techniques are just as important as the rhetorical ones, in the sense that they aim to transform and reshape discourse (here understood in both visual and linguistic terms), and not merely marshal it through its most effective communicative means. They push audiences to see and listen differently, and in doing so, they allow them to encounter difference differently. In this sense, we can see how they not only reframe bodies on a representational level in the works themselves but also potentially reframe the relationship between witness and viewer. Queer AIDS media push viewers to relinquish their normal positions of narrative identification and voyeuristic mastery in favor of entering an intersubjective space in which spectatorship may constitute an ethical encounter with an other. The viewer can become a witness herself or himself, a secondary witness, with the responsibility that the position accrues.

In positing the possibility of an ethical encounter produced by queer AIDS media, I am not trying to simply override the political value of these films and videos with an ethical one. Queer AIDS media do not function as a kind of individualized moral pedagogy in which becoming a secondary witness to historical trauma is to learn to care for the other or even to recognize a normative moral duty to the other. Rather, my understanding of the ethical dimension to such bearing witness is indebted to Emmanuel Levinas's philosophy and its inscription of the ethical relation at the heart of the encounter between subject and other. In a radical philosophical move, Levinas argues for ethics as the "first philosophy" before ontology or epistemology.[57] Paralleling other post-Holocaust critiques of the Enlightenment and of modernity, Levinas's philosophy stands as a profound challenge to rethink the subject in a way other than as the "ego-logical center of power" that it subsumes in modernity.[58] Levinas contends that subjectivity is formed in the asymmetrical encounter with the other—the other calls or commands us. The ethical self is formed in being *for* the other. I take responsibility for the other without any guarantee of reciprocity; the other's responsibility for me cannot enter the equation, as I then cease to be constituted as an ethical subject, that is to say, I revert to the ego-logical subject of ontology centered in self-preservation and self-interest.

Moreover, Levinas argues that to encounter the other is to encounter the "face" of the other. Because of Levinas's alignment of visual perception with the "ontological imperialism" of the Western philosophical tradition that ties being to knowing, many readers of Levinas have consequently argued that the face is solely a metaphysical trope in his philosophy and that it cannot signify the physical face of a person.[59] Since Levinas continually employs the visual discourse of phenomenology to describe the encounter with the face, despite his continued critique of vision, other readers have remained committed to the understanding of the encounter with the other's face in the embodied, experiential sense. David Michael Levin persuasively argues that this fundamental ambiguity in Levinas's use of the face is constitutive of his project. He argues that Levinas is neither merely literal nor merely metaphorical in his use of the face. Levin draws on the Greek etymology of *metaphor* to clarify his position (words used in a way that deeply moves us, carrying our experience forward into its transformation): "But in this sense of the word 'metaphor' his words are being used literally, but in such a way that they may alter that to which they are referring in the very process of referring. In this way, we can understand his words as quite 'properly' phenomenological, albeit truthful only to that dimension of our experience that they bring out from its ordinary, conventional concealment."[60] Levin ultimately understands Levinas's philosophy as performative since it transforms our experience as it explains that experience. Similarly, the queer films and videos that I discuss in this book performatively transform the mediated space of witnessing precisely as they bear witness. The direct address of their talking heads, for example, achieves its testimonial effectiveness—that is to say, its ethical address to its viewer—through the ways in which such direct address comes to be reframed, both formally, in the works themselves, and institutionally, in the alternative modes of distribution and exhibition in which they have been placed.

The real revelation of Levinas's conception of the other's face is his argument that the face signifies the uniqueness and singularity of the other, its ultimate alterity. Alterity is here distinguished from difference, which ultimately folds back into the "Same" since it is rooted in a binary relation, whereas alterity points to an infinite number of differences. It is in this sense that Levinas can argue that the face signifies both "the Unique" and "the Infinite."[61] It is through these two characteristics that the face of the other can resist the objectification of the gaze that places it within the grasp of knowledge.[62] Levinas presents this encounter with the other as face (unique and infinite) as the concealed dimension of our experience that needs to be revealed. This is precisely where Levinas proves useful to an understanding of the ethical dimension of bearing witness through moving-image media, a process that necessarily involves the reframing of direct address. The high degree of visual mediation occurring in the intersubjective encounter of film or video spectatorship clearly creates problems for any systematic application of Levinas's philosophy to mediated acts of bearing witness through moving images.[63] Yet his redemptive understanding of the ethical encounter between subject and other offers a promising way into a comprehension of how queer film- and videomakers can bear witness to AIDS in a media landscape saturated with objectification and pathology.

The films and videos that I examine in this book employ various reframing strategies of defamiliarization, interruption, displacement, and anachronism to open up a revelatory space for the intersubjective encounter of bearing witness, and they thereby interfere with the objectifying mechanisms of pathology and spectacle, themselves visual forms of mediation rooted in modernity and its ego-logical subject. Throughout the almost quarter century since the discovery of AIDS, recurrent references to "giving a face to AIDS," "the changing face of AIDS," and "the new face of AIDS" have provided a persistent discursive framework of faciality for the mainstream documentary representation of AIDS. Such recourse to the human face has been taken up both by the disciplinary gaze of popular media, eager to identify and pathologize the deviance of infected bodies, and by the humanistic gaze of documentary photographers and filmmakers, who seek to exploit the human face's presumed ability to engender universal identification.[64] By contrast, queer

AIDS media have sought to construct a discursive space in which one may encounter the face of an other without doing such violence to that other's alterity, that is to say, without reducing that other to the humanistic Same or the pathological other through the binary structure of difference. Whether produced by the visage of a talking head or the auditory call of a voice-over, the ethical encounter with the face of the witness—with his or her alterity— is maintained in queer AIDS media through the various reframing strategies that I have described above. In recognizing the alterity of a testifying witness, the viewer of queer AIDS media comes to respect the singularity of that witness, not as a transcendental subject beyond the social and the political, but as a subject embedded in an infinite set of social and political relations—relations that must be engaged in any effective response to the historical trauma of AIDS.

Although I have already mentioned the multiplicity of such an ethical address across various indices of difference (sexuality, gender, race, nationality, serostatus, health, and generation), it is important to recognize how the address of queer AIDS media could also change as they moved across different viewing contexts, from an activist meeting to a lesbian and gay film festival to a museum to a classroom. These moving images traveled extensively and as much within queer communities and networks as beyond them. I can trace this mobility in my own initial encounter with queer AIDS media in 1990 as an undergraduate at Oxford who had just come out in my second term of college. My first boyfriend, Chris, an American graduate student and ACT UP/Philadelphia activist, brought a tape of Robert Hilferty's *Stop the Church* (1990) to show at a regular meeting of the university's lesbian and gay student alliance. Hilferty's video about the notorious demonstrations by ACT UP and WHAM! (Women's Health Action and Mobilization) at St. Patrick's Cathedral in 1989 generated much discussion at our meeting about the ethical and political legitimacy of the radical queer tactics presented by the video. For many of us in the group, the video opened up a new strategic horizon for our own local lesbian and gay activism in the city and the university.

Initially sheltered by the relatively lower (and later) rates of HIV infection among young gay men in Britain and thus, at the time, not personally knowing anyone living with AIDS, I felt moved by the tape to take further action, to respond to its political and ethical address from across the Atlantic. The tape offered an image of queer community at once radical and intimate, as well as a queer identity promising liberation but also responsibility. Along with my relationship with Chris, my encounter with *Stop the Church* and other works of AIDS cultural activism led me to get involved in ACT UP, confirming Cvetkovich's claim that ACT UP constituted an affective public sphere in which emotional investments and personal relations were deeply entangled with political ones.[65] The tape certainly moved me, but not in the straightforward emotional sense that media scholars have long found ideologically suspicious. Infused with anger, political conviction, and camp pleasure, *Stop the Church* produced an ethical address to join the "new" social movement of AIDS activism.[66] It was able to move me with the dynamic of a social movement, that is to say, to draw the individual into a collective struggle for social transformation through the construction of a new identity position. *Stop the Church* proved to be the kind of moving image that both affectively moves and politically mobilizes.

To describe such moving images in terms of *queer* AIDS media invokes the often tumultuous cultural politics of nomenclature. *Queer* is a promiscuously polysemic term, but that is precisely what makes it so useful. AIDS cultural activism emerged in a historical period characterized by the dynamic contestation in lesbian and gay communities over the meaning of the word *queer*. This "queer moment" between the late 1980s and early 1990s marked the convergence of developments in the intellectual, political, and cultural practices of lesbians and gay men.[67] While queer theory sprung from the freshly institutionalized field of lesbian and gay studies to interrogate the epistemologies of sexual identity through psychoanalytic and poststructuralist theory, queer political groups like Queer Nation in the United States and Outrage in the United Kingdom challenged the orthodoxies of identity politics that had dominated lesbian and gay political movements since the early 1970s. In the realm of cultural production, B. Ruby Rich famously announced the arrival of a "New Queer Cinema" in the early 1990s with the independent film circuit's critical recognition of a group of narrative feature films that used formal innovation to repudiate the positive images approach to representation generally adopted by lesbian and gay cultural politics in the early 1980s.[68]

While Rich cited the AIDS crisis as an important factor in the emergence of New Queer Cinema, José Arroyo argued that AIDS in fact constituted its political unconscious, marking the "epistemic shift" in gay culture caused by the epidemic through the depiction of fragmented subjectivities, temporal dislocations, and melancholia in film narratives that elided the direct representation of AIDS (such as Gus van Sant's *My Own Private Idaho* [1991] and Derek Jarman's *Edward II* [1991]).[69] *Safe* (1995), Todd Haynes's miminalist narrative about Carol White (Julianne Moore), a rich white California housewife suffering from environmental illness, is arguably the most sophisticated and complex example of such films, as it critically engages the regime of visuality and queer structures of feeling around AIDS without directly addressing either the syndrome or queer sexuality.[70] Although *Safe* and other fictional narrative films in the New Queer Cinema canon simultaneously interrogated the dominant representation of AIDS and thematically embraced the testimonial imperative of the epidemic (albeit often allegorically), I have chosen, for several reasons, not to incorporate them in this book, nor to utilize Rich's framework of New Queer Cinema.

In focusing on the question of how the mediated space of the moving image can be transformed into a testimonial encounter, I prioritize works that function outside the dynamics of mis/dis/identification produced by fictional narrative filmmaking (the one narrative feature film covered in this book, John Greyson's *Zero Patience* [1993], is analyzed in relation to the direct address of its musical spectacle rather than to its narrative engagement with the audience).[71] I am interested in films and videos that acknowledge an intersubjective space between the screen subject and the viewer, rather than those that disavow it to facilitate forms of identification, whether with the camera gaze or the screen subject. In addition, the film industry context of New Queer Cinema and the scholarship developed around it (with its concentration on theatrical distribution, critical recognition, crossover, niche marketing, and auteur-stars) provide an unsuitable framework to address the multifarious contexts in which queer AIDS films and videos were produced, distributed, and exhibited—contexts in which collectivity, collaboration, and the intermixing of artistic practice, media production, and political activism flourished.

Despite setting aside New Queer Cinema, I do nevertheless want to retain its middle word. As queer theory has amply demonstrated, the term *queer* invokes an appropriative dynamic: it twists, bends, and mutates the codes of normativity, deforming them in the process. Much of its potency as a form of political affect derives from its reclamation of phobic discourse, its playful arrogation of the word as a shaming interpellation.[72] From painful psychic terrain, queer practice mines pleasure. Moreover, queer cultural practices exploit the mutual interdependence of the heteronormative center and the sexual margin, blurring the boundaries that distinguish them.[73] Embodying a dynamic of such interruptive transformation and semiotic recoding, *queer* thus perfectly resonates with the poetic and rhetorical techniques of reframing used by lesbian and gay media makers to bear witness to AIDS. The notion of the "queer moving image" signals the process through which the normative uses of moving-image media themselves become queered. Furthermore, *queer* offers the opportunity to conceptualize community, politics, and cultural production across different identities. Referencing the 1991 arrest of queer ACT UP activists in New York for running a needle exchange program, Crimp contends that "once engaged in the struggle to end the crisis, these queers' identities were no longer the same. It's not that 'queer' doesn't any longer encompass their sexual practices; it does, but it also entails a *relation* between those practices and other circumstances that make very different people vulnerable both to HIV infection and the stigma, discrimination and neglect that have characterized the societal and governmental response to the constituencies most affected by the AIDS epidemic."[74] Queer, in this sense, functions as alterity, that is to say, as an openness to relationality, rather than an index of difference that permits a specific form of identification.

Arguably the most significant of these queer relations in AIDS cultural activism occurred between women and gay men. Feminist body politics and aesthetics proved enormously influential on AIDS activism in both its political and cultural manifestations. Lesbians and other women activists were key players within ACT UP, bringing strategic knowledge about political organizing from their substantial involvement in second-wave feminism, the reproductive rights movement, the feminist sex wars, and other leftist struggles of the early 1980s.[75] Although the term *queer* has now been thoroughly domesticated as consumer style (for example, *Queer Eye for the Straight Guy*), I aim to retain its sense of transgressive relationality across differences. Similarly, I also continue to use the term *gay* to acknowledge the historically specific identities, communities, and practices developed in post-1960s culture that the AIDS crisis has imperiled on numerous levels.

Mourning, Militancy, and the Archive

As the pandemic has changed, so too have the testimonial dynamics of queer AIDS media. The comparatively small corpus of works produced since the mid-1990s has sought fresh means to bear witness to the contradictions of the post-AIDS era. A case in point is Gregg Bordowitz's *Habit* (2001), which bears witness to the economic, political, and affective differences between the videomaker's normalized life on antiretrovirals in Chicago and the lives of South African AIDS activists fighting for access to them. The ethical questions posed by the dialectical structure of *Habit* considerably complicate any straightforward conception of either post-AIDS or global AIDS. In addition to the production of new works, earlier queer AIDS films and videos have undergone a variety of transformations with age. An AIDS activist video made in the late 1980s as a mobilizing tool would become a memento mori by the mid-1990s and an archival object by the end of the millennium. But it would be a mistake to render these historical transformations as a linear progression from politics to mourning to historical memory.

One of the central themes to run throughout this book is the evolving function of the archive in queer AIDS media. From the time of their original production and exhibition, queer AIDS media already articulated the political and psychic exigency of the present moment through a complex engagement with archives that range from the personal and the local to the popular and the official. The concept of reframing here takes on an additional meaning related to time and not just space. To reframe is to transform the present by illuminating its relation to the historical past. The space of witnessing constructed by queer AIDS media has therefore always been inscribed by multiple temporalities. In fact, Marshall's *Bright Eyes*, one of the first documentary works of AIDS cultural activism, examines the conditions of possibility for a person with AIDS to speak within mass media by investigating the discursive archive of homosexuality and disease in modern medicine, documentary representation, and popular culture going back to the nineteenth century. I will be discussing *Bright Eyes* in more detail in the following chapter, but for now, I want to offer a later example by the Canadian experimental filmmaker Mike Hoolboom, *Letters from Home* (1996), which illustrates how a complex engagement with the archive facilitated witnessing dynamics in queer AIDS media.

Made just before the introduction of antiretroviral combination therapies, *Letters from Home* mines old home movies, science fiction B-movies, early nonfiction films, songs by Billy Holiday ("You've Changed") and Leonard Cohen ("Waiting for a Miracle"), Hermann Hesse's *Steppenwolf*, and Russo's "Why We Fight" speech to articulate the specific queer structures of feeling around AIDS at that particular historical moment, one layered with attenuated hope, emotional burnout, and political despair.[76] Immersed in the aesthetic conflicts of the Canadian avant-garde when he was diagnosed as HIV-positive in 1988, Hoolboom was a relative latecomer to AIDS cultural activism, and, as Thomas Waugh notes, one of the first male artists of the movement not to have emerged from gay cultures and communities.[77] Since the mid-1990s, when he began making films that specifically address AIDS, Hoolboom has refused to pin down his own sexual identity, preferring a queer fluidity reflected in the crystalline aesthetics of his films.[78] *Letters from Home* finds its origins in a trip Hoolboom made with his fellow experimental filmmaker

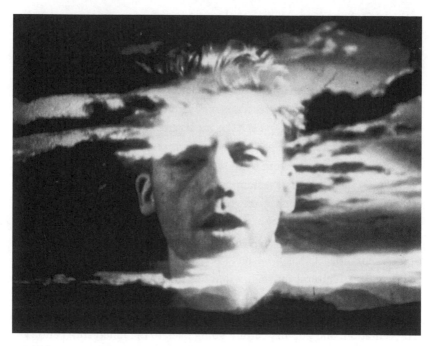

1. Still from *Letters from Home* (Mike Hoolboom, 1996). Courtesy of the artist.

and collaborator Tom Chomont to New York City to participate in an ACT UP rally where he heard Russo speak and first experienced a sense of an AIDS community. Hoolboom decided to use sections of Russo's "Why We Fight" as the foundation for the script of *Letters from Home*, supplementing the political address of its testimony with new material that amplified attention to the physical and psychosocial aspects of living with AIDS.

Hoolboom constructed both sound and image in *Letters from Home* around an aesthetics of fragmentation and dispersal. The text is spoken by a multicultural array of speakers differentiated by sex, ethnicity, and age (mostly Hoolboom's colleagues in the Toronto art scene) and shifts between voice-over and talking head (figure 1). Rather than merely illustrate the spoken text, the images abide more by the logic of a dream, with its tendency toward metaphorical condensation and metonymic displacement. For example, in one sequence early in the film, a young woman speaks in voice-over of the psychosocial barriers experienced by a person living with AIDS: "If I'm dying from anything, it's from the way you look when I see that funny kind of half smile on your face, like you've farted or something. Like there's a bad smell in the room and it's coming from me."[79] The accompanying hand-held shots depict a young woman in various domestic settings but always through forms of visual refraction or interference—orange flare-outs, double exposures, mirror reflections, silhouetted figures, and a facial close-up shot through lace curtain. The brief sequence with Hoolboom himself is similarly marked by visual interference. Superimposed on a shot of waves, he appears as a talking head with words adapted from Russo's original speech, "I'm here to speak out today as a person with AIDS who is not dying from, but for the last three years successfully living with . . . AIDS." Irony frames Hoolboom's testimonial utterance on several levels. Performatively, the pause before AIDS unsettles the affirmation of the line. Visually, the superimposition of the two shots thins out the visual presence of the testifying body that claims to be "here." And finally, on a historical level, the fact of Russo's death in 1990 qualifies the words' attestation of survival—both Russo's words and his death would be well known to queer audiences in the mid-1990s.[80] The rhetoric of combat and survival that Russo had employed so inspiringly in 1988 had become in only a few years a potential means of denying the psychic burden of loss. Letters from Home thus bears witness to the activist affirmation to live with AIDS, but also to the memory of loss and anticipation of death by AIDS that would haunt any such enunciation in the mid-1990s. Previous acts of bearing witness, such as Russo's, would necessarily have to be reframed if they were to engage the testimonial imperative of a new historical moment.

In its deeply ambivalent structures of feeling, Letters from Home engages with the fierce debate among queer critics, activists, makers, and artists in the decade between the mid-1980s and the mid-1990s: What should the function of cultural practice be in the midst of an epidemic? Often crudely reduced to a set of binary oppositions—political/psychological, public/private, individual/collective, active/passive—the debate most frequently focused on the distinction between memorial and activist responses to AIDS in cultural production. In its performance of mourning the loss of friends, lovers, or community members, memorializing work tended to focus more on individual lives and responses to the epidemic. There were notable exceptions, such as the early candlelight vigils begun in 1983 and the AIDS Quilt, in which the collective act of memorializing a large number of individuals in public space performed political acts.[81] But to many activists and artists, acts of memorializing appeared an altogether too passive response to the crisis, even if performed collectively in an ideologically charged space such as the Washington Mall, where the AIDS Quilt was displayed in 1992.[82] By contrast, these artists and activists posited the collective production and function of activist work as moving beyond the expression of loss, as Grover notes, to "make the social connections, touch the anger and harness it to social purposes."[83]

In a highly influential article written in 1989, Crimp warned against the danger in essentializing this distinction between mourning and militancy.[84] Elaborating on their interrelation, Crimp indicated how mourning often becomes militancy for gay men in a cultural environment that consistently imposes a shaming silence on gay male bereavement. Yet Crimp also cautioned against the militant understanding that the social violence related to the AIDS epidemic is all externally imposed, in which case "we disavow the knowledge that our misery comes from within as well as without, that it is the result of psychic as well as social conflict" (16). While deeply aware of the risk of pathologizing gay men in their responses to the epidemic, Crimp nevertheless insisted on addressing this problem of making all violence external, of only objectifying it in "enemy" institutions and individuals. He thus concluded with the call for AIDS cultural activism to acknowledge the necessary interrelation of both mourning and militancy: "There is no question but that we must fight the unspeakable violence we incur from the society in which we find ourselves. But if we understand that violence is able to reap its horrible rewards through the very psychic mechanisms that make us part of society, then we may also recognize—along with our rage—our terror, our guilt, and our profound sadness. Militancy, of course, then, but mourning too: mourning *and* militancy" (18; emphasis original).

The testimonial power of *Letters from Home* lies precisely in the film's embrace of that necessary duality through the very same principle: its fragmentary aesthetic of dispersal. On the one hand, we may read the dispersal of the film's testimonial voice across multiple bodies as the centrifugal dynamic of Hoolboom's response to Russo's political act of bearing witness. We must all become witnesses to the epidemic; we all bear the responsibility to end the AIDS crisis.[85] On the other hand, the film itself is dispersed across many types of images (home movies, archival ephemera, superimpositions, haptic handheld shots, black-and-white, sepia, and color shots) and across many images of fragmentation, dissolution, and disintegration (explosions, crashes, fires, and ghostlike figures). This visual dispersal bears witness to the psychic and corporeal experience of living with (and dying from) AIDS.[86] *Letters from Home* exemplifies how queer AIDS media have consistently approached the archive not merely as the site of cultural and material preservation but also, and more important, as a tool to bear witness to the exigencies of AIDS in the present moment. These exigencies paradoxically include the articulation of its historicity, given that one of the principal traumatizing effects of AIDS has been the difficulty of positing any notion of beyond or after AIDS that does not incorporate death.

❑ In the first two chapters of the book, I analyze the talking head, the most rudimentary form of mediated acts of bearing witness in film and video. As the most prevalent enunciative form in nonfiction audiovisual media, this device performs a substantial function in contemporary disciplinary power, especially given its historical roots in the dynamics of modern photographic portraiture. In the context of AIDS, the conventions of the talking head have reinforced the codified and limited enunciative positions available in public discourse to those directly affected by the epidemic, namely, as victim, patient, sinner, criminal, or caregiver. Chapter 1 focuses on films and videos that use self-consciously performed talking heads to reconfigure the discursive space within which bearing witness to AIDS may take place. Moreover, Bright Eyes, No Regret, Sadness, and Jack Lewis's and Thulanie Phungula's Sando to Samantha, aka, The Art of Dikvel (1998) all challenge the confessionalizing function of the talking head by connecting the historical trauma of AIDS to prior historical trauma, namely, the Holocaust, African American slavery, Australian anti-immigrant violence, and South African apartheid. To permit these earlier traumas to serve as redemptive resources for AIDS witnessing, these films and videos explicitly draw from the cultural archives produced by the earlier traumas.

Chapter 2 continues the focus on the talking head by examining how activist videos produced in the context of ACT UP/New York, such as Stop the Church, Like a Prayer (DIVA TV, 1991), and Voices from the Front (Testing the Limits, 1992), contested the shadow archive of AIDS representation by queering the spatial dynamics of television broadcast news, the most influential medium for shaping popular conceptions of AIDS. These "direct action videos" combine direct address and hand-held camerawork to generate the effect of what I call "embodied immediacy": the urgent, visceral sense of the here and now. This effect situates the viewers' encounters with the talking head in the midst of the public and community spaces occupied by AIDS activists, a position that places them in proximate relation to a community of political witnesses, rather than as detached spectators positioned to look at the activist spectacle from the outside, like television news journalists (and their viewers). My concern in this chapter is not only with the videos' testimonial transformation of mediated space but also with their physical movement through different exhibition spaces. Yet not only the videos themselves moved from one context to another; so did the raw footage as it became reused in new contexts. I consequently examine two such reframings, namely, the memorial tapes made for deceased activists and James Wentzy's retrospective chronicle of the movement, *Fight Back, Fight AIDS: Fifteen Years of ACT UP* (2002), both of which rework the relation between mourning and militancy.

The autobiographical use of video constitutes the central concern of my third chapter, which principally discusses Joslin's and Friedman's *Silverlake Life: The View from Here* (1993) and Bordowitz's *Fast Trip, Long Drop* (1993). In turning the video camera on themselves to bear witness to their experience as people living with AIDS, Joslin and Bordowitz necessarily had to negotiate the idioms of what Jon Dovey has called "first person media," the panoply of media texts committed to the articulation of subjectivity, including talk shows, video diaries, Webcams, and the continually burgeoning genres of reality television programming.[87] First person media are saturated with the confessional imperative, pushing Joslin and Bordowitz to develop specific means to ensure that their autobiographical acts retain the intersubjective dynamics of bearing witness. Both videos create doubled autobiographical subjects, but in different ways and to different ends. Whereas Joslin's sharing of the camera with his lover provides an unflinching bifurcated perspective on living with the late stages of AIDS that resists the confessional trope of the isolated moribund homosexual, Bordowitz creates an alter ego to articulate what has become ineffable for an activist living with AIDS in the early 1990s. The historicity of these two groundbreaking videos becomes even sharper as I close the chapter with a discussion of *Habit* (2001), Bordowitz's sequel to *Fast Trip, Long Drop*, and Juhasz's *Video Remains* (2005), two autobiographical videos by long-standing AIDS activists that rigorously contemplate the transformed structures of feeling of the twenty-first century pandemic.

The importance of space to mediated acts of bearing witness returns in chapter 4 as I turn my attention to how film and video can reframe the performance of song and render the kind of discursively privileged space on which effective testimony relies. I focus this chapter around Greyson's *Zero Patience* (1993), an AIDS musical about Gaetan Dugas (the alleged Patient Zero of the North American epidemic) and *Fig Trees* (2003), Greyson's video opera installation with David Wall about the South African AIDS activist Zackie Achmat. By bringing Dugas and Achmat into contact with several queer historical figures, these works use the incongruity of anachronism to challenge the mythologization of these two gay men in the history of AIDS—Dugas as a villain and Achmat as a hero. Songs become spaces that enact resistance to such roles but keep in tension the affective and political aspects of these two men's lives. I am also interested in how Greyson's movement from feature film to gallery installation reveals the complex dynamics between the *discursive* space produced by testimonial song and the *physical* space in which the viewer encounters it.

The final two chapters of the book ask what happens when the visual inscription of the enunciating witness to AIDS is displaced or resisted altogether. Examining the experimental AIDS cinema of Michael Wallin, Matthias Müller, and Jim Hubbard, chapter 5 illuminates how these filmmakers tap into the rich tradition of gay cinephilia by fashioning a "cinema of small gestures" out of the archive of industrially produced film. Visual details and devices seized from classical and ephemeral cinema—including Technicolor, widescreen cinema, shots from instructional films, and fragments of film musicals—provide an oblique aesthetic vocabulary for bearing witness to traumatic loss. The films address their viewers through poetic and testimonial voice-overs of grief, mourning, and physical and psychic alienation. Rather than provide narrative or documentary illustration of the testimonial discourse on the soundtrack, the image tracks to these films stress the affective intensity of gestures and visual fragments that resonate with the structures of feeling articulated by the voice-overs. In performing the habeas corpus inherent to bearing witness, the films complement strategies of visual embodiment and embodied vision seen elsewhere in queer AIDS media with the metaphor of film as body—a body subject to damage and decay, but also to love and care.

Chapter 6 examines arguably the most radical reframing of moving-image aesthetics to be found in queer AIDS media. By presenting a monochrome blue screen for its entire seventy-six minutes, Jarman's autobiographical Blue (1993) completely rejects the very "language" of film as moving pictures. The body of the witness is thus not merely reframed in the image but it is completely displaced from visual to aural perception through the soundtrack's complex mix of closely miked voices, music, and sound effects. Without cinema's conventional anchor of visual figuration, both sound and image operate in Blue in radically differently ways. Jarman's film, I argue, opens up the potential for a radical reconfiguration of the relation between witness and spectator by constructing a different kind of intersubjective space that implicates the spectator's own body in the process of bearing witness to AIDS. But it is not just the radical reframing of film form in Blue that makes it such an important work of queer AIDS media, for *Blue* is also a profoundly multi-media work that has existed in numerous forms, each promising a further opportunity to reframe its witnessing dynamics.

In the book's afterword, I reflect on the historicity of queer AIDS media by considering their relation to the new media ecology that has developed over the past decade. As my brief discussion of the ACT UP Oral History Project and Ultra Red's SILENT|LISTEN project illuminates, this new media ecology is now creating new witnessing dynamics through the logics of the database and the remix.

□

CHAPTER ONE

Historical Trauma

and the Performance

of Talking Heads

Queer AIDS media abound with talking heads, that is to say, with speech acts performed before the camera and embodied by the face of the speaker. The talking head arguably constitutes the most straightforward manifestation of direct address in moving-image media. Yet queer makers have persistently subjected this long-standing device of nonfiction film and television to various kinds of transformative adaptation, playful deconstruction, and even iconoclastic violence. Let me briefly offer a few examples from several historical moments in the gay AIDS epidemic to illustrate the multiplicity of such engagements.

In *Some Aspects of a Shared Lifestyle* (1986), one of the earliest videos to present a sustained critique of dominant AIDS representation in the United States, Gregg Bordowitz consistently messes with the conventions of the talking head. Framed in a medium shot, he appears in several scenes in a white doctor's coat as he reads dense medical information about AIDS at an accelerating speed. His increasingly garbled speech is gradually overridden by a woman's voice-over reading an excerpt from Cindy Patton's book *Sex and Germs: The Politics of* AIDS which discusses the political and cultural position from which she writes. Through this and other distortions of the talking head convention, the video exposes the ideological construction of authority and transparency in early media coverage of AIDS. In contrast to Bordowitz's surplus of discourse, Nino Rodriguez's seven-minute video *Identities* (1991) collects all the interstitial, extradiscursive moments of a conventional talking

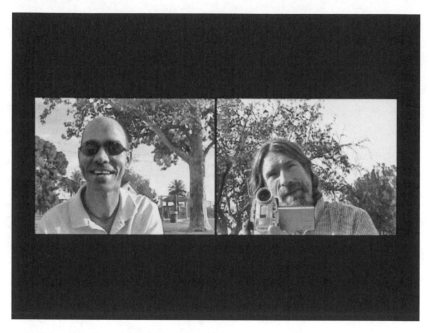

2. Frame capture from *Overdue Conversation* (Charles Lum, 2004).

head interview with Thomas Padgett, a gay man living with AIDS. With the narrative context of his testimony completely elided, our attention can only focus on Padgett's sighs, gulps, tears, facial twitches, and hand gestures. Rather than reduce his testimony to pure sentiment, the video reveals the ineffable psychic dimensions of trauma, which become registered through the body.

The question of the ineffable also structures Charles Lum's *Overdue Conversation* (2004), a ten-minute split-screen conversation about HIV disclosure between Lum and an unnamed friend as they sit in a park cruising area. Each man is holding the camera that films the other (figure 2). Lum recalls their first sexual encounter in the park back in 1998 and reveals that he failed to mention "something" at the time. His friend replies, "Probably the same thing I didn't tell you." As the conversation circles around the still unnamable issue of serostatus, both men reveal and explore the continuing challenges of sexual communication between gay men in the third decade of the epidemic. In the epilogue, Lum's friend affirms the value of their exchange: "I think four years from now we'll probably sit and talk about that video we made four years ago and the first time that we ever mentioned to each other that we were positive." The reciprocity of the two cameras not only facilitates the mutual disclosure between two friends but it also explicitly opens up the conversation to a public audience, since both men directly address the viewers of the video at the same time that they address each other through the camera.

Queer media makers understood the need to challenge the documentary conventions of the talking head, which are deeply implicated in the disciplinary function of dominant media representation. These conventions regulate the visible identification of specific bodies and identities, their authority to speak, and the possible forms of address they may perform. Although the talking head first emerged in early sound documentaries, such as Harry Watt's Housing Problems (1935), and only became a documentary convention in the television era, the visual aspects of its conventions and their ideological underpinnings involve a genealogy that extends back into the nineteenth-century history of photographic portraiture. Both the photographic portrait and the talking head have played significant roles in the cultural visibility of male homosexuality in the nineteenth and twentieth centuries, providing visual forms in which the homosexual body is made to confess its pathological identity. But these visual conventions have also provided queers with valuable opportunities for self-definition, collective identity, and performative politics, as seen, for instance, in Word Is Out (1977), the Mariposa Collective's landmark gay-liberation documentary that consists almost entirely of talking head interviews with a range of lesbians and gay men.[1]

In this chapter, I examine four queer AIDS documentaries that explicitly use forms of performance to reframe their talking heads: Stuart Marshall's Bright Eyes (1984), Marlon Riggs's No Regret (Non, je ne regrette rien) (1992), Tony Ayres's Sadness (1999), and Jack Lewis's and Thulanie Phungula's Sando to Samantha, aka, The Art of Dikvel (1998). The self-consciously performative elements of these documentaries provide the very means for bearing witness to the historical trauma of AIDS. Each of these videos staves off the confessional imperatives of dominant AIDS representation, specifically those bound up in the conventions of the talking head, through a different set of techniques, namely, Brechtian distantiation, performative styles of oral culture, explicit theatrical staging, and dramatic reenactment. Moreover, these performative elements contribute to the documentaries' attempts to frame the historical trauma of AIDS through its relationship to prior historical traumas.

As the first British AIDS documentary produced by a gay man, Bright Eyes culminates, unsurprisingly, with a series of interviews with British lesbian and gay community activists, followed by a complete speech given by the American AIDS activist Michael Callen. Yet these seemingly straightforward talking heads are thoroughly contextualized by the preceding forty minutes of the video, which interrogate the historical conditions of possibility for gay public testimony about AIDS. To this end, *Bright Eyes* employs various forms of historical reenactment and archival investigation to situate AIDS in relation to the history of scientific photography in the nineteenth century and to the Nazi persecution of homosexuals during the Holocaust. Taking up quite different archives, *No Regret, Sadness,* and *Sando to Samantha* all frame the individual and collective trauma of AIDS for different groups of queer men of color through the optic of earlier racially defined historical trauma and their legacies, namely, U.S. slavery, Australian anti-immigrant violence, and South African apartheid. These works thus stress the need to understand not only how race and sexuality intersect in the experience of the epidemic by different constituencies of queer men around the world but also how the historical trauma of AIDS reaps its social and psychological destruction through reopening or intensifying the wounds of prior historical trauma. The incorporation of performance not only allows a representational space in which these prior historical traumas may be brought into sight but it also engenders a certain working through of trauma, both prior and ongoing. The chapter concludes with a brief consideration of Matt Wolf's *Smalltown Boys* (2003), a short experimental video that explores the intergenerational challenge of working through the loss of AIDS cultural activism itself by reframing its archive through the self-conscious performance of the mockumentary.

Although each of the documentaries discussed here employs different forms of explicit performance, they all rely on such performance to ensure that the film or video emphatically produces a testimonial address to the viewer, retaining the intersubjective potential of the moving image in the act of bearing witness. We can thus understand such use of performance as performative, in J. L. Austin's sense.[2] Too often, talking heads are marshaled by the discursive structure of the documentary into serving as merely another form of evidence in the rhetorical and narrative construction of an argument. Testimony subsequently loses its performative function in constituting the ethical address at the heart of the act of bearing witness and recedes into the realm of the constative, where the utterance serves only to represent the world rather than engage it. I want to distinguish my discussion of documentary performativity from the one offered by Stella Bruzzi in her influential book, *New Documentary*, since she is more interested in how the self-reflexive presence of the filmmaker in the "performative documentaries" of Nick Broomfield, Molly Dineen, and Michael Moore draws "attention to the impossibilities of authentic documentary representation." She uses such films as the clearest expression of her argument that documentaries are fundamentally "a negotiation between filmmaker and reality and, at heart, a performance."[3] My understanding of performativity in documentary media is closer to that of Bill Nichols, despite his decision not to engage with an Austinian framework. Nichols argues that the "performative mode" emerged as a new mode of documentary in the 1980s, responding to the critique that self-reflexive documentaries were increasingly becoming formalist exercises disengaged from the social worlds they represented. Nichols writes, "Unlike reflexive documentary, performative documentary uses referentiality less as a subject of interrogation than as a component of a message directed elsewhere. . . . Performative documentary attempts to reorient us—affectively, subjectively—toward the historical, poetic world it brings into being."[4] *Bright Eyes*, *No Regret*, *Sadness*, and *Sando to Samantha* are clearly "performative documentaries" in Nichols's sense, in that they use performance not only to politically interrogate dominant AIDS representation but also to produce the embodied knowledge of experience and memory, which provides the affective ground for the intersubjective encounter of bearing witness to AIDS.

The Talking Head in the Shadow Archive

The talking head has become a foundational practice in documentary films that bear witness to historical trauma or systematic oppression. With its nine hours of interviews with survivors, bystanders, perpetrators, and historians, as well as its deliberate absence of any archival images, Claude Lanzmann's *Shoah* (1985) arguably stands as the benchmark for this commitment to the power of the talking head in documentary film. There is a pervasive belief among documentary makers that testimony performed before the camera produces a more powerful effect on its viewers than any comparable strategy for presenting testimony to historical trauma.[5] What is the power or efficacy of this particular form? Film and television studies have largely divided analysis of the talking head into considerations of its distinct practices— principally the documentary interview, television news reporting, and the talk show—rather than assess how these practices function in relation to each other in the larger "discourse space" of direct address that structures so much of contemporary audiovisual media.[6]

In one of the earliest attempts to theorize the talking head interview and its use in documentary film, Julia Lesage defends the political aesthetics of feminist documentaries from the 1970s against the charge that they naïvely bought into the idea of realist transparency.[7] She argues that feminist documentaries such as *Janie's Janie* (Geri Ashur, 1971) and *Union Maids*

(Julia Reichert and Jim Klein, 1976) drew directly from the deep structure of the consciousness-raising group, which itself had been a principal strategy of second-wave feminism. These films both record and stimulate politicized conversation among women, thus transforming conversation, an older tool of women's subcultural resistance, into a self-conscious political act. Such testimony allows women to recognize their experiences in relation to those of other women, facilitating the emergence of a collective consciousness. But as Alexandra Juhasz has argued in the context of alternative AIDS media, this use of documentary as a political organizing tool also permits viewers to "recognize how their other loci of identity must necessarily sever them from other viewers in the room."[8] Rather than extinguish the political efficacy of documentary, such possibilities for disidentification in fact intensify it, opening up the difficult question of forging community across difference.

Following second-wave feminism, the political understanding of the talking head would be assumed (and expanded to incorporate the performative incitement to come out) in political documentaries of gay liberation, such as Mariposa's Word Is Out. Although Lesage's analysis explains the efficacy of the form in the context of feminist organizing practices at a particular historical juncture, it does not address the risk that politically committed documentarians who use the talking head must negotiate: how to avoid the confessional functions of the form? We should not forget that the convention of the talking head is as much part of hegemonic media discourse as it is of politically committed documentary. As this chapter elucidates, the talking head convention plays a significant role in the power relations constituted by documentary film and television journalism, which are themselves rooted in the disciplinary mechanisms of modern portraiture.[9]

Allan Sekula argues that modern portraiture be understood in terms of "a double system" of representation that has functioned both honorifically and repressively.[10] The development of photography in the nineteenth century realized that double system more fully than ever before. Photographic portraiture expanded and popularized the ceremonial presentation of the bourgeois individual, which had been the modern function of portraiture since the seventeenth century. While largely undoing the economic privilege of access to the apparatus of portraiture, photography did not dismantle portraiture as an apparatus of power: it merely allowed honorific conventions to proliferate downward in the social hierarchy.[11] At the same time, photographic portraiture performed an increasingly vital role as a new representational technology in medical, criminological, and anthropological discourses. It functioned in such scientific contexts not to individualize but to classify and

categorize. Scientists used photography to develop new physiognomic technologies, such as Francis Galton's application of composite photography to
visual pathology and Alphonse Bertillon's anthropometric system of classi-
fication for identification photographs.[12] Sekula thus argues that "photography came to establish and delimit the terrain of the *other*, to define both
the *generalized look*—the typology—and the *contingent instance* of deviance and
social pathology" (7; emphasis original). Moreover, he insists that the double
system of photographic portraiture—as ceremonial presentation and scientific categorization—should not be understood as individual and opposing
traditions; rather, he contends that photography welded its honorific and
repressive functions as a function of the panoptic principle of everyday life:
"Every portrait implicitly took its place within a social and moral hierarchy.
The *private* moment of sentimental individuation, the look of the frozen gaze-
of-the-loved-one, was shadowed by two other more *public* looks: a look up,
at one's 'betters.' And a look down, at one's 'inferiors'" (10). In speaking of
"a generalized, inclusive *archive*, a *shadow archive* that encompasses an entire
social terrain while positioning individuals within that terrain," Sekula delin-
eates the semiotic interdependence between the actual physical (and seemingly separate) archives at each end of this double system (10). For instance, a
photographic portrait of a criminal type shown in a nineteenth-century illustrated lecture would derive its ideological significance from its contrastive
relation to the daguerreotype or *carte-de-visite* portraits of loved ones tucked
away in the pockets of the bourgeois audience at such an event.

In his conception of the archive as both a concrete institution and "an
abstract paradigmatic entity," Sekula provides a useful framework for understanding how the visual representation of individual bodies, and in particular of their heads and faces, participates in the course of modern panoptic
power. In the convention of the talking head so prevalent in contemporary
documentary media, we can see a similar double system to the one of modern
portraiture. The honorific portrait of the bourgeois subject finds its correlate
in nonfiction media in the authoritative figures of the newscaster and the expert witness, while the repressive portrait of the pathological subject finds its
equivalent in the objectified other of documentary film and television news,
which incorporates an array of figures including the pauper, the primitive,
the immigrant, the refugee, the nonwhite, the criminal, the sexual deviant,
and the sick person.[13]

This double system has been in place within documentary film since the
1930s and 1940s when the Griersonian movement in Britain and later in
Canada pioneered the rhetorical form of the talking head in documentary

film.[14] Although the difficulties of recording synchronous sound fostered a reliance on voice-over narration in much early sound documentary film, the steady development and improvement of synchronous sound technologies soon increased the prevalence of the talking head. Early television's reliance on the presentational format for nonfictional programming also further consolidated its conventionality in postwar moving-image media. Sekula's conceptual framework of a shadow archive offers documentary studies the opportunity to analyze more fully how the embodied voices of the talking head convention come to signify, since it understands this process of signification in a broad intertextual manner, one not confined to the discursive parameters of any particular film, program, or even genre. How we come to understand the meaning and significance of talking heads and their enunciation in contemporary audiovisual culture is framed precisely by their placement within this all-inclusive shadow archive.

The archive became a central concern for queer AIDS media right from their very beginnings in the mid-1980s. On the one hand, it constituted the intertextual matrix for situating the ideological value and meaning of each specific talking head or photographic portrait in dominant AIDS representation, while on the other hand, it allowed queer makers to explicitly reframe their talking heads historically, often in highly creative ways, and thereby challenge the disciplinary function of the device.[15] My invocation of the archive throughout this book lies somewhere between the archive as the empirical accumulation of representation and the ideality of the archive posited by Michel Foucault in his *Archaeology of Knowledge*.[16] For Foucault, the archive should not be understood as "the sum of all texts that a culture has kept upon its person as documents attesting to its own past."[17] Rather, it is an entirely abstract conception, "the general system of the formation and transformation of statements" (130). Fundamentally, it contains the limits and the forms of the sayable: "What is it possible to speak of? What is the constituted domain of discourse? What type of discursivity is assigned to this or that domain (what is allocated as matter for narrative treatment; for descriptive science; for literary formulation)?"[18] Foucault insists that we can never describe the archive of our own historical time: "It is the border of time that surrounds our presence, which overhangs it, and which indicates it in its otherness; it is that which, outside ourselves, delimits us."[19]

Although the domain of the visual stands outside Foucault's conception of the archive, the analysis of visual representation gains much from his historicizing insights into the formation and transformation of discourse. Like other forms of representation, images rely on signification through language to produce meaning. The question of the archive may consequently be reformulated to ask: What are the forms and limits of the visually representable in a given historical time? While the empirical archive of visual representation presents us with the historical sum of images that produces the dense intertexuality regulating their signification, the Foucauldian archive pushes us to consider what lies outside the empirical archive, delimiting it. The act of bearing witness through moving-image media engages with precisely those forms and limits of the sayable and of the representable that concern the Foucauldian question of the archive. How can the media of film and video communicate the magnitude of historical trauma in ways that do not render the witness an individual victim, domesticate magnitude's excess, or abrogate the ethical address to respond?

Illuminating the Shadow Archive

Marshall took up the question of AIDS representation and its shadow archive in his eighty-minute video Bright Eyes, which was commissioned in early 1984 by Britain's newly established Channel Four for its Eleventh Hour series, a late-night showcase for new independent work.[20] Taking full advantage of the new institution's initial openness to innovative and experimental forms of television, Marshall chose to make one of the very first independent videos about AIDS in "the form of a collage of different historical discourses, images, and meanings about homosexuality and disease."[21] Marshall took the stipulation for a segmented structure to the documentary (to facilitate commercial breaks) as an opportunity to produce a video of three thoroughly autonomous parts. However, Bright Eyes resists the imperative of commercial broadcasters to regularize the length of its parts. The duration of each part increases throughout the video—from fifteen to twenty-five to forty minutes. Moreover, the video refuses to pursue, as Martha Gever notes, either a straightforward chronological development or a linear rhetorical argument.[22] Part 1 draws together archival photographs, contemporary press clippings, voice-over commentary, and carefully staged talking heads to trace the discursive continuities between contemporary AIDS representation and the nineteenth-century development of medical photography as a disciplinary technology.[23] Historical reenactments predominate in part 2, which examines the fate of Magnus Hirschfeld's sexual reform movement in Wilhelmine and Weimar Germany and the subsequent use of eugenic discourses by the

Nazis in their persecution of homosexuals. Part 3 returns to the explicit concern with dominant AIDS representation and its impact on gay communities through extensive interviews with activists and medical professionals.

Constructing the video as "a series of temporal juxtapositions of textual units," Marshall aimed "to collide different historical episodes in such a way that the viewer would be presented with the problem of assembling their mutual relationships" (67). Ian White has read this structural characteristic as Marshall's engagement with the dynamics of televisual flow: "Its juxtapositions and variety of registers emulate the variety of an evening's viewing while staging its own disjunctions as a brilliant seduction into and activation of the viewing experience."[24] Although *Bright Eyes* emphatically plunders the generic diversity of television programming—from hospital soap opera and historical costume drama to news programming and historical documentaries—its experimental form allowed it to circulate beyond the documentary circuit of public broadcasting and film festivals. Framed in the context of video art, *Bright Eyes* was thus also screened at the Tate Gallery in London, the New Museum in New York, and during the eighth Documenta in Kassel.[25] The video's peripatetic circulation would not only set a precedent for AIDS activist videos produced a few years later in the context of ACT UP (which I discuss more fully in the following chapter) but it also helps explain how *Bright Eyes* came to have such a wide formal influence on later queer AIDS films and videos.[26]

Part 1 of *Bright Eyes* opens with anachronism and juxtaposition. In the midst of what appears to be the high melodrama of a contemporary hospital soap opera (with medical staff loudly and urgently clearing the path for an incoming patient with AIDS), two doctors engage in an impassive conversation about diagnostics that bears the distinct resonance of nineteenth-century positivism: "Sometimes a symptom is invisible, and we need to hunt it out quite aggressively. Sometimes a symptom is visible, but we just don't see it" (figure 3). Stark stylistic juxtaposition continues in the second sequence with the silent contemplation of the textually "loud" AIDS hysteria found in tabloid articles with headlines such as "Fear over Sex Bug 'Killer'" and "Exclusive: Pictures That Reveal the Disturbing Truth of AIDS Sickness." The video repeatedly returns to this latter headline and to a photo featured in one of the tabloid articles, which shows a gay man, Kenny Ramsaur, before the onset of AIDS (figure 4). Each subsequent appearance of Ramsaur's photograph in *Bright Eyes* is framed differently, first, with a black matte to isolate it on the screen, second, in the full context of the article, which places it next to a later photograph of Kenny as an "AIDS victim," and finally in a close-up that fills

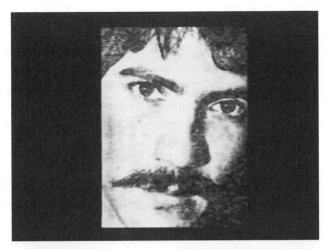

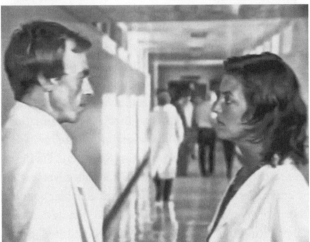

3–4. Frame captures from *Bright Eyes* (Stuart Marshall, 1984).

the screen. The third sequence then returns to the discourse of nineteenth-century medicine with an actor playing a Victorian doctor who painstakingly reads a letter he wrote to the *Lancet* in 1859 lamenting that medical science has not yet exploited the new medium of photography for its capacity to render true likeness (figure 5). The fourth sequence then presents a series of nineteenth-century photographs labeled by their pathological diagnosis: "a mad woman," "an hysteric," "an intermediate type," "a moral imbecile" (figure 6).

In their autonomy from each other, these first four sequences of part 1 establish the modus operandi of the whole video by demanding an interpretative labor on the viewer's part to figure out the relationship between these sets of still and moving images of the past and the present. Yet clues are given. Actors play multiple roles throughout the video. The same actor plays the roles of the Victorian doctor and of one of the doctors in the hospital scene. He also will appear again in part 2 as Heinz Heger, a young Viennese man imprisoned for homosexuality under Paragraph 175 (of the German Criminal Code) in 1939 and later sent to the Sachsenhausen and Flossenbürg concentration camps, and in part 3 as a television presenter interviewing a person with AIDS and as a police officer involved in the entrapment of a gay man.[27] Gever rightly points out how this Brechtian distantiation device frustrates the normative mechanisms of televisual transparency and viewer identification, but there is, I would argue, more at work here. On the one hand, the actor's presence across generically and historically diverse scenes in all three parts of *Bright Eyes* encourages the viewer to consider connections between these disparate scenarios. On the other hand, the device's emphasis on his role-playing foregrounds how historically constituted identities function as discursive positions, both enabling and delimiting enunciative possibilities for their subjects. *Bright Eyes* repeatedly indicates the function of photographic portraits, and later of talking heads, in this production of modern subjects.

In the later sequences of part 1, a voice-over commentary begins to draw together the connections between nineteenth-century medical photography and the contemporary journalistic images of AIDS and homosexuality: "It seems that the *Sunday People* has taken up a question that has troubled the medical profession since the last century: How does one form a true picture of an illness? The media's answer to this question is similar to the one first suggested by medical science: identify and isolate certain groups and then describe them as inherently ill." The tracing of this discursive genealogy culminates in the final sequence of part 1, in which an actor portrays a middle-aged gay man being interviewed about his coming out. Although the man de-

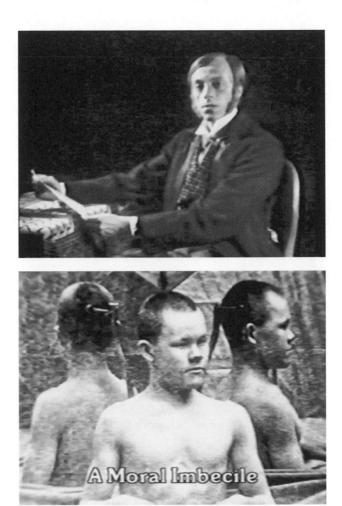

5–6. Frame captures from *Bright Eyes* (Stuart Marshall, 1984).

scribes how he rejected the pathologizing pressure both of his family and of his doctor, his body is cast into shadow by backlighting, a technique used by television producers for the confessional presentation of homosexual talking heads in the decades before gay liberation.[28] Marshall indicates the discursive line of continuity between such talking heads and photographic portraiture by immediately preceding the interview scene with a nineteenth-century medical photograph entitled "A Group of Sexual Perverts." By bringing the shadow archive of AIDS representation into the light of scrutiny, Bright Eyes denaturalizes its mechanisms for producing the truth of the epidemic.

The Question of Historical Continuity

The discursive lines of continuity between the past and the present become more complicated in part 2 of Bright Eyes, as the attention shifts to Hirschfeld and the Nazi persecution of homosexuals. Although Marshall's video was one of the first queer cultural productions to posit a relationship between the historical trauma of Nazi persecution and the AIDS crisis, he later insisted at the "How Do I Look?" conference in 1989 that he never intended for Bright Eyes to draw a direct parallel between the Holocaust and the AIDS epidemic.[29] Following gay liberation's earlier appropriation and resignification of the pink triangle, numerous AIDS activists and artists made various and often highly disputed allusions to Nazi Germany and the Holocaust during the 1980s and 1990s.[30] The sociologist Arlene Stein reads such allusions as attempts to construct a "social movement frame" that would function to produce both historical analogy and revisionism.[31] Frequently drawing parallels between AIDS service organizations and Jewish councils in the wartime ghettos, the activist and playwright Larry Kramer arguably framed the AIDS epidemic through the genocidal analogy of the Holocaust more vociferously than anyone else, first in his 1985 play The Normal Heart and later in numerous speeches and essays, collected in his book Reports from the Holocaust.[32] Yet the original New York projects of the ad hoc art collective that later became Gran Fury were far more complex in their engagement with the Holocaust frame. The "Silence=Death" poster campaign (with its plain, upturned pink triangle above the slogan) and Let the Record Show . . . (a gallery installation that combined images of the Nuremberg Trials, quotations from contemporary politicians, and the "Silence=Death" logo) created both the analogy of genocide as the specter hanging over the AIDS crisis and the invitation to reconsider the historical connections between Nazi persecution, gay liberation, and the AIDS crisis.[33] Marshall's Bright Eyes similarly posed questions about the potential historical continuity between the Third Reich and the AIDS crisis in the 1980s, namely, about the ideological function of the homosexual body in the state's regulation of desire throughout the entire population.

Bright Eyes first broaches the subject of Nazi persecution in part 2 by implying its continuity with the nineteenth-century pathologization of homosexuality elaborated in part 1: an intertitle quotes Heinrich Himmler's 1936 speech in which he framed homosexuality as a symptom of racial degeneracy in need of extermination. The next scene presents the exiled sexual reformer Hirschfeld (played by an actor) sitting alone in a Paris movie theater in May 1933 as he watches a newsreel report the Nazi destruction of his Institute of Sexual Research in Berlin. Looking despondently at the screen, Hirschfeld glumly recounts his life's work. Once a prolific producer and collector of scientific images dedicated to social reform (including photographic portraits), Hirschfeld is here reduced to a helpless spectator witnessing the rapid transformation of those images into the political spectacle of degeneracy as they are burned by Nazi activists. The transformation of images continues in the next reenacted scene, which depicts Heger's arrest and interrogation in 1939. An innocuous snapshot portrait of Heger with his lover, Friedrich Müller, becomes evidence of "degeneracy" due to Heger's affectionate inscription to Müller on the back of the photograph. A silent zoom-in on Heger's face in one of the snapshots suggests a continuity with the earlier shots of Ramsaur and the voice-over commentary in part 1 that noted how every image of a gay man risks becoming two pictures of a homosexual: "A member of an exotic species and a case history of a pathological sickness."[34] Part 2 concludes with a fictionalized talking head interview in contemporary Germany that consolidates the video's imperative to trace the discursive continuities between past and present. A woman interviews Heger about his experiences in the Flossenbürg concentration camp while she drives along the autobahn to Nuremberg. The same actor plays Heger as in the 1939 reenactment of his arrest, yet no attempt is made to make him look like the old man he would be by the mid-1980s. The past cuts through the present, defamiliarizing both of them for the viewer, who is thrown into considering their lines of historical continuity.

The return to the AIDS crisis in the third and final part of Bright Eyes is initiated by a dramatized scene set in a television studio where a man with AIDS is about to be interviewed on live television about his personal experiences of discrimination. But the sound technician refuses to wire the guest, leading the latter to suggest using a telephone hookup, a demeaning compromise he feels compelled to make if his voice is to be heard at all. A newspaper clipping about such an incident at a San Francisco television station subsequently reveals the scene's historical foundation. The following, self-contained short interviews with John Weber, a doctor and AIDS researcher; Richard Wells, a nursing official; Tony Whitehead, the chair of Britain's first AIDS service organization; Nick Billingham, a gay activist; and Linda Semple, the manager of Gay's the Word bookstore, progressively situate the AIDS crisis within the larger context of regulating sexuality in contemporary Britain. The interviewees counter the AIDS hysteria generated by the dominant media by carefully and calmly explaining the function of media discourse in public perceptions of deviance and disease. Although these interviews lack the formal self-reflexivity of the talking heads in the earlier parts of the video, they nevertheless deviate from conventional documentary form because Marshall eschews crosscutting between them to build an argument.[35] Each given his or her own successive sequence, the interviewees appear as witnesses speaking from a specific position, rather than as chunks of accredited talking head discourse marshaled by the documentary's rhetorical system.

Bright Eyes concludes with the PWA activist Michael Callen standing outdoors in front of a verdant trellis as he rereads the whole eleven-minute speech that he gave before a New York State Senate Committee hearing on AIDS funding in June 1983. Callen begins by specifying the position from which he speaks, acknowledging that he cannot speak for the Haitian immigrant or the child of poverty living with AIDS, nor even for all gay men with AIDS. The value of his testimony, he asserts, lies in its potential opportunity to illuminate what links all people living with AIDS: "We are human beings suffering from an illness whose cause remains unknown and for which there is no known cure." However, Callen moves quickly from speaking in the first-person singular to speaking in the first-person plural as he describes what he and the members of his AIDS support group talk about at their meetings — the day-to-day physical challenges of living with AIDS, its psychological toll, the social stigma attached to the syndrome, the personal economic burden borne, and the demand for sufficient funding of all potential avenues of treatment research.[36]

The directness of Callen's words is matched by the manner in which he is shot. The static camera fixes on Callen for the whole duration of the speech, with only two cuts shifting from a medium shot to a facial close-up. Yet the directness of the speech is reframed by two crucial strategies of displacement. First, as Gever notes, Callen makes no attempt to hide that he is reading from a piece of paper. The intertitle preceding the speech specifies its original date in 1983, and a subtitle at the end of it indicates that it was recorded in London in September 1984. Second, the speech is not only re-performed at a later date but is also spatially relocated from the state capitol in Albany to Hampstead Heath in London, thus reclaiming a well-known public cruising space as a site for gay male enunciation rather than state and dominant media surveillance. Whether or not Marshall had access to an archival recording of the original speech (if one existed), his decision to re-stage the speech in a different time and place both reaffirms the significance of its content outside its immediate context and self-consciously resists the notion that testimony is most effective when it is completely transparent, spontaneous, and seemingly unmediated. Callen's ability to bear witness in Bright Eyes is thus achieved by the temporal and spatial reframing of his direct address. The deliberate formal tensions between directness and mediation and between the present and the past that characterize Bright Eyes and its critical engagement with the shadow archive of AIDS representation would be taken up by many other queer makers who sought differing means to resist its confessionalizing pressure. Moreover, by tracing the lines of continuity between the double systems of nineteenth-century photographic portraiture and documentary talking heads, Bright Eyes established very early in the epidemic the political imperative not merely to contest but also to historicize the discursive construction of AIDS in dominant media representation.

The Palimpsest of Historical Struggle

The conventional documentary portrait furnished the formal model for many of the earliest works of queer AIDS media produced in the United States, including Tina DiFeliciantonio's Living with AIDS (1986), Tom Brook's Hero of My Own Life (1986), and Mark Huestis and Wendy Dallas's Chuck Solomon: Coming of Age (1986). All three of these early documentary portraits focus on individual gay men living with HIV/AIDS: Todd Coleman, David Summers, and Chuck Solomon, respectively. Each follows the standard conventions of the television documentary portrait, editing together observational footage of daily life with talking head interviews in which the documentary subject relates both his life narrative (coming out, diagnosis, disclosure, and illness) and the philosophical and psychological insights derived from the life-altering experience of AIDS.

By consistently depicting the community of lovers, friends, family, and volunteers that afforded crucial support for the person living with HIV/AIDS, these independently produced documentary portraits successfully countered the dominant media trope of the isolated and lonely homosexual AIDS victim. Yet they nevertheless failed to transcend the notion of AIDS as primarily an individual trauma. In his critique of these works, Timothy Landers acknowledged their clear capacity to elicit a sympathetic identification with the main character, but he also warned that "by using AIDS as a dramatic catalyst in a familiar format of heightened emotion saturated with the rhetoric of personal heroism, these videotapes tend to overlook the specifics of AIDS."[37] Landers further argued that merely celebrating the heroism and courage of the gay man battling AIDS ends up as the flip side of blaming him for his illness. As the remainder of this chapter will elucidate, subsequent documentary portraits of people with AIDS have sustained their ability to effectively bear witness by developing three main strategies for overcoming the tendencies of the documentary portrait to individualize and dehistoricize experience: first, multiplying the number of documentary subjects; second, framing the documentary portrait as an encounter between maker and subject(s); and third, articulating the experience of AIDS in relation to the other historical coordinates of the documentary subject's identity.

In making No Regret (Non, je ne regrette rien), Riggs aimed both to transcend the individualizing dynamic of these earlier documentary portraits of gay men with AIDS and to situate the collective trauma of AIDS in the longer history of African American political struggle. After the widespread acclaim and notoriety of Tongues Untied (1989), his groundbreaking articulation of African American gay identity, Riggs was invited to produce a video for the Fear of Disclosure Project, which the artist and AIDS activist Phil Zwickler had initiated in 1989 to explore the issue of HIV disclosure in different communities.[38] No Regret is ostensibly a documentary portrait of five black gay men living with HIV/AIDS: Assoto Saint, Joseph Long, Donald Woods, Michael Lee, and Reggie Williams. Riggs skillfully reworks the conventions of a traditional talking heads portrait to explore the complex dynamics of sexuality and intersubjectivity at work in African American communities around the public disclosure concerning HIV/AIDS. The primary material for the video is the taped interviews with these five men who passionately and eloquently relate their experiences of living with the virus, progressing from a discussion of infection through familial and social disclosure to community building and activism. Yet Riggs presents these interviews in ways that continually undermine the audience's ability to read these talking heads through the shadow archive of dominant AIDS representation. Through its use of mattes, nonsynchronized sound, inset images, on-screen text, and superimposition, the video disrupts and reframes the familiar conventions of nonfictional televisual media, opening up the space to bear witness to the

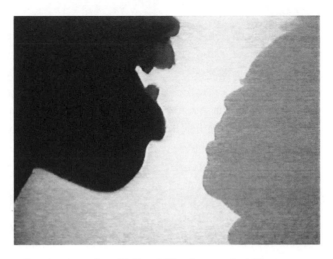

7. Frame capture from *No Regret* (*Non, Je ne regrette rien*)
(Marlon T. Riggs, 1992).

very issues that dominant U.S. media has consistently neglected, disavowed, or distorted.

No Regret opens on a black screen to the refrain of a spiritual song, "Oh Freedom!" The first image one sees is the partial silhouette of a woman singing against a blue screen: "I'll never be a slave / To go in silence to my grave / When I go home / I'll be strong / And I'll be free." Another image appears with another voice: the partial silhouette of a young black man performing an elegy is superimposed onto the existing image: "No point in crying injustice / shooting off in public places / they are slack-handed and wet-eyed / with sympathy."[39] All one sees of the young man is a close-up of his mouth, offering a glimpse of the physical rhythm to the lyric. Both superimposed over a blue screen, these human figures convey an ephemeral, ghostly presence as they speak to one another, both visually and aurally (figure 7). The superimposition in this opening scene constructs a palimpsest that effectively places the video in the African American tradition of oral culture. Like Riggs's celebrated earlier work *Tongues Untied*, which used rap, blues, soul, poetry, and pig Latin in its articulation of black gay identity, *No Regret* consciously draws from various strands of African American oral culture to address its audience.

When Riggs opens his video on a freedom song from the tradition of African American spirituals, he appropriates this cultural form with a specific function in mind. He situates the testimonies of the video in a longer history of black struggle and cultural articulation. Spirituals are considered the earliest body of vernacular folk literature that expresses African American religious feeling. They derived from the African technique of reshaping bits of preexisting songs into new ones. Within the plantation society during slavery they constituted a space for resistance, celebration, and community building.[40] The political character of the spiritual continued into the civil rights era, when the movement turned to spirituals as a means of organizing, bringing people together, forging a sense of purpose and faith, and diffusing violence.[41] The lyrics of the original spiritual songs (principally the freedom songs) were either directly adopted or, in keeping with the African American tradition of cutting and mixing, adapted to the context of the civil rights movement. Martin Luther King Jr. called these songs "the soul of the movement."[42] As Jon Michael Spencer points out, the freedom songs of the civil rights movement chronicle a palimpsest of historical struggle, recalling the antislavery movement while also chronicling the various forms of protest and personal reflections of the civil rights movement itself: "Those songwriters involved in the movement were both history makers and historians" (104).

Riggs continues that tradition in his use of spirituals in No Regret, including an original spiritual (in this opening scene) and later adapting a freedom song from the civil rights movement for the struggle against AIDS: "Ain't Gonna Let No Virus." The spiritual "Oh Freedom!" also returns in a later sequence, sung this time by the gay performer Blackberri, accompanying a montage of still and moving images that depict black gay community and mobilization, specifically video footage of marches and political activism. Such montage strategies indicate the degree to which the video addresses a broad African American audience by tracing the lines of historical and political continuity from antislavery discourse through civil rights culture to black gay and AIDS activism. This strategy encourages such viewers to understand the strong relation between AIDS activism and black activism, rather than continue to insist on their differentiation. Asserting such continuity would prove vital at a time in the early 1990s when the New Right was strategically trying to hinder political solidarity and coalition building between African American communities and lesbian and gay ones.[43] As in his earlier works, especially Tongues Untied, Riggs is working here to build on and strengthen the historical consciousness of his audience.

The video brings in the adapted freedom song "Ain't Gonna Let No Virus" right at the end when the interviewees are finally named by subtitles imposed over their portraits. By withholding the names of his documentary subjects until the end, Riggs inverts the conventional introduction and discursive placement of talking head subjects. Usually when a new documentary subject is introduced, the narrational structure provides a name and a status to authenticate and authorize that subject's discourse. A subject's claim to truth may be his or her status as an expert witness (with institutional credentials) or his or her very ordinariness (the media trope of vox populi: the person asked impromptu on the street). But this process of naming consistently frames such discourse as a matter of prior authorization or permission to speak. It stands as the speaker's alibi, but also confines him or her to a specific enunciative role. Thus Riggs's decision to withhold the names of his subjects for most of the video provides them with a less restricted discursive space within which to bear witness.

In naming his interviewees at the very end, Riggs emphasizes the performative nature of their presence in the video, as though the sequence were a cast list preceding the end credits. It also allows the names of the dead seen in the opening credits' dedication to remain foregrounded in viewers' minds.[44] The video thus suggests the continuity of struggles partaken of both by survivors and by the dead. No Regret is in fact less interested in sharing individual stories and articulating particular subjectivities for their own sake than in giving expression to a community-constituting relationality across various indices of difference—the living and the dead, documentary subject and viewer, infected and uninfected, homosexual and heterosexual, self and other. The individual interviews are edited together in a poetic and rhythmical fashion that breaks up the interviewees' testimonial narratives into "verses" woven into a larger narrative of collective struggle. Although the video's editing continually moves among its subjects, constituting them in the conventional terms of what John Corner calls "part characters, part presenters," Riggs carries this technique beyond its normal bounds, creating a lyrical texture for the video.[45] The resonances established among the five testimonies builds up across No Regret, shaping the video into a kind of poetic conversation, a palimpsest of historical struggle built around African American forms of oral culture.[46]

Undoing the Confessional Screen

The question of individual deemphasis is further invoked by one of the video's principal aesthetic strategies—the use of black video mattes during interviews. Riggs deploys them in a complex manner, alluding to their conventional use in mainstream media to simultaneously "protect" the identity of interviewees and to produce their discourse as a confession of guilt. The use of black mattes that obscure large portions of the frame and thus disguise the identity of the documentary subject derives from the tradition of silhouetted talking heads alluded to in *Bright Eyes*. With the emergence of the AIDS epidemic and the ensuing media hysteria around it, black mattes and silhouettes once again became common devices in media interviews with gay men and other "guilty victims" of the epidemic.[47]

As *No Regret* first introduces each of the five interviewees, viewers only have visual access to one part of their talking head—either their eyes or their mouth—indications of their presence as they speak yet ones insufficient to identify them. As we hear the interviewees relate the experience of stigma around HIV/AIDS and its silencing pressure in African American communities, the initial visual blocking of these documentary subjects suggests the continuance of their stigma as they appear to "confess" their condition. Indeed, the aesthetic arrangement of the matte and its concealment of all but an expressive body part invokes precisely the structure of vision within a confessional box, where the grille provides the only space of visual contact between confessor and confessant. Consequently, the role of confessor is offered up to the viewer. As we listen to these five interviewees, however, their sophisticated understanding of internal and external perceptions around AIDS and the everyday negotiation of stigma becomes clear. These very articulate men do not just describe the effects of stigma but they unpack its psychological dynamics, explaining how it comes to be internalized by those affected. They relate and analyze stories of panic, denial, repression, and recovery. A distinct tension arises between the confessional connotations of the video's visual effects and the sophisticated analysis produced by its supposed confessants.

Once all the interviewees have been introduced using black mattes, Riggs switches techniques, maintaining the interviewees' anonymity through the use of close-up shots on their hands. He also significantly breaks down the synchronization of sound and image. Although one hears the continuing testimony, the image is reduced to slow motion, emphasizing the expressive gestures of the subjects' hands, which convey a complex affective range from prayerful contemplation to gentle-hearted queeniness (figure 8). In this sequence, Donald Woods speaks of his initial inability to tell his mother of his serostatus as she was dealing with the trauma of his brother's murder and another brother's drug addiction, while Assoto Saint recounts how his mother's grief over her recently deceased dog delayed his disclosure: "I imagined how she would react to my death." This experience of dissociation is effectively articulated through the way in which the speaker's discourse is severed from the visible body that has enunciated it. The bodies may correspond to the voices with which they appear, but their sense of presence and stability is undermined by the desynchronization of sound and image.[48] There is something delicately erotic about the way Riggs's camera slowly moves across Assoto Saint's body as he gestures with his hands. At one point, his mouth appears in the frame—closed, even though one hears his voice, thus fully confirming the performative nature of his presence on the screen. The eroticism of these shots interferes with their signification as markers of anonymity and confession. When the video subsequently returns to using black mattes in the following sequence, it is done playfully: the matte quickly fades away as each interviewee is called on to relate his story of disclosure, thus self-consciously drawing attention to it as a rhetorical device. Riggs's skillful use of black mattes allows him to invoke the confessional pressure of mainstream AIDS coverage while playfully disrupting and dismantling it. Understood in the specific context of the video's address to African American communities, it also points to the power of stigma and secrecy, only to triumph the inverse power of disclosure, visually articulated through the series of unmaskings (as the interviewees relate how they told their families and communities about their serostatus).[49] No Regret is, as its title declares, a refusal of shame that engenders identity-affirming pride. But as the supplemental reference to Edith Piaf's classic queer torch song suggests, it is one that resists heteronormative black masculinity.

As the interviewees narrate their disclosure of their condition to family, friends, and community, Riggs employs another technique invoking mainstream news coverage—the inset photo window (figure 9). When Michael Lee relates how he told his mother, family photographs appear in the upper left-hand side of the screen behind Lee's head. The use of such windows in conjunction with the conventionally posed talking head is the staple format for broadcast news programs, where a news photo or visual symbol cues the viewer's attention to a recognizable public issue. Such photographs need to be instantly recognizable, either as identifiable signs (such as the caduceus) or iconic photographs (the U.S. Capitol). Yet Riggs undermines the clear distinction of public images by inserting personal and family photographs into this device. The conventions of documentary film practice tend to favor shooting personal photographs in full frame (often with a slow zoom-in) accompanied by a testimonial voice-over to convey a sense of intimacy, producing a kind of revelation of the private to the audience. It is often figured as a moment of opening up on the part of the speaking subject, as though

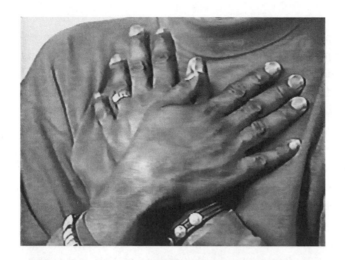

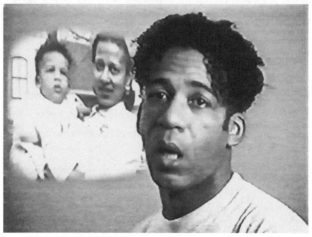

8–9. Frame captures from *No Regret* (*Non, Je ne regrette rien*)
(Marlon T. Riggs, 1992).

the camera's movement closer to the image constituted an intimacy with its referent (usually the speaking subject caught at some significant moment in his or her past).

Although Riggs utilizes this convention several times in No Regret, his predominant strategy with personal photographs is to insert them via a technique that consciously recalls the context of public images and their dissemination (i.e., broadcast news), thus encouraging the viewer to interrogate the distinction between private and public spheres. Riggs is here able to personalize discursive structures that normally depersonalize what they reference in that they tend to reduce the signification of photographs used as inset images to generic themes and tropes, such as the "terror" or "panic" of AIDS. Moreover, the strategy wittily invests the interviewees with the newscaster's presumed authority—to situate images as they speak, rather than to be situated by the text's narration. A sense of the performative agency of testimony rather than the subjection of confession is clearly apparent in this sequence.

No Regret is not merely an exercise in the critique of media conventions around the talking head, for it is also driven by the imperative to generate discourse—its interviewees devote their testimony to the proliferation of PWA discourse. The video is performative in the sense that its focus on and discussion of the power of discourse produces a space for its viewers to embrace the opportunity to speak. Such an insistence on the need to speak publicly (whether infected or uninfected) indicates the value of Riggs's video as a pedagogic tool for HIV/AIDS education in African American communities, where the stigma of the virus has historically maintained an intense shaming pressure to silence and marginalize. No Regret moreover constituted a clear attempt to reframe AIDS as an urgent political issue of marginalization, discrimination, and stigma in African American communities after a decade of neglect and avoidance by black political and media elites. Cathy J. Cohen argues that such elites uncritically accepted the Centers for Disease Control and Prevention's (CDC) initial emphasis on high-risk groups, which allowed black political leaders, clergy, and reporters to engage in what Cohen calls the "secondary marginalization" of HIV-positive African Americans through discourses condemning "immoral behaviors"—homosexuality and drug use—that allegedly undermined "the black family" and "the black community."[50] No Regret articulates a strong resistance to such increasing ideological normativity at the heart of contemporary black politics by simultaneously bearing witness to the historical continuity of collective struggle and the right to sexual diversity.

The pedagogic impulse of *No Regret* could also be found in Richard Fung's *Fighting Chance* (1990), a group portrait of Asian gay men living with AIDS in North America. *Fighting Chance* shared several aspects with *No Regret*, including the integration of talking head interviews with performative scenes, the extensive discussion of the significance of family support, and a sustained engagement with particular challenges of silence and denial with communities of color. However, Fung's video articulated a more explicit connection between discourse-proliferating testimony and the prevention and treatment of HIV/AIDS. Toward the end of *Fighting Chance*, its witnesses living with HIV/AIDS offer specific, pragmatic advice to fellow Asians living with the disease, thus constructing a direct address to others in their own communities.[51]

The Aesthetics of Intimacy

Like *Fighting Chance*, Ayres's *Sadness* presents a documentary group portrait addressing the relationship between AIDS, homosexuality, and Asian diasporic identity, yet rather than examine the lives of Asian gay men living with AIDS, *Sadness* reframes the collective trauma of AIDS for Sydney's gay community through the optic of a racialized trauma experienced by the family of the Chinese Australian photographer William Yang. *Sadness* adapts Yang's critically acclaimed "monologue with slides" of the same title, which Yang began performing in 1992 in Australia, and later internationally. Yang established himself in the 1970s as one of the most important chroniclers of the Sydney arts and social scene. He was also one of the first photographers to document Sydney's liberation-era gay community. In his performance piece *Sadness*, Yang explored the interrelationship of personal, familial, and community trauma and loss through the parallel narration of two sets of experiences: the loss of numerous gay friends and lovers to AIDS and the investigation of his uncle's murder in the 1920s. Presenting color and black-and-white photographic slides accompanied by narration and reflection by Yang himself, *Sadness* counterposed the effects of trauma in two sets of intimate community: his family and his network of friends.

Ayres saw the production in Sydney and approached Yang, believing it could work well on film. The film was produced by the Australian Film Institute and broadcast nationally on the independent SBS television channel in November 1999. *Sadness* is not the only queer performance piece about AIDS to be adapted for the screen. In fact, *Sadness* formed part of a larger tendency in the 1980s and 1990s toward adaptation and intertextuality across media in queer cultural production, particularly work concerning AIDS, a trend initiated by films like *The AIDS Show: Artists Involved in Death and Survival* (1986), Peter Adair and Robert Epstein's documentary about an acclaimed community theater project organized around various testimonial sketches and vignettes about AIDS.[52] Decisions to adapt works for the screen were often partially motivated by a desire to widen the audience for the artist or performer, allowing the circulation of his or her work to extend beyond the limits of live performance and benefiting from the developing infrastructure of queer public culture, particularly the growing international network of lesbian and gay film festivals, which became an important exhibition network for queer AIDS media.

Perhaps the most significant work to parallel *Sadness* in this regard is *I'll Be Your Mirror* (1996), Edmund Coulthard's documentary collaboration with the photographer Nan Goldin. Also produced for public television (in this case the BBC), *I'll Be Your Mirror* explores the dynamics between artist and subject for a photographer considered one of the major figures of the "aesthetics of intimacy" prevalent in contemporary photography.[53] In summarizing such aesthetics of intimacy with reference to Goldin's work, the critic Liz Kotz argues: "Presented under the guise of an 'intimate' relationship between artist and subject, these images relegitimize the codes and conventions of social documentary, presumably ridding them of their problematic enmeshment with histories of social surveillance and coercion."[54] Challenging the widespread critical acclaim for Goldin's work, Kotz's critical skepticism questions whether even a photographic practice with such an insider's perspective as Goldin's—she portrays her own intimate circle of friends, often inscribing herself as a subject—can escape the power relations that structure social documentary. Like Goldin, Yang developed a photographic practice driven by a strong narrative impulse. His pictures are produced in the service of storytelling, facilitated through the performance of a slide show, a predominantly temporal structure, rather than the normal spatial structure of the gallery exhibition. Whereas Goldin principally uses recorded music to frame and bind her images in her slide show performances, Yang performs his own accompanying monologue in front of the screen onto which his slides are projected. He stands to the side of these projected images but remains prominent in the mise-en-scène of the piece.

Both the visual and the verbal aspects of *Sadness* constitute acts of bearing witness. Yang's photographs are strongly rooted in the practice of social documentary. Ever since he first came to Sydney in 1969 he has sought to document a scene, a community, a social milieu—his first exhibition in 1977 was the ethnographically titled Sydneyphiles. Yang continued to photograph his social life and community as the AIDS epidemic hit Sydney in the 1980s and 1990s, creating a record of how gay men responded to the crisis on an individual and a social level: "My main document of AIDS happened with one or two friends of mine, one in particular called Allan, and I'd always photographed Allan and I felt that I shouldn't stop photographing him just because he had AIDS so that's how I got a continuous record of him in his last years. And I felt that he'd have felt rejected if I stopped photographing him. But, there is that record of AIDS, but also I photographed the social way in which the gay community has come to terms with AIDS."[55] From this interview we can see that Yang wants to frame his AIDS-related photography both as a natural continuation of his ongoing social documentation of Australian gay life and as a form of support in his personal relationships with PWAs. The usual ethical dilemma of the social documentarian is reversed—not, should I begin to photograph the subject, rather, how can I not continue? His photographs of Allan bear witness (in the historical sense) to an Australian gay man's life and death. But they also bear witness (in a more involved, psychological sense) to the difficult and painful experience of seeing a close friend suffer terminal illness. As I indicated in the introduction, the photographic witness in Sadness appears to oscillate between the roles of external witness (testis) and internal witness (superstes). Yang did not immediately embrace the subjective aspect of this latter role in his social documentary practice. The relational aspects of his photographic practices thus evolved over time.[56]

It was only after he had lost beloved friends that he began to use his photographs to work through his own experience of the AIDS epidemic. He began to write on his photographs, articulating his feelings toward his subjects and toward what they were going through (figures 10 and 11). This discursive supplement to the image eventually developed into the performance pieces as he worked with the photographs to narrativize what the pictures had recorded. In the years following Allan's death, Yang reworked his telling of Allan's story several times before it reached its final form in Sadness. The long creative process leading to the production of the performance piece illuminates the difficult work of bearing witness to trauma. The subject's desire to bear witness is problematized by the trauma's challenge to narrativization—it is an event not properly incorporated into the psyche as an experience since it resides beyond the realm of our normal cognitive and affective framework. It evades the subject's control by denying it the power to consciously recollect and relate the complete story. Thus the work of narrativization constitutes the foundation to bearing witness, for it is a task never self-evident or unhindered for the traumatized subject.

Yang's performances powerfully reframe his photographic practice to enable a fluid movement between the roles of external and internal witnessing, between the recording of another's life and death and an articulation of one's own experience of those events. This kind of witnessing dynamic was first seen in queer AIDS media in Stashu Kybartas's groundbreaking documentary portrait, *Danny* (1987), which openly constructed its discursive framework around the intersubjective relationship between Kybartas and Danny Sbrochi, a friend living with AIDS, who died during the making of the video.[57] In a moment that breaks the frames of dis/identification that conventionally subtend documentary portraiture, Kybartas reveals his erotic attachment to Danny as a significant dynamic in their documentary encounter. Like Yang's, Kybartas's self-inscription in his work engendered a fluid movement between internal and external forms of witnessing. Characteristic of much queer AIDS media, such movement points not to the distancing difference of subject/object relations, but to the proximate intersubjectivity of queer intimacies.

Yang has professed to the influence of Spalding Gray's work on his performance methods, but the structure of his exhibition practice can be historicized in a much older photographic (and protocinematic) tradition that uses a talking head to structure its presentation of images: the illustrated lecture.[58] Recent historiography of early cinema has emphasized the need to place the medium in the longer history of what Charles Musser calls "screen practice," thus tracing cinema's lineage in the magic lantern traditions of projected images accompanied by voice, music, and sound effects.[59] I want to invoke this history in discussing Yang's *Sadness* because it explains how the work already represented a protocinematic performance even before it was adapted for the screen. This history also illuminates a particular tension at the heart of the film's use of the talking head as a mode of performance.

Although disguised by the mantle of its pedagogic function, the nineteenth-century illustrated lecture offered the middle class spectatorial pleasures similar to those of the more popular form of the magic lantern. The lecturer's speech not only contextualized the images he or she presented but, more important, it performed the work of narrativization. In the travel lecture, for example, the monologue animated a series of autonomous photographic images into a journey, a movement through space and time that could be conveyed as story. Although these images had yet to attain the impres-

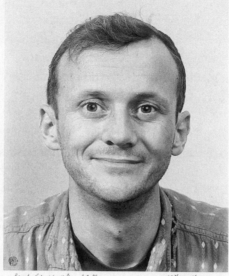

4. "Allan". From the monologue "Sadness."

Bronte Rd, Waverley Oct 99.   William Yang

He started to improve. He got his appetite back and he
began to put on weight. He came to visit me when I lived
at Waverley and after lunch I took him upstairs, put
him under the studio lights and I took this photo. It was
the best he ever looked during this period.

3/6

10. William Yang, "Allan," from the monologue *Sadness* (1992). Courtesy of the artist.

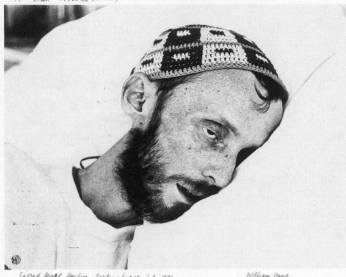

17 "Allan" From the monologue "Sadness"

Sacred Heart Hospice, Darlinghurst July 1990   William Yang.

He went into a coma. I saw the nurse give him a
glass of water but the water just ran out of his mouth.
He didn't respond to touch. I half expected him to be
cold but he was burning with fever. His pulse was
racing. Later this evening Jeffrey rang me up and
told me he had died.

3/2

11. William Yang, "Allan," from the monologue *Sadness* (1992). Courtesy of the artist.

sion of physical movement, their arrangement and framing by the lecturer's speech achieved the narrative movement that would prove so central to the development of cinema.[60] The talking head of the lecturer beside the screen proved a crucial source in the development of cinematic narrative by producing narrative continuity between successive images. As cinema developed its own forms of visual continuity, the film lecturer's role became more ambiguous. Noël Burch argues that the film lecturer actually offered the opportunity for the cinematic illusion to be unmasked rather than disavowed by the structures of visual and narrative continuity (154–55). He contends that this modernist possibility for the film lecturer was realized most fully in Japan, in the tradition of the *benshi*, whose elaborate and self-conscious verbal performance in front of the screen continuously acknowledged the material presence of the filmic image. The *benshi* stood in stark contrast to the Western film lecturer, who increasingly served as an inobtrusive guide through the narrative.[61]

I want to argue that Yang's presence and role in the film *Sadness* function in an ambivalent and complex manner similar to the historical function of the film lecturer—he both defamiliarizes and narrativizes the succession of images he offers up to the audience. I am not, however, suggesting that Yang is deliberately engaging with this tradition. Rather, by situating the performance and the film in this historiography of screen practice, I can illuminate precisely how the film reframes the conventional dynamics of the talking head in the service of witnessing. Yang's inscription within the film as a talking head continually emphasizes its very theatricality, its origins in live performance. This strategy certainly imbues the viewing experience of the film with the sense of the photographer's presence, which is the affective linchpin of the performance and its production of a testimonial address to its viewer. Yet the film's theatricality also produces a self-consciousness that encourages the viewer to consider the actual construction of the work, particularly its narrative structure. The film moves back and forth between the narration of the two themes of Yang's family history and his dying friends, but Yang does not explicitly articulate the relationship between them until the very end, when he speaks of his mother's death, which acts as a sort of dénouement and revelation: "The two strands of my story—the gay and the Chinese side—had come together over the experience of grief." Throughout the film, however, the viewer is compelled by the "parallel editing" of narratives to work through the connections between them by him- or herself. By the end of the film, the connections and meanings actively produced by the viewer resonate far beyond Yang's understated conclusion.

The Undoing of Identity

Sadness opens with an image of a white screen that turns out to be a photographer's light box onto which a stack of color and black-and-white slides are thrown. A hand arranges the slides into rows, and then we see successive close-ups of individual slides as a magnifying glass is gradually passed over each slide, momentarily enlarging its image. In voice-over we hear Yang describe the very process of his artistic practice: "All my performances begin with photographs. First I take the slides which I push around my light box and then words come." He explains how he wanted to explore two themes in his third show: the loss of friends and a family murder. In his opening lines of Sadness, Yang explicitly frames the project as an act of bearing witness: "I felt compelled to tell these stories of my friends. To unburden myself of what I have seen." He is a survivor psychologically driven by the experience of trauma to share its burden. We then see the slides gathered up and placed in a slide projector, followed by a close-up of the lens and its projection beam. The opening credits appear, succeeded by a close-up of a hand pressing a button on the slide projector's remote control, accompanied by a distinct mechanical click that introduces the first topic with a new intertitle ("allan") as though it were a title slide in the projector. The film consistently returns to this shot and sound of the remote control button throughout Sadness as a means to punctuate the transitions between narratives.[62] It is one of the film's several self-conscious devices that sustain its theatricality. Indeed, Sadness makes no attempt to conceal the staginess of its moving images, employing two major devices to this end: back projection in the theatrical reconstructions of Yang's journey to North Queensland and of his uncle's murder, and a proscenium mise-en-scène in Yang's shots as a talking head "lecturer."

After the first intertitle, Yang appears smartly dressed and framed above the waist before a red theatrical curtain as he addresses the camera directly. We subsequently also see him in medium long shots where he is standing on a proscenium stage in front of a large screen onto which his slides are projected (approximating the mise-en-scène of the original performances). As his monologue progresses, the image track cuts and dissolves between shots of Yang in direct address, full frames of his photographs, and reenactments resembling tableaux. The method of using sound bridges to suture the embodied voice of the talking head with a disembodied voice-over (framing images and scenes) has by now become a very common convention in documentary film and television. However, in its self-conscious and dialectical theatricality, Sadness resists using this convention to produce a seamless rhetorical and narrative flow. Rather, the film uses sound, editing, and mise-en-scène to accentuate Yang's complex shifts between the positions of internal and external witness.

In *Sadness* Yang narrates and discusses his repeated experience of witnessing five of his close friends—Allan, Nicholaas, Scotty, Peter, and David—struggle with illness and eventually death. Each one of his friends seems to cope with his illness and mortality in his own way, and Yang pays tribute to each of their lives by sharing cherished moments from before and during their illness. These anecdotes speak of friendships, relationships, and community, thus the identities of these individual gay men are always considered within the context of their relationship to others—lovers, friends, those also living with HIV/AIDS, or those caring for them. *Sadness* underscores the intimate bonds that constitute contemporary gay identity by paralleling these relationships with those of Yang's extended biological family. The second thematic strand of the film concerns Yang's literal and metaphorical journey to undercover the truth of his family's darkest trauma: his uncle's murder. Yang explains that his mother had always been extremely reticent about precisely how and why his prosperous uncle, William Fang Yuen, had been murdered in the 1920s in rural North Queensland. Yang recalls interviews that he conducted with relatives and other individuals who might shed light on the murder, but the stories they offered seemed to conflict. Fang Yuen was stabbed; he was shot; he was murdered over a gambling dispute; he died because he discovered an employee's extortion. Yang finally pins down the circumstances of the murder from court records: a racially motivated murder tolerated in a rural community steeped in racialized anti-immigrant sentiment. Yet the court records also reveal a family secret that actually proves more important than the details of the murder itself: his mother was a witness at the trial in which Fang Yuen's murderer was acquitted (figure 12). Throughout his investigation, Yang reveals the profound ambivalence he felt for most of his life about his ethnic identity, which he is eventually able to trace back to his mother's conscious decision to assimilate her family in light of witnessing the traumatic murder and seeing her own juridical act of bearing witness, as an external witness, fail to matter at the trial. She would consequently refuse to bear witness, as an internal witness, within the family. She figured that "you could be murdered and your killer go free, just because you were Chinese." Yang further assumes that "the legacy of this murder came down to me in the way my Chineseness was denied."

The film suggests that the facts of the traumatic event of Fang Yuen's murder are not the truth that Yang's journey discovers; rather, it is its long-term

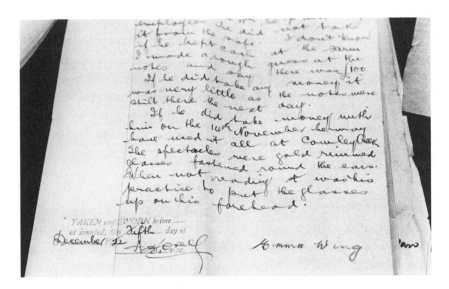

12. William Yang, "Mother's signature," from the monologue *Sadness* (1992).
Courtesy of the artist.

effects on his family members and their relationship to their own ethnicity.
The trauma of Fang Yuen's murder produced a powerful undoing of identity
in Yang's family. A story that could not be fully narrativized in the family history pulls its ethnic identity into crisis. In the conscious comparison of two
distinct traumas, *Sadness* suggests that the lesson Yang learns from the family
trauma is the imperative to bear witness, to endure the difficult narration of
painful experience, for to evade such an undertaking risks the potential undoing of identity. What is at stake here for gay men in the age of AIDS often
seems painfully apparent. As Simon Watney has warned, the devastating collective loss faced by gay men endangers the very fabric of gay identity itself:
the sense of social belonging formed through bonds of friendship and shared
personal histories.[63]

Throughout *Sadness*, Yang relates the stories of his friends' illnesses and
deaths in terms of his particular relation to the subject. He speaks of having
not seen Allan for several years, of his emotional reactions to Allan's deterio-
rating condition, and of his own romantic relationship with him many years
earlier. The narrativization of the images Yang performs in his monologue is
not just the story of a young gay man's illness and death but, more significantly, a recounting of the relationships that sustained him and his intimate
community.[64] Unlike the social documentary of certain AIDS photography,
such as Nicholas Nixon's controversial People with AIDS exhibition, Yang's

practice is always embedded in an articulation of the relationship between subject and photographer. It attests to how subjectivity is constituted through intersubjective relations, particularly those of family and queer intimates. The undoing of identity caused by historical trauma may thus perpetuate itself across and among generations. Yet *Sadness* also demonstrates how belatedly bearing witness to one historical trauma may furnish a redemptive opportunity to challenge the undoing of identity by a more recent one.

Witnessing at the Historical Crossroads

Lewis's and Phungula's *Sando to Samantha, aka, The Art of Dikvel* begins with a straightforward written text that situates the video's portrait of the HIV-positive drag queen Sando Willemse (aka Samantha Fox) precisely in a period of considerable national transformation: "In 1994, South Africa held its first democratic election. In the same year, Samantha Fox and friends went to Steinkopf, 600 km north of Cape Town for a drag show." In the precredit sequence that follows, the video presents selected moments from that trip. With its alternation between scenes on and off the drag show floor and its on-screen translation of the queer colored patois used by the Cape Town drag queens, the sequence distinctly recalls the ethnographic gaze of Jennie Livingston's *Paris Is Burning* (1990) on the Harlem drag ball scene. We are introduced to the term *moffie* (translated as "fag, fairy, fruit"), which Willemse later repeatedly uses as an appropriative label of self-identification, an indispensable part of being *dikvel* ("thick-skinned" in Afrikaans).[65] This opening sequence diverges from *Paris Is Burning* in the inclusion of scenes in which the drag queens engage with local people in the rural backwater of Steinkopf (Livingston's camera remains tightly focused on the interiority of the drag scene). The drag queens elicit a range of positive and negative responses to their queer presence in the town. In an important scene one of them asks a group of local women, "It's a New South Africa. It's going to be a New South Africa. Do you think that we as gays deserve a place in the New South Africa?"[66] It is not a woman's immediate affirmative response that is significant here, but the way in which the question posed renders a historical frame for the whole video. South Africa's past, present, and future are all invoked in this utterance. The current arrival of a "New South Africa" implies a differentiation from the old one, one rooted in the apartheid state and presumably now located in the past. Yet the drag queen's revision of her initial assertion hesitantly defers the transformation into a "New South Africa" onto the future, implying the continued legacy of apartheid in the present.

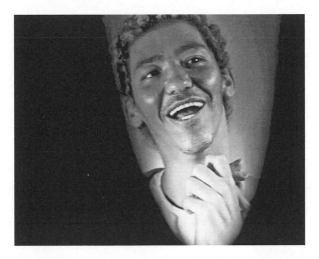

13. Frame capture from *Sando to Samantha, aka, The Art of Dikvel* (Jack Lewis and Thulanie Phungula, 1998). Courtesy of Idol Pictures.

The video consequently frames Willemse's testimony to his queerness and experience of living with HIV/AIDS in the context of South Africa during a complex period of transition, in which comprehending the continuities and discontinuities between past, present, and future becomes increasingly exigent. To further reinforce the issue of temporal framing, the videomakers embedded the moving images of this 1994 sequence in a static visual frame consisting of ephemeral material from Willemse's life, a mixture of personal photographs and official state documents, such as the infamous passbooks that restricted freedom of movement in the apartheid state.

Following the title credits, Willemse appears literally as a talking head — a black matte covers the majority of the frame, revealing only his head and thus completely obscuring the mise-en-scène of the interview (figure 13). He opens with a surprising assertion that sets off his testimony and the re-enacted scenes of his life: "My life in the army before I was diagnosed was just wonderful." As he begins to recall the circumstances of his military call-up in 1991, a wipe cut shifts the mode of representation from Willemse's talking head narration to a reenactment of the event with an actor (Ashraf Johaar-dien) performing the role of Willemse. The video subsequently alternates between these two representational modes, allowing for an unusual doubling of the witness's body, a device through which we are reminded of the temporal gap between the recent past (of Willemse's story) and the present (of the story's telling).

The black matte remains in place throughout the talking head scenes until the moment at which Willemse relates how the military establishment involuntarily tested him for HIV and callously informed him of his seropositive diagnosis without counseling or any other form of support. Whereas Riggs's *No Regret* dissolves its black mattes at the moments when its witnesses recount their empowering decisions to self-disclose their HIV status to their families and their communities, *Sando to Samantha* removes the matte precisely at the moment at which Willemse recalls the subjugation of involuntary disclosure. At this point in the video we come to see the position and space from which Willemse bears witness — dressed in an institutional bed gown, he sits alone in a sparse hospital ward. By withholding such information for much of the video, *Sando to Samantha* self-consciously resists the pervasive ideological trope of the homosexual AIDS victim who is embedded in a teleological narrative of self-inflicted fatality. According to this trope, the ill homosexual relates in the now his life before diagnosis, but the image of his present emaciated and hospitalized body recasts that prior life as a perilous lifestyle, the precondition, if not causation, of his current mortality. By contrast, from the moment at which we finally see Willemse in full frame in the hospital ward, his testimony and the reenacted scenes from his life focus on his tenacious struggle to survive in the face of institutional abjection and the inadequate state provision of social and medical support. As the temporal gap between his story and its telling closes, the final reenacted scene presents the actor playing Willemse alone in a hospital ward. A wipe cut then pulls the frame back to Willemse's talking head testimony; the doubled body of the witness thus comes to be reintegrated. In the final section of the video, Willemse relates his politicization and transformation into an AIDS activist after the diagnosis, which provides him with a self-empowering relation to his HIV status deliberately denied him by the South African military (figure 14).[67]

Unlike white South African men, black, Indian, and colored men were not subject to conscription into the South African Defence Force (SADF) under the apartheid regime. Thus Willemse formed part of a minority of colored South Africans who served in the segregated colored regiment of the Cape Corps (Kaapse Korpse). Willemse's mother had in fact volunteered him for the force to "make a man out of him."[68] Nevertheless, *Sando to Samantha* avoids explaining the circumstances that triggered his military service, allowing the video to frame the SADF as an institution standing in for the larger apartheid system. In light of the militarist masculinity at the heart of Afrikaaner national identity, the gender subversion of Willemse's drag persona Samantha Fox persistently articulates resistance not only to gender norms but also to

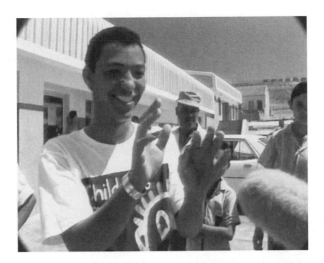

14. Frame capture from *Sando to Samantha, aka, The Art of Dikvel* (Jack Lewis and Thulanie Phungula, 1998). Courtesy of Idol Pictures.

the political system that relies on their continued performance. The video parodically draws parallels between the ritualized gender performances of the drag floor and the drill yard. Similarly, as a reflection of the larger racial segregation of South African society, the exclusively colored regiment in which Willemse serves actually generates a space of community that proves considerably accepting of Willemse's queerness, just as Cape Town's colored communities have long supported richly diverse queer subcultures.[69] On learning of Willemse's HIV diagnosis, the men in his unit express support and respect for him and frustration with the military command that orders his quarantine and eventual discharge from his unit. While policies of quarantine for people with HIV/AIDS have been called for and indeed practiced in many parts of the world, in South Africa they clearly resonated with the country's long history of imbricating discourses of epidemiology and race.[70]

Sando to Samantha concludes with Willemse defiantly refusing to regret anything about the life that he has chosen to lead: "I would live it all over again, only better." This defiant spirit, the art of *dikvel*, is captured visually in three photographs of Willemse spliced into the final scene, showing him as a child in the township, as a soldier in the Cape Corps, and as a drag queen activist at a gay rights demonstration. The subsequent written dedication communicates Willemse's death: "For Sando, 1974–1996." After the end credit sequence that presents an outtake of Willemse chatting and joking around with the cameraman, a rolling text addresses the viewer with a list of services and conditions that "You Have a Right To," including voluntary HIV testing, pre- and posttest counseling, HIV confidentiality, sexuality education, and job protection against HIV/AIDS discrimination. Funded by the AIDS Foundation of South Africa, the Levi Strauss Foundation, and the Western Cape Health Department, Sando to Samantha was clearly designed to serve as an outreach tool for HIV/AIDS education in postapartheid South Africa, yet it approaches the task by recognizing the necessity to frame it not only through the perspectives of South Africa's present and future but also through its complex past, particularly the historical trauma of apartheid and its continued legacy.

Queer Memory and the Archive of AIDS Cultural Activism

Despite its systematic destruction of the individual body, on the one hand, and its global prevalence, on the other, AIDS, like other historical trauma, is never merely an individual experience, nor universal in its effects. The value of Bright Eyes, No Regret, Sadness, and Sando to Samantha lies in their ability to situate their queer subjects and the trauma of AIDS firmly within the historical contexts that have constituted both. They resist the disciplinary function of the talking head in the shadow archive of AIDS representation by self-consciously using performance to bear witness to AIDS through the specific cultural archives of prior historical trauma, namely, the Holocaust, U.S. slavery, Australian anti-immigrant violence, and South African apartheid. These documentaries acknowledge that the historical trauma of AIDS may open up the wounds of prior historical trauma, but they also reveal the potential for the latter to provide the kind of historicization that facilitates rather than forecloses the political dimensions of bearing witness to AIDS.

But now that AIDS cultural activism of the 1980s and 1990s has itself entered the material archive, what value can it hold for queer AIDS media in the early twenty-first century? Matt Wolf's witty fake documentary Smalltown Boys addresses this very question through the optic of queer generational memory. Smalltown Boys functions simultaneously as a biographical homage to the queer artist and AIDS activist David Wojnarowicz and as an autobiographical sketch of Wolf's millennial queer generation and its relationship to the AIDS cultural activism that preceded it. The video alternates between three distinct strands: Wojnarowicz performing monologues on video tapes drawn from the artist's archive at New York University (NYU); Wolf's contemporary restaging of well-known Wojnarowicz projects; and talking head interviews with a fictional character named Sarah Rosenburg, a sullen lesbian

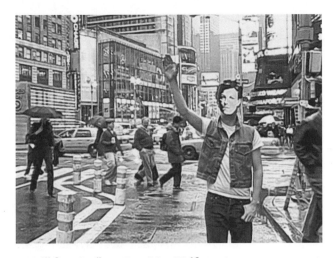

15. Still from *Smalltown Boys* (Matt Wolf, 2003).
Courtesy of the artist.

teen, whom the video fantasizes as Wojnarowicz's biological offspring (facilitated by the artist's anonymous deposits at a Manhattan sperm bank). In an
interview with the NYU archivist Marvin J. Taylor in GLQ, Wolf explains that
the imaginary relationship constructed between Wojnarowicz and Rosenburg "marks a generational transition and shifting ideas about activism in
queer culture."[71] Fictionalizing Wolf's own queer adolescence, the Rosenburg scenes are set in 1994 as the Upper West Side teen becomes involved in
online fan communities trying to save the queer-friendly teen drama *My So-
Called Life* from cancellation by its network, ABC. The earnest, radical intensity
of Wojnarowicz's performative address to the camera contrasts sharply with
Rosenburg's studied disaffection and the deliberate artifice of her talking
head interviews, thus rendering the former an object of nostalgic desire and
the latter an apparent degradation of the former's cultural activist legacy.

Despite Wolf's desire to produce an aesthetic intervention that "reacti-
vates Wojnarowicz's political rage in a culture where AIDS had become mainstream and visible," his contemporary restaging of works by Wojnarowicz
are marked by a silent, citational blankness (661). Reenacting Wojnarowicz's
masked queer flâneur from the photographic series *Arthur Rimbaud in New
York* (1978–79) in a cleaned-up subway train and a sanitized Times Square
merely highlights the historical distance of the recent past from the normalized present (figure 15).[72] Wolf's anonymous stenciling of Wojnarowicz's
famous burning house over subway posters for corporatized AIDS benefit
concerts becomes merely an act of tagging. Like Rosenburg, his fictional-

ized surrogate, Wolf is just a fan, and he knows it. Yet in the GLQ interview, Wolf argues that we need to reconsider how contemporary forms of queer fandom may in fact constitute new modes of activism and archiving: "Like the sexually charged corners of ACT UP meetings, the more abstract zones of fandom host a peculiar intersection of fantasy, desire, and community-based need for organization and preservation" (667). Smalltown Boys does not fully bear out that assertion, but it does suggest how queer fandom and its archival impulse may constitute a vital chance to build a queer intergenerational memory of AIDS. Maintaining a queer collective memory of the trauma of AIDS poses a specific challenge that differentiates the disease from other collective traumas that have produced extensive testimonial practices such as the Holocaust and the Hiroshima-Nagasaki bombings. Jewish collective memory of the Shoah, for instance, has been significantly grounded in the initial familial transfer of memory through "second generation witness."[73] Sons and daughters of survivors grew up in families in which the trauma of the Holocaust was still very present, either consciously through testimonial practices or unconsciously through traumatic repetition and transference. Marianne Hirsch proposes the notion of "postmemory" to describe the psychological specificities of such "passing on": "Postmemory most specifically describes the relationship of children of survivors of cultural or collective trauma to the experiences of their parents, experiences that they 'remember' only as the narratives and images with which they grew up, but that are so powerful, so monumental, as to constitute memories in their own right."[74] Although lesbians and gay men have developed alternative forms of familial and intimate bonds, it is precisely these bonds that have been endangered by the AIDS epidemic. In the face of such threats to queer intersubjectivity, the intergenerational "passing on" of the collective memory of AIDS as historical trauma produced by the works discussed in this chapter becomes all the more important. Now themselves reframed by time, such queer AIDS media may therefore come to serve as a repository of collective memory, "an archive of feelings," to borrow Ann Cvetkovich's phrase, which preserves the acts of bearing witness to the historical trauma of AIDS by many of those who have not survived: Stuart Marshall, Michael Callen, Marlon Riggs, Assoto Saint, Reggie Williams, Donald Woods, and Sando Willemse.[75]

□

CHAPTER TWO

The Embodied Immediacy

of Direct Action:

Space and Movement in

AIDS Video Activism

On 22 January 1991, the writer and AIDS activist John Weir jumped in front of the camera at the beginning of the CBS *Evening News*, shouting "AIDS is news. Fight AIDS, not Arabs!" (figure 16). As Weir's head was yanked from the frame by studio security, a surprised but generally unflappable Dan Rather immediately cut to a commercial break. Rather apologized dourly after the break for the "rude people" who had interrupted the beginning of the program and promised to return to the network's coverage of the Gulf War. That night, the eve of ACT UP's Day of Desperation, a massive nationwide demonstration against the continued neglect of the AIDS crisis, fourteen of the group's members were arrested as they tried to disrupt the broadcast of the news programs of CBS, NBC, and PBS.[1]

As Paula A. Treichler notes, this piece of direct action realized, if only momentarily, the powerful fantasy among AIDS activists of hijacking the evening news, something that had already been wittily articulated in *Rockville Is Burning* (Bob Huff and Wave 3, 1989), a video inspired by ACT UP's highly effective demonstration against the Federal Drug Administration in October 1988.[2] Documenting a collaboration between La Mama Experimental Theater Company and Wave 3, an ACT UP affinity group, the video presents a fictional guerilla group, the New Center for Drugs and Biologics, taking over and reprogramming the evening news to serve the needs of people living with HIV/AIDS (figure 17). Three activists in white doctors' coats storm the

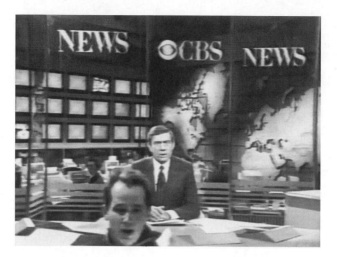

16. Frame capture from *Voices from the Front*
(Testing the Limits, 1991).

studio, overrunning the self-satisfied news anchor. They immediately link up
via video feed to other activists and people with AIDS all around the United
States, thus replacing the regular national network of news reporters. Although the video invokes the particular spatialized discourse of broadcast
news, it blatantly rejects or inverts its hierarchal dynamics. For instance,
when a scientist from the National Institute of Allergy and Infectious Disease is interviewed, he is shown in silhouette, shaming this institution's representative for its inaction with precisely the same confessional device used
by broadcast news to shame people with HIV/AIDS. In *Rockville Is Burning*,
the collective authority of the activists displaces the individual supremacy of
the anchor. Rather than address the general population, they speak for and
to the constituencies most directly affected by the AIDS crisis: video activism
as direct action.

The commitment to interrogate and challenge the discursive operations of
broadcast news runs through AIDS activist video production from the 1980s
and 1990s. Understanding the considerable ideological power of television
news in shaping the representation of the AIDS epidemic, video activists
created diverse means to appropriate, parody, and analyze the mechanisms
of television news, particularly its reliance on the talking head. In their radical transformation of the discursive space in which activists and people with
HIV/AIDS could speak, videos produced in the culture of ACT UP smashed
the liberal pieties of "giving a face" and "giving a voice" to the person with
HIV/AIDS. In fact, they often demonstrated how such seemingly affirmative

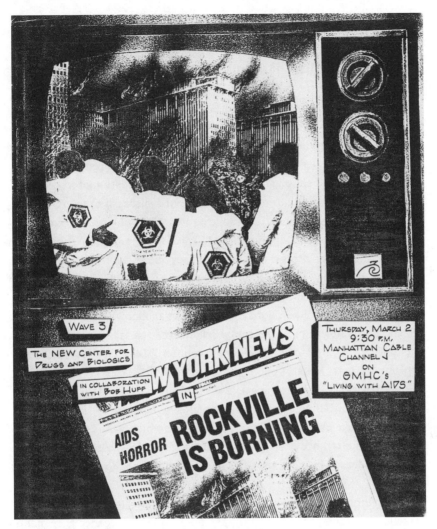

17. Photocopied flyer for *Rockville Is Burning* (Bob Huff and Wave 3, 1989). Phil Zwickler Collection, no. 7464. Courtesy of the Division of Rare and Manuscript Collections, Cornell University Library.

goals were undoubtedly implicated in keeping people in their ideologically predetermined roles. In this chapter I examine how AIDS activist video production in ACT UP/New York sought to transform discursive space along two simultaneous lines.[3] Like the action at CBS *Evening News*, one part pursued an intervention in the dominant media representation of the epidemic, while the other part, like *Rockville Is Burning*, aimed to participate in the lesbian and gay counterpublic and the networks that supported the social movement of

AIDS activism.[4] A number of videos, including Robert Hilferty's *Stop the Church* (1990) and *Voices from the Front* (1992) by the video collective Testing the Limits, were produced and distributed with both lines of interventions in mind. Yet all of them grappled with the challenge of reconfiguring the possibilities of the talking head as the means to forge a discursive space in which effective political testimony could be enacted.

Nowhere is the contrast between the honorific and the repressive functions of the talking head, which I outlined in the previous chapter, more apparent than in news broadcasting, which has arguably been the most important medium for shaping the dominant public perception of AIDS in the United States. News anchors sit at the apex of a discursive hierarchy; they are, in Robert Stam's words, "symbolic figures who will keep us from going adrift on a stormy sea of significations."[5] Speaking straight into the camera, the news anchor performs the pseudointimacy of television's direct address, which simulates face-to-face communication. This invocation of the face-to-face situation in the discursive address of television news lends it both authority and intimacy. Television news frames its anchor within a set of reality effects that simulate both the temporal and the spatial sense of presence necessary for a simulated face-to-face encounter. "The telecaster is not *here*," explains Margaret Morse, "but the impression of presence is created through the construction of a shared space, the impression of shared time, and signs that the speaking subject is speaking for himself, sincerely."[6] Using the teleprompter, the anchor reads the news as if it were not read, as if it were the spontaneous utterance of a speaker in conversation, which produces a sense of the broadcast's liveness and an impression of the anchor's discursive authority.

The anchor, most often male, plays a sovereign role in the discursive construction of the news as he seemingly summons the heterogeneous elements of the news program: on-site correspondents, interviews, and news footage. With a glance to the side that frequently precedes a correspondent's report, the anchor sutures the shift in discourse as though he were in spatial proximity to the reporter, yet also paradoxically invoking a movement in perspective to the correspondent in the world "out there." In fact, broadcast news relies on the discursive construction of a studio-bound "here" (correlated with a predominantly home-bound viewer) and a world out "there."[7] As a talking head, the anchor has his discursive sovereignty rest in his ability to situate the other talking heads that make up the news program, marshaling them as evidence in his narration of significant events. The correspondents are necessarily situated in the particular geographical or social location of the news event, but ultimately their enunciation is not defined by that situatedness. They will stand outside that location to speak (in at least part of the report) either through voice-over narration or the convention of the stand-up. The stand-up situates them in front of the particular location — away from it while simultaneously borrowing from its indexical presence — but speaking in direct address to the camera and thus affecting a pseudoconversation with the anchor.[8]

Direct address is deployed in broadcast news as a structure of power. The subjects of news do not speak directly to the television audience via the camera, but to an off-screen interviewer whose presence is implied by the news subject's line of vision. Or if the news subject is in a studio, he or she may speak directly to the camera, but the discursive structure of the broadcast positions that dialogue as one between the anchor and the subject. Although the subjects of news, whether politicians, business people, or the urban poor, are positioned by the discourse of broadcast news to speak indirectly through its apparatus, the manner of that placement determines the degree to which they are discursively enfranchised or disenfranchised. The mise-en-scène of professional expertise includes the case full of books behind the speaking subject and often a desk to situate him or her in a professional (as opposed to a domestic) environment, while political mise-en-scène predominantly deploys the podium as the sign of power and the authority to speak. Whereas a politician or professional needs only a few props to situate his or her enunciation, a working-class woman living in a housing project, as Harry Watt's *Housing Problems* illustrates, tends to be obscured by the very plenitude of detail that situates her speech. In such instances, the enunciation of the subject becomes overwhelmed by the reality effects that situate them.

Containing "Them" out "There"

The history of AIDS representation in broadcast news demonstrates the pervasiveness of these spatialized power relations around the talking head, and nowhere was this more apparent than in the U.S. television coverage of the epidemic in its first decade. Unlike newspapers that picked up on the initial Centers for Disease Control and Prevention (CDC) report in June 1981 of a rare pneumonia affecting gay men, television news media did not begin to cover AIDS until a full year later. Television's attention to AIDS reflected neither the empirical indicators of the epidemic's development nor the professional concern with AIDS.[9] Compared to the steady rise in AIDS cases reported by the CDC throughout the 1980s and the simultaneous growth of medical literature on AIDS, television news coverage remained unstable, peaking sporadically in 1983, 1985, and 1987, during periods of public alarm over the potential threat of AIDS to the so-called general population. Moreover, news media proved highly reticent in the early years of the epidemic in reporting a subject that mixed references to blood, semen, sex and death, which might offend the norms of taste for its presumed audience: the middle-class family. Gay men were deemed outside this all-important category. Thus the news media tended either to ignore AIDS stories or present them in the reassuring terms of a threat contained in several highly marginalized groups (including homosexuals, Haitians, intravenous drug users, and hemophiliacs). Such containment involved the discursive delineation of boundaries, in which the normative healthy center of the general population is maintained through the separation and abjection of an infected margin. In his explanation of this spatialized othering process, Simon Watney contends that the discourses of containment in mainstream news media during the 1980s participated in the neoconservative project of reducing the social to the scale of the family, which would subsequently function as its "monolithic and legally binding category."[10] By understanding the social solely in terms of the family, governments could ignore the needs of gay men who, like other affected groups, were considered outside the social.

But containment always carries the feared risk of leakage and even collapse. These fears are precisely what fueled the three principal periods of media hysteria over AIDS: the initial "epidemic of fear" in 1983, the disclosure of Rock Hudson's illness in 1985, and the panic over "heterosexual AIDS" in 1987. In 1983 news media began to report on an "epidemic of fear" around AIDS, covering stories of the potential threat caused by AIDS to social institutions such as prisons, schools, and hospitals. In what would set a precedent for future periods of intense media attention to AIDS, reports adopted the common "alarm and reassurance pattern" used by news media to cover ongoing crises. News reports would provoke alarm by focusing on the spreading fear, often including interviews with "ordinary" citizens who frequently offered misleading information about the risks around AIDS. The reporter would then offer reassurance, often in the tag line, that the threat of contamination from the abjected margins was still contained. Rather than mitigate and dispel fear and ignorance about AIDS, such television news reports actually increased them.

The disclosure of Hudson's AIDS-related illness in 1985 led to the second period of media hysteria around the epidemic. His illness proved a pivotal moment in AIDS media representation, but not for its presumed effect on his friend, President Ronald Reagan, who would not utter the "A-word" in public for another two years. Since Hudson's image had long been a staple of rugged but clean-cut American masculinity, his star persona after the disclosure of his illness was haunted by a doubling effect as he came to embody the dangers to the normal body posed by the contagion of homosexuality, rendering it an abnormal and sick "anti-body."[11] The long discursive history of homosexuality as itself a contagion, continually haunting and threatening the healthy social body, resurfaced with a vengeance during the months following Hudson's hospitalization in Paris. The inert weight of his star persona produced, however, a complex set of contradictions around the reporting on his illness. Even the most lurid and sensational tabloid coverage was marked by a defensive mixture of sympathy and fear. The event of Hudson's illness finally lent AIDS a certain legitimacy as a newsworthy issue. For a brief period around Hudson's illness, gay men living with AIDS and lesbian and gay activists were given opportunities in interviews, albeit limited ones, to speak their concerns and articulate perspectives outside the heteronormative general population.

The third and most intense period of media hysteria erupted in 1987 when rising infection rates among nonmarginalized groups became unavoidably visible in the monthly figures produced by the CDC. An inadvertent comment by Rather during a CBS News Special entitled "AIDS Hits Home" and broadcast on 22 October 1986 explicitly demonstrates the subtext of media discourse that would explode in the following year: "The scary reality is that gays are no longer the only ones getting it." The epidemic of fear returned as file footage of gay men was replaced by footage of the general population, whose prophylactic normality had now been penetrated by its diseased margins. Although these new visual discourses swirled around the fear of an unseen heterosexual threat, such invisibility was haunted by the shadow archive of the diseased antibody, figured in the dying homosexual in his hospital bed and the prostitute soliciting on the street at night. The intense media coverage finally pushed Reagan to make his first public statement on AIDS in April 1987. As both political and media elites began to address AIDS in that year, it finally gained a regular place on the public policy agenda.

Although the following decade saw the diversification of AIDS representation into other areas of television programming, broadcast news continued to maintain the binaries established in the first decade of the AIDS epidemic.[12] Kevin B. Wright's analysis of AIDS coverage on Nightline (ABC) and The MacNeil/Lehrer News Hour (PBS) from 1992–94 demonstrates how these agenda-setting news elites persisted in excluding or marginalizing those people and communities most affected by AIDS.[13] The shadow archive that distinguished body from antibody continued to be produced in the studio forums that these media programs favor. Inscribed by an ideology of "balance" rooted in the liberal construction of the public sphere, studio forums become the valorized space of public discussion, lending credibility to the discourse of their guests. Wright points to a tendency to exclude community activists and people with AIDS from the studio discussions altogether, or, if they were invited, to restrict their opportunity to speak. Frequently, when activists or PWAs were included in the program, they were shown in video footage speaking at demonstrations. At best, such inclusion in debate positioned their perspectives as out there (on the street), outside the "true" public sphere for "rational" debate (in the television studio); at worst, this footage continued to position gay men and people with AIDS as a dangerous (and highly politicized) volatile mass threatening public order. Such protracted exclusion from the dominant media discussion of the epidemic would prove a decisive incentive for the production of alternative AIDS media.

The Alternative Space of Direct-Action Video

Responses to the mainstream representation of AIDS began to emerge in the mid-1980s as community organizations involved in AIDS prevention and support services for people with AIDS began to organize the production of alternative media for their specific pedagogic functions. For these videos to successfully fulfill their intent of imparting vital information about prevention and caregiving, they were first compelled to unpack many of the ideological assumptions about AIDS produced by the dominant media. They needed to present affirmative counterimages of people with AIDS, whose lives and identities were neither to be reduced to pathology nor to be confined merely to the context of their illness. Independent queer film- and videomakers followed suit in the subsequent years with a mixture of portrait pieces documenting the courageous struggle of people with AIDS—such as *Chuck Solomon: Coming of Age* (Mark Huestis and Wendy Dallas, 1986), *Living with AIDS* (Tina DiFeliciantonio, 1986), and *Hero of My Own Life* (Tom Brook, 1986)—and experimental works aimed at deconstructing the discourses of AIDS in the mainstream media, including Stuart Marshall's *Bright Eyes*, Emjay Wilson's *A Plague Has Swept My City* (1985), and Barbara Hammer's *Snow Job: The Media Hysteria of AIDS* (1986), and Bob Huff's *AIDS News: A Demonstration* (1988).[14]

In March 1987, at the height of the third wave of media hysteria around AIDS and amid the anger generated among lesbian and gay communities by the U.S. Supreme Court's decision in *Bowers vs. Hardwick* to uphold state sodomy statutes, the establishment of ACT UP in New York triggered a major transformation in alternative AIDS media.[15] The group defined itself as "a diverse, non-partisan group united in anger and committed to direct action to end the AIDS crisis."[16] By shifting from the mobilization of public demonstrations to the practice of direct action, in which specific institutional bodies were directly confronted to demand change, ACT UP radicalized and widened AIDS activism from its initial base in PWA groups, who had begun to stage marches, candlelight vigils, and other public memorials as early as 1983. Following Cindy Patton's account of AIDS politics in the early 1980s, David Román argues that it is vitally important that early AIDS activism not be forgotten or dismissed by revisionist historical analysis that privileges the establishment of ACT UP as the "real" beginning of AIDS activism. While I concur with Román and Patton on this point, this chapter will address the activism around ACT UP, since it marks the first major convergence of direct action and video activism in the context of AIDS.[17]

Like so many other grass-roots AIDS organizations, ACT UP was formed and organized predominantly by gay men and lesbians. However, in its desire to forge a broad-based inclusive movement, the group often oscillated in its negotiation of the complex connections between AIDS and homosexuality. As the sociologist Josh Gamson notes in his analysis of ACT UP/San Francisco's activities, "AIDS activists find themselves simultaneously attempting to dispel the notion that AIDS is a gay disease (which it is not) while, through their activity and leadership, treating AIDS as a gay problem (which, among other things, it is)."[18] Many ACT UPers came to AIDS activism from lesbian and gay politics and thus saw ACT UP as an urgent and necessary development of lesbian and gay activism, whereas others, especially women, came also from the context of reproductive rights and women's health movements, leading them to understand AIDS politics within a larger framework of healthcare issues, which eventually brought many of them into conflict with the gay male activists focused primarily on treatment access.[19] Influenced by the media expertise of an initial core membership that included artists, designers, and media professionals, ACT UP adopted an activist practice grounded in the exploitation of media spectacle and graphic publicity.[20] The group was not only professionally but also theoretically informed as its practice drew from various intellectual sources, ranging from popular culture to situationism and postmodernism.[21]

AIDS activist video practice emerged from the need felt by a number of individuals and newly formed video collectives, namely Testing the Limits and DIVA TV (Damned Interfering Video Activists), to document and disseminate the explosion in AIDS activism through alternative forms of media production and circulation.[22] Like other affinity groups in ACT UP, these video collectives operated relatively autonomously within the movement. They insisted on maintaining a fluid, process-oriented method of production that balanced the freedom of individual videomakers to choose how they shot their footage with the collective decision making of the editing process.[23] Despite some initial resistance and skepticism from fellow ACT UP members who were most concerned with getting attention from the mainstream media, video activists like Gregg Bordowitz firmly understood their practice as a form of direct action itself. Bordowitz and David Meieran saw themselves as the "Dziga Vertovs of our revolution," videomakers whose media production formed part of the revolutionary process, not merely of its post facto representation.[24] Bordowitz has argued that "it became clear that the production of documentary overlaps with the efforts of political organizing. In order to tear down the structures that house the 'public discussion' of AIDS, we have to build alternative structures."[25]

The video activism around ACT UP was influenced by a wide range of developments in politically engaged media over the previous thirty years. In summarizing these influences, Alexandra Juhasz argues that they all revolved around an opposition to dominant media production and circulation, stressing "the significance of self-expression, the politics of self-definition, the power of speaking 'in our own voices.'"[26] The major influences on AIDS video activism included the decolonizing culture of Third Cinema, the community circulation of the American Underground Cinema, the reflexive turn in recent ethnographic film, the identity politics of feminist and lesbian and gay film, and the developing infrastructure of alternative television. Technological innovation in film and video have of course contributed significantly to all these movements, but the major developments in video technology in the 1980s with the so-called camcorder revolution played a particularly crucial role in facilitating new movements of media activism. The increased access to media production and circulation provided by the cheap technologies of the camcorder and the VCR revitalized alternative television practices after the waning fortunes of guerilla television during the late 1970s.[27] AIDS video activists also found creative ways of accessing production resources, from exploiting the professional media facilities available to a number of them at their jobs to buying expensive new cameras, shooting protests, and then returning the cameras for a refund. Veteran videomakers like Dee Dee Halleck, an important member of the influential Paper Tiger media collective, also provided the experiential bridge to the younger generation of video activists, urging them to constitute their intervention through the production of videos for targeted audiences and with specific purposes in mind. This type of intervention thus required using alternative modes of circulation, rather than aspiring to break into the distribution structure of dominant media (207).

The videomakers involved in Testing the Limits and DIVA TV understood their practice in terms of three primary functions: to produce their own news service that could distribute coverage of actions within activist communities and to progressive independent media outlets; to generate their own archive so that communities affected by the epidemic would not need to rely on commercial news services to write their own history in the future; and to serve as a video witness whose presence might guard against any police misconduct or abuse.[28] These functions articulate three different manifestations of bearing witness: to facilitate the testimony of the internal witness addressed to others affected for the purpose of affirmation and empowerment; to generate testimony and evidence dedicated to future collective memory; and to serve as an eyewitness or external witness in the juridical sense.

Since alternative AIDS media engendered a set of practices as diverse as AIDS activism itself, an examination of the video practices connected to ACT UP requires a more specific term than AIDS *activist video*, which appropriately encompasses a wide range of media production, including works dedicated to HIV prevention, civil rights advocacy, community outreach, and self-health promotion. I have therefore chosen to name the body of videos analyzed in this chapter "direct-action videos," as they are all engaged in some form of representational practice around the direct-action practices of ACT UP. Moreover, their makers understood such video production as itself a form of direct action, not merely as its audiovisual documentation. Although each of the direct-action videos bears its own specific visual and rhetorical logic, all of them demonstrate a sustained critical engagement with the media convention of the talking head. Most significantly, these videos adopt a striking proliferation of talking heads. They introduce many more speaking subjects than are commonly employed in contemporary documentary practice. We see a great variety of speakers in terms of sex, sexuality, race, ethnicity, age, and profession speaking in a wide array of registers and framed in a number of different situations (e.g., interviews in offices and at demonstrations, discussions at the Monday night meeting of ACT UP/New York, and speeches and addresses recorded at public events and actions).

On a general level, this multiplication of voices produced two effects crucial to the project of AIDS activism. First, it decentered authority and dispersed it among the numerous speaking subjects. This decentering of authority is also reflected in the collective authorship of many of the works. Embodying the radical democratic and anarchist ethos of ACT UP and its organization, direct-action video resisted the hierarchical structures of broadcast news and television documentary, which use anchors, presenters, reporters, and omniscient off-screen narrators to structure and frame the speech and events recorded by the camera. It also rejected the more subtle use of talking heads as "part characters, part presenters," which John Corner sees as a major strategy of discursive organization in contemporary documentary practice, where the film or program continually returns to a particular set of interviewees who gradually become both characters and presenters.[29] Second, the very proliferation of subjects given the opportunity to articulate their perspectives, expertise, and opinions constructed an image of emergent community that remained vitally important as a counterimage to the phobic iconography of dominant representation, which consistently framed PWAs in isolation and outside their social contexts (either alone in hospital beds or returned to the fold of the nuclear family). Moreover, these videos offered the opportunity for people affected by the epidemic to recognize their relation to others also affected. Testing the Limits, for instance, produced its very first video called *Testing the Limits: NYC* (1987) precisely to connect disparate groups and constituencies affected by AIDS. As Bordowitz declared: "Video puts into play the means of recognizing one's place within the movement in relation to that of others in the movement. . . . The most significant challenge to the movement is coalition building, because the AIDS epidemic has engendered a community of people who cannot afford *not* to recognize themselves as a community and to act as one."[30] To ensure the collectivism of their first project, Testing the Limits determined each edit of the video through a consensus decision among the group.

In their emphasis on community building and the articulation of empowering relations between people directly affected by AIDS, these videos refused the structures of address that the dominant representation of AIDS, particularly in broadcast news, had maintained, where the audience is constructed as an exclusionary general population. The activists who constitute the vast majority of speakers in direct-action video are invariably presented in such a way that their speech can be understood as a direct address to those most affected by the epidemic. Activists are therefore framed in two predominant speaking positions. Much of the footage captures their speech in the context of a group meeting or action where they are seen addressing other activists and people assembled in public spaces. The camera frequently

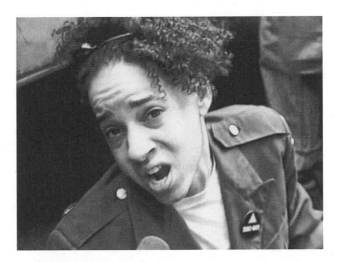

18. Frame capture from *Voices from the Front*
(Testing the Limits, 1991).

cuts from this observational mode to a more interactive mode where activists speak directly to the camera, often right in the middle of an action, demonstration, or meeting (figure 18). Patricia Zimmermann argues that this latter mode of framing activist speech is not interactive in the traditional documentary sense that can be traced back to *cinéma vérité* and the ethos of Jean Rouch's *Chronicle of a Summer* (1960). Rather than privilege the camera as the epicenter of action, out of which political confrontation and articulation are produced, "these works figure cameras and representations as social and political actors together with the subject."[31] In direct-action videos, the camera is seen to work alongside politicized subjects who clearly need neither the provocation of the camera's presence nor the inquiry of a media reporter to enable and generate their testimony.

Many of the activists interviewed in these tapes speak directly into the camera lens, which differentiates their testimony from the structures of address normally used in media interviews, in which the speaker's address is mediated through his or her implied conversation with an interviewer who stands alongside the camera. Compelling the speaker's line of vision to be directed either slightly to the left or to the right of the camera, such indirect address to a media audience facilitates the containment of minority speech through the regulated discursive space of conventional documentary and news forms. In other words, the subject's speech is mediated through his or her discursive and spatial relations to a reporter, interviewer, or news anchor. However, the presentation of many speakers in direct address to the camera in direct-action video occurs, I would argue, for two reasons. First, most activists interviewed adhere to their media training in ACT UP, which stressed the need to bypass or neutralize the mediation of the mass media machine as much as possible. As the activist and former network television producer Ann Northrop is heard reiterating at one point in *Stop the Church*: "Not to the media, but through the media!" Direct address was understood in ACT UP and its video collectives as itself a manifestation of the direct-action ethos. The second reason for this prominent use of direct address would seem to stem from more practical considerations. Videomakers recording demonstrations frequently found themselves to be the ones holding the camera and asking the questions of the activists they encountered, thus creating a speaking situation in which direct address was virtually inevitable.[32]

This construction of an imagined spatial relation of copresence between speaker and viewer in direct-address testimony points to the significance of space in AIDS activist video. As I have discussed earlier in this chapter, television news and documentary forms construct spatialized power relations in which a hegemonic "here" is pitted against a threatening "there." In the context of AIDS, this binary has all too often been played out as the white heteronormative general population, embodied by the presumed normality shared by the newscaster in his (or sometimes her) studio and the viewer at home, needing to protect itself from contamination by an abject abnormality, out "there" in the inner city (the locus for infectious urban queerness, dangerous femininity, and threatening blackness) or in Africa (the imagined cradle of the epidemic).[33] The various textual mediations of television reporting allow that threatening otherness to be kept at bay from the general population and contained "out there." Direct-action video, on the other hand, explicitly rebukes such spatialization by insisting that the construction of a textual "here" be grounded in a public space that the activists defiantly occupy, whether it be St. Patrick's Cathedral, Wall Street, or the National Institutes of Health (these were three of ACT UP's major actions). By making a spectacle of their speech in public space, AIDS activists testified against the reduction of the social by neoconservative politics, which continues to push for the privatization of not only culture but also social provision.

Through its use of hand-held cameras that function as fellow social actors in the activist body, direct-action video produces its own particular form of mimesis, which I will call its effect of "embodied immediacy." Such a sense of immediacy in the here and now of ACT UP's occupation of symbolically and institutionally powerful public spaces demonstrates a liberating resistance to the discourse of containment. This juncture between the use of public space and the discursive mediation of the public sphere is critical to an understanding of how direct-action video functioned performatively.[34] Although we understand the public sphere to be an increasingly dematerialized and by now largely imagined space in postmodern, late capitalist societies, the occupation of material public space by living bodies continues to be a critical political strategy in that dematerialized public sphere. In its embodied immediacy and recording of the dynamic occupation of public space, direct-action video participates in what Jane Gaines terms the "political mimesis" of committed documentary.[35] In working through one of documentary film's perpetual mythologies—that it has "the power to change the world"—Gaines concludes that we need to examine the sensual aspects of politically committed documentary as much as its analytical ones: "The whole rationale behind documenting political battles on film, as opposed to producing written records, is to make struggle visceral, to go beyond the abstractly intellectual to produce a bodily swelling" (91). While careful to retain the imperative to foster political consciousness through intellectual means, Gaines argues for the need to value the potential affective power of images that depict the bodily movement and struggle of those involved in political direct action.

Gaines's conception of political mimesis points to the performative aspect of direct-action video. The activists' demands articulated as a form of political testimony emanate from bodies that physically put themselves on the line for their own survival. People with AIDS and their fellow activists are seen risking arrest and possible police brutality by literally laying down their bodies to occupy public space and disrupt its functioning (figure 19). By bringing viewers into the midst of the activist body through its effect of embodied immediacy, direct-action video both implicates viewers in the maintenance of the social and, in the process of political mimesis, affectively moves them to take action. A segment of DIVA TV's *Target City Hall* (1989) illustrates this particularly well: the camera follows CHER, an ACT UP affinity group, as it collectively decides exactly when is the right moment to initiate acts of civil disobedience by blocking traffic in front of City Hall.[36] Positioned in the center of the circle of activists, the camera spins around to catch each new voice that enters the deliberation. The momentum to act is viscerally felt through the embodied immediacy of the camera at that moment. Having learned well the lessons of earlier social movements, ACT UP always vitally understood the magnitude that grounds speech when the body that articulates it acts up in civil disobedience and disrupts "business as usual."[37] In ACT UP demonstrations, the specific demands of the group were explicitly underwritten by activists' bodies simultaneously bearing witness to their continued

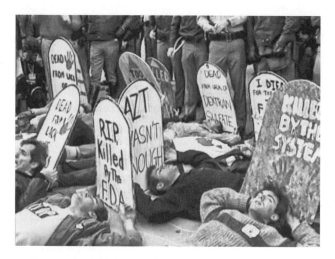

19. Frame capture from *Voices from the Front*
(Testing the Limits, 1991).

survival (against the pervasive phobic fantasy of a world after the homosexual) and to the risks posed to their lives by the inaction that was denying
them the fullest opportunities for survival. Such activism reminds us of the
profoundly somatic dimension to bearing witness in which bodily presence
has the capacity to produce the kind of extradiscursive excess that constitutes
the affective and ethical dimensions of magnitude. The challenge to direct-
action video has been to find means to communicate such magnitude to its
viewers, while communicating the specific political imperatives of the action
documented by the video.

Recording the Action

Although both DIVA TV and Testing the Limits grounded their practice in a
combination of direct-address testimony and political mimesis, their completed works demonstrate noticeably divergent applications of such strategies. Their differences attest to the various means by which magnitude could
be articulated. Like Hilferty's *Stop the Church*, DIVA TV's videos showed a
greater propensity to replicate ACT UP's irreverent attitude and boundary
crossing, whereas Testing the Limits, though far from conventional in its
documentary practice, tended to rely more heavily on what Bill Nichols has
called documentary's "discourses of sobriety."[38] Both *Stop the Church* and *Like
a Prayer* (DIVA TV, 1991) examine AIDS and abortion rights activists' massive
demonstration against New York's Cardinal John O'Connor and the Catholic

Church at St. Patrick's Cathedral on 10 December 1989. The videos' use of camp, parody, and black humor effectively imitates the tone of many strategies used in the actual demonstration. More than forty-five hundred people showed up at St. Patrick's for the action carrying signs rich in appropriative word play: "Stop This Man, Curb Your Dogma!" "Danger, Narrow-Minded Church Ahead!" and "Public Health Menace: Cardinal O'Connor." Inside the cathedral, activists disguised as regular Catholic churchgoers staged a "die-in" in the main aisle during O'Connor's sermon, and several of them yelled out their protests and blew whistles as they were carried out by the police. O'Connor responded by handing out printed copies of the sermon. Forty-three activists were arrested inside the cathedral and sixty-eight in the streets. Acting on his own decision, one activist (and former seminarian) broke the consecrated communion wafer and threw it on the floor. In what would become an overwhelmingly negative media reaction, reporters made most of this last protest, turning it into a desecration of the host by legions of "homosexual activists."[39]

The seven separate sections of Like a Prayer were each made by a different member of the collective and addressed a different "deadly sin" committed by the Catholic Church in the AIDS crisis. The video's diverse parts are woven together by Madonna's song "Like a Prayer," interviews with Catholic members of ACT UP, and the DIVA member Ray Navarro's reporting from the scene in Jesus Christ drag. The video appropriates and resignifies both the music video form and the discourse of broadcast news as its principal structuring devices. Navarro performs as Jesus Christ, a news reporter for FBN (Fire and Brimstone Network), positioned with his microphone in front of the crowd outside the cathedral, parodically invoking the authority of the field reporter: "This is Jesus Christ. I'm in front of St. Patrick's on Sunday. We're here reporting on a major AIDS activist and abortion rights demonstration." When he ends his report with the comment, "We're here to say, we want to go to heaven too," he is not just being sarcastic. This tongue-in-cheek remark produces a shift in the use of "we" from the conventional address to a news audience (outside the events) at the beginning of his report to an inclusive assertion of his participation in the demonstration at the end. This subtle play in address points to a major issue raised by the demonstration— whether activists themselves were speaking out within the Catholic Church (as Roman Catholics) or outside it (as activists criticizing an institution and its policies).[40] In the actual demonstration this metaphorically spatialized debate becomes mapped onto the real spatial dynamics of inside versus outside the cathedral, which Like a Prayer emphasizes. The appropriation of the

Madonna song worked in a similar fashion, invoking a figure who had herself been performing a comparable critique of the Catholic Church from the position of someone also within it.

Hilferty's *Stop the Church* similarly makes much of the inside/outside distinction, both thematically and visually. While there is plenty of campy humor in the video about ACT UP's pseudomilitary planning, including a strategy session focused on the cathedral's blueprints, *Stop the Church* devotes much of its time to the debate within the group about how the demonstration should be positioned rhetorically in the public sphere. The video opens with a montage of paintings depicting pain and suffering by Masaccio, Caravaggio, and others, then cuts to a forceful soundtrack that mixes the "Dies Irae" section of Hector Berlioz's *Symphonie fantastique* with whispering voices muttering the question, "What is the Catholic Church?"[41] (figure 20). A number of different talking heads follow, each offering their own answers, which mostly express alienation and bitterness at the church.[42] When Hilferty inserts one response from an "ordinary" parishioner outside the cathedral, who says, "It's a communion, a oneness, all across the world," it serves less as an attempt to institute so-called media balance and more as a reminder, when placed in relation to the other responses, of the failure of the church to actually foster an inclusive communion. The montage of talking heads becomes far more dialectical when the focus shifts to the actual debates held during ACT UP meetings in early December 1989 as the action was being planned. In further moments of embodied immediacy, the camera cuts between various speakers debating the rhetorical position from which ACT UP should speak out in protest (figure 21). The name of the action, Stop the Church, raised the question of what constituted the church. The debate recorded by Hilferty indicates how the issue had become far more complex than the initial talking heads in the video implied.

The arguments heard in the video testify to the explicit spatialization of the discussion as activists debated whether they could speak as insiders or outsiders in relation to the church, if they should verbally protest inside the cathedral, and even where one might locate the church as a body. As one female activist argues: "Either the church is alive and well in this room, or it doesn't exist at all." Although Hilferty's own position seems clear elsewhere in the video (e.g., in his satirical musical sendups of Cardinal O'Connor using Tom Lehrer's "The Vatican Rag"), he does retain a dialectical structure to this sequence of talking heads in debate, mirroring ACT UP's policy of free and open debate at meetings. We hear, for instance, one male activist argue against disruptive verbal protest during the service in St. Patrick's on the

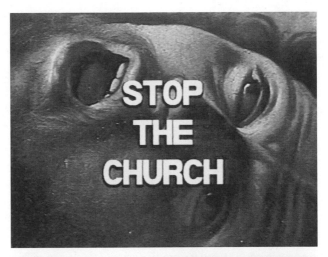

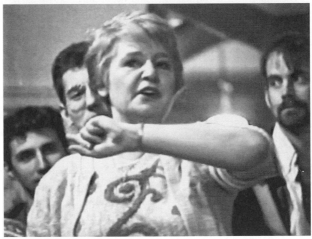

20–21. Frame captures from *Stop the Church* (Robert Hilferty, 1990).

grounds of honoring free speech: "We wouldn't want them bursting into an ACT UP meeting and celebrating mass." This is countered a little later by another male activist who argues that the cardinal has already politicized the space of the cathedral, treating it as his personal power base: "O'Connor, try keeping *my* life out of *your* church!" *Stop the Church* clearly figures the ACT UP demonstration as a secularized form of the type of Christian witnessing that extends back to the public protestation of individual conscience and faith against the institutional power of the established church during the Reformation.

In comparison to the coverage the video gives to the preparation and internal debate leading up to the action, the demonstration itself is covered quite swiftly. A fast moving montage sequence edited to the "Hallelujah" chorus of G. F. Händel's *Messiah* produces a strong sense of "political mimesis" in its depiction of the mass mobilization outside the cathedral as thousands of people gathered in protest, barely able to be contained by the police (figure 22). The visual register shifts abruptly as the tape switches to cover the actions within the cathedral. The jerky movements of the hand-held camera, the low-level light, and the rough, directly recorded sound all contribute to the effect of embodied immediacy in the sequence. While the camera certainly implicates the viewer in the here and now of the demonstration, it constructs an ambivalent position in the pews from which the protest is witnessed. It is with both the activists and the churchgoers, prioritizing neither spatially. The camera records bewildered and upset churchgoers as much as it does angry and solemn protesters. Since the actions inside the cathedral prompted the substantial number of political and media responses following the demonstration, the address and identificatory structures of this sequence remain deliberately ambivalent, forcing the viewer to momentarily examine the ethical stakes in the situation. As the congregation leaves the cathedral after the mass, Hilferty interviews churchgoers offering countertestimony, which he edits so that its rhetoric gradually increases in vehemence and homophobia, from the simple comment, "Blasphemous!" to the snide suggestion, "You'd think if they behaved themselves, they wouldn't get into this mess," and culminating in the explicit condemnation by an old man proclaiming that "sodomy and abortion are evil" (figure 23). Since Hilferty was misrecognized in the cathedral as a cameraman doing police surveillance, he was able to elicit candid vitriol from these churchgoers and subsequently use the camera to bear witness on another level—to the pervasive manifestations of institutionally sanctioned homophobia and intolerance.[43] But Hilferty refuses nevertheless to completely homogenize the attitudes of the congregation by

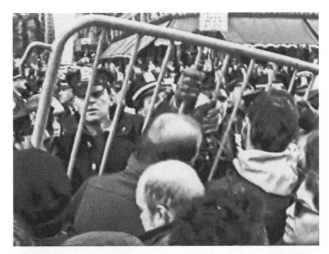

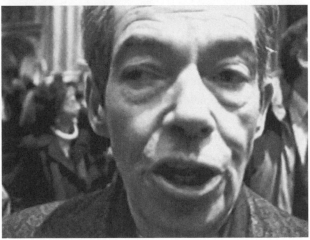

22–23. Frame captures from *Stop the Church* (Robert Hilferty, 1990).

including one final talking head of a young man as he leaves the cathedral who, when asked what he thought of the demonstration, responds with a wry smile and the bemused endorsement, "Oh, it was pretty good."

Stop the Church skillfully develops various functions for its use of the talking head, which include establishing the affective and political investment of its subjects, fostering a dialectical engagement with the issues faced by the activists, and providing the counterwitnessing of the very attitudes that necessitate such intervention and protest. These functions would indicate a high degree of use value for the tape as a mobilizing and organizing tool. In fact, like several other direct-action videos, it was widely distributed in ACT UP groups. Shown in group meetings and passed around informally, it supported the continuing discussion of activist tactics and assisted in sustaining the momentum and morale of the group by providing a crucial affirmation of direct action, which proved critically important when mainstream media reporting of AIDS activism was negative and misleading. The video's circulation beyond AIDS activist networks involved the common exhibition sites for queer independent media in the 1990s: museums, galleries, college classrooms, and film festivals. The discussion and criticism around the tape on the alternative media circuit generated sufficient interest that a recently established public television series, P.O.V., arranged to air it on PBS and its affiliates in August 1991. PBS pulled the broadcast at the last minute, citing the video's "pervasive tone of ridicule," despite P.O.V. having been specifically commissioned to create a venue for committed documentary practice outside the ideology of media balance, which still continues to stifle distribution opportunities for socially critical media.[44] While an analysis of the ensuing controversy around the broadcast and its cancellation is beyond the scope of this chapter and has been well covered by other scholars, I would like to briefly consider the question of the tape's effectiveness in generating discourse.[45] Although I would agree with Adam Knee's conclusion that the controversy did bring the video and ACT UP "far more into the public eye," it is also important to acknowledge that the controversy displaced issues, shifting focus from the Catholic Church's policies on AIDS and abortion to the question of censorship and the politics of public television.[46] Such a shift may in fact have been inevitable, since many of those protesting from the Right viewed these battles of the "culture wars" in the early 1990s as opportunities to weaken institutions of public culture such as public television. Hilferty did, however, make consistent efforts to exhibit the tape in the context of a public discussion of the issues and appeared in person to discuss the video at numerous screenings.

Voices from Another Space

The problems of access to public television continued to hinder the circulation of direct-action video in the case of Testing the Limits' *Voices from the Front*, though it was specifically produced with such an audience in mind. Unlike *Stop the Church* and DIVA TV productions, it explicitly aspired to broadcast standards of production and avoided the mimicry of ACT UP's theatricalization of anger and the satirical appropriation seen in the former works. Testing the Limits had been striving to produce a mass-release AIDS documentary for a broad audience since it got a five-minute pilot video off the ground in early 1987. The failure to get a public television broadcast for their thirty-minute documentary *Testing the Limits: NYC* pushed the collective further toward greater institutionalization, causing several members to leave.[47] Testing the Limits intended *Voices from the Front* to be a broadcast-formatted sixty-minute show on the PWA empowerment movement. By the time it was completed in 1992, it had expanded to ninety minutes and covered the huge developments in AIDS activism in the United States between 1988 and 1991. *Voices from the Front* was never broadcast on PBS, although it did gain an airing on HBO following its moderately successful run as a documentary feature in independent film theaters. The producers Robyn Hutt and Sandra Elgear have suggested that their perspective as fellow activists as well as videomakers and the sense of intimacy it produced in the video generated a textual address that PBS was unwilling to sanction (63). The network was also very wary of any controversial queer-related material following the protests from the Religious Right over the plans to broadcast *Stop the Church* and Marlon T. Riggs's *Tongues Untied* on public television stations across the country. However, what proved so difficult for PBS about *Voices from the Front* was not only its intimacy and use of low-grade video footage of demonstrations but, more significantly, its fundamental challenge to the socially sanctioned roles of patients and experts. Engendering the politics of PWA empowerment, *Voices from the Front* conveys the authority of PWAs and other community activists and criticizes the production of expert knowledge in dominant media representations of AIDS.

Hegemonic AIDS discourses and the power relations they constitute have consistently positioned people in particular roles, each with their own authorized position from which to speak. In her critique of the power relations produced by the institutionalization of an "AIDS service industry," Cindy Patton articulates how these interpellated roles played out: "The emerging social roles within the industry were each believed to possess unique forms

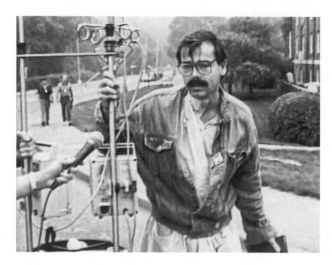

24. Frame capture from *Voices from the Front*
(Testing the Limits, 1991).

of knowledge—the 'experts' knew about the virus and treatment, the 'person living with AIDS' knew about suffering and death, the 'volunteer' knew about the courage of the human spirit."[48] Although the discourses that defined these various identities rarely corresponded with the lived, multiple, and intersecting experiences of the epidemic, speaking outside the limits of a designated role usually produced a silencing effect. By the late 1980s, however, AIDS activism had significantly challenged the maintenance of these roles. Many activists sought out AIDS knowledges outside their assigned roles (as patients and volunteers), gaining medical competence to participate in community-run trials of experimental treatments that were "based on the methods of clinical science, but grounded in an ethics of community survival, rather than in future-oriented altruism" (51). *Voices from the Front* repeatedly highlights how activists challenged such discursive roles, including through an interview with Jim Jensen, who had left his hospital room at the National Institutes of Health (NIH) to join the ACT UP protest outside (figure 24).

Similar to other direct-action videos, *Voices from the Front* combines talking head testimonies with the political mimesis of demonstration footage. But whereas *Stop the Church* recorded individual actions and narrated them in the present tense, *Voices from the Front* attempted to document the movement over a period of time. This historicizing function necessitated the frequent use of past-tense narration as activists reflected on the significance of particular actions and events in the movement's history. The video is in fact driven by this tension between contrasting desires to document the history of AIDS activism and its achievements and to articulate the urgency of the present situation and the subsequent need for action. *Voices from the Front* negotiates this tension through a narrative logic of incompleteness. As each ACT UP demonstration is documented, its particular successes are qualified by the related issues that the protest revealed but could not contemporaneously address. For instance, while the action against the Federal Food and Drug Administration centered on speeding up the final stages of drug approval, it also raised the issue of new drugs further up the development process, which necessitated the ensuing focus on the NIH. In the protest directed at that institution in Bethesda, Maryland, ACT UP protested the collusion between the NIH and the major pharmaceutical companies, which then explained the logic of the next major protest in New York City directed at those multinational corporations on Wall Street.

Voices from the Front insists on the authority of embodied voices, avoiding the kind of unseen voice-over narrator employed in Robert Epstein's and Jeffrey Friedman's *Common Threads: Stories from the Quilt* (1989). *Voices from the Front* starts and ends with PWA activists speaking to public audiences. Its narrational voice is distributed among the activists who speak before the camera. Unlike *Stop the Church*, which never names any of its talking heads (possibly as means to maintain that video's embodied immediacy), *Voices from the Front* persists in presenting all its speaking subjects with their name and affiliation or self-description. As Jack Ben-Levi points out in his review, the video alternates between the articulation of individual and collective voices through its sustained parallel montage of talking heads and demonstration footage, "each drawing considerable authority from the other."[49] Many of the activists relate their experiences of coming into consciousness and acting on their politicization, which included gaining a sophisticated understanding of the latest medical research, providing access to experimental drugs yet to be sanctioned by the state, and undertaking community organized research initiatives. These narratives of personal transformation in a collective context establish the authority and expertise of these activists as documentary subjects. Challenging the conventional distinction between witnesses inside an event (the documentary victim of the Griersonian tradition as *superstes*) and witnesses outside it (the expert witness as *testis*), *Voices from the Front* presents witnesses who are able to speak within *both* the discourses of subjectivity by relating the embodied experience of the epidemic and the discourses of objectivity by analyzing the epidemic in various fields of scientific knowledge.

Furthermore, the expert-witness testimony provided by the activists con-

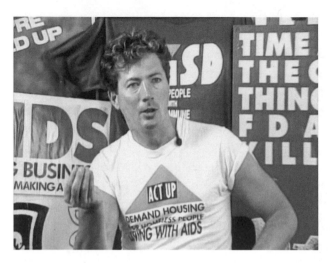

25. Frame capture from *Voices from the Front*
(Testing the Limits, 1991).

tributes to the video's critique of the dominant media's production of knowledge. Unsettling the conventional documentary use of newspaper headlines
to summarize and establish the objective reality of narrative events, the talking heads in *Voices from the Front* consistently undermine the authority of print
media by deconstructing the very language within which the reporting is performed. When shots of newspaper headlines are inserted into talking head
sequences, the critical analysis of the activist speaker deflates rather than re-
inforces the authority of the dominant media. Television coverage is similarly
targeted for criticism, with one sequence performing a detailed critique of
the supposed inclusion of activist perspectives on an edition of ABC's *Nightline*.

In its reporting of the Sixth International Conference on AIDS in San Fran-
cisco in 1990, *Nightline* organized a satellite discussion among Forrest Sawyer,
Nightline's news anchor (in the studio), Anthony Fauci, the director of the
NIH, Louis Sullivan, the secretary of Health and Human Services, and Aldyn
McKean, an ACT UP treatment activist (all via satellite). *Voices from the Front*
revisits this broadcast with McKean (as a talking head) offering a firsthand
account and a retrospective critique of it. This critical analysis performed by
McKean from the "present tense" of his interview with Testing the Limits
historicizes the *Nightline* discussion, robbing it of its sense of liveness (figure
25). The sequence inverts the power relations, so that McKean gets to situate
the anchor's speech, rather than the other way around. Intercutting between

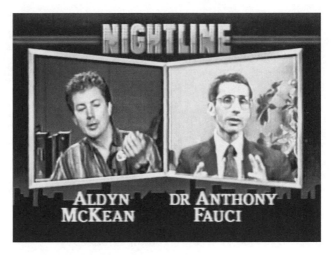

26. Frame capture from *Voices from the Front*
(Testing the Limits, 1991).

McKean's talking head (in the present) and the Nightline footage breaks down
and subsequently reveals the imagined spatial dynamics that naturalize such
broadcast discourse. McKean's analysis carries over in a sound bridge from
his appearance as a talking head (in the present) to a voice-over commentary
on his participation in the Nightline discussion.

We see images of the special effects used to construct the space of the
debate as a two-dimensional split screen of two talking heads (McKean and
Fauci) is rendered three dimensional with these images of the two talking
heads appearing to partially recede in the middle, giving the impression that
the two speakers could be facing one another in conversation (figure 26).
Such digital effects uphold the ideological construction of balance and debate that McKean systematically unpacks in his voice-over as he reveals the
real conditions of speech in the satellite discussion: Sullivan refused to participate in the program unless McKean's microphone was turned off when-
ever Sullivan spoke: "If I had a microphone that was working while he was
saying all that stuff, I could have said, 'You doubled the budget several times,
but when the budget, when started, was zero, doubling it doesn't really do
much.'" McKean goes on to correct inaccuracies and misleading comments
made by Sullivan, including his ignorance of the basic global mortality statis-
tics for AIDS at the time. McKean's critique is not restricted to the politician.
Following a shot of Sawyer complaining after McKean's satellite contribution
that he's "getting lost in all these terms," McKean's voice-over summarizes

the ethos of such dominant media with regard to the authority of talking heads: "They would rather provide platforms for researchers and scientists that they feel comfortable with."

In a confirmation of Wright's analysis of agenda-setting news coverage during the early 1990s, which he argued marginalized perspectives from those most affected by AIDS, McKean comments, "So what does America get? The impression that is created is that here's Louis Sullivan saving the world and here's this angry activist. Basically, I was allowed to speak three times." The sequence in *Voices from the Front* concludes with a manipulation of Sullivan's speech; as he claims to be doing everything possible, the image and soundtrack slow down to a gradual halt, distorting his voice and bringing his speech visibly to a standstill, offering a potent device to represent the inaction of George H. Bush's administration.

Direct-action video consistently worked to break down the regulatory binaries governing dominant AIDS representation, such as here/there, honorific/repressive, normal/abnormal, expert/victim, innocence/guilt, and general population/risk group. Accomplishing this end entailed not only challenging concrete instances of dominant AIDS representation from broadcast media but also reconfiguring the discursive space within which one could speak of AIDS. Direct-action videos achieved this through a complex reworking of rhetorical conventions, including the powerful combination of direct address and the political mimesis of demonstration footage. When that discursive space was mapped onto the physical spaces of distribution and exhibition, the possible limits of such reconfiguration became more apparent. Videomakers fought hard to screen their work in both mainstream and alternative contexts, yet they found far greater success in reaching the latter. Ultimately, most direct-action videos functioned more effectively in building and sustaining activism in communities already most affected by the epidemic than in directly influencing the discursive space of mainstream media in the United States. The latter consistently rejected any reconfigured discursive space as unreadable within its own signifying system—the work supposedly lacked the ideologically charged requirements of broadcast standard production values, media balance, and authoritative sources.

The usefulness of direct-action video for AIDS activists themselves increasingly became a focus of debate as the structures of feeling in the movement shifted from the optimism of the late 1980s to the despair of the early 1990s. In a 1994 speech entitled "De-moralizing Representations of AIDS," Douglas Crimp criticized *Voices from the Front* for what he saw to be its continued reliance on a discourse of heroic militancy at a time when it had become imperative to acknowledge the psychic toll of sustaining optimism in the face of an epidemic by then recognized as permanent, at least for his generation's lifetime. In valorizing Gregg Bordowitz's autobiographical video *Fast Trip, Long Drop* (1993) for its "self-representation of our *demoralization*," Crimp noted that "the rhetorics we employ must be faithful to our situation *at this moment* rather than what seemed true and useful last time we set to work."[50] The practices of direct-action video had in fact waned by the mid-1990s as chapters of ACT UP across the United States fractured under the stress of multiple loss, activist burnout, and the rising conflicts between professionalized treatment activists, universal healthcare advocates, and HIV dissidents.[51] However, the direct-action strategies of ACT UP and its video collectives did influence the burgeoning social movements for global equity that came together most visibly in the 1999 Seattle protests.[52] While global activist video productions like *The Fourth World War* (Big Noise Films, 2003) borrowed many of the formal strategies developed by AIDS activist video collectives, the Independent Media Center (Indymedia) exploited both the media convergence and the participatory networks of the Internet to revolutionize the nonconventional forms of media distribution used by AIDS video collectives.[53] Direct-action videos specifically focused on AIDS would eventually reappear after the turn of the millennium as part of a new global movement of AIDS treatment activism that connected activists across the global North/South divide in the fight for equitable access to effective antiretroviral therapies.

The influence of earlier direct-action videos is apparent in *Pills, Profits, Protest: Chronicle of the Global AIDS Movement* (2005), produced by U.S.-based activists Anne-Christine d'Adesky, Shanti Avirgan, and Ann T. Rossetti. The embodied immediacy of scenes shot at demonstrations, rallies, and protests situates the viewer within the space of political action. The discursive authority of the video's talking heads is shared among a diverse range of activists, community health workers, NGO officials, politically engaged doctors, lawyers, and journalists. When institutionally powerful voices are heard, such as Peter Piot (the director of UNAIDS) and Colin Powell speaking at the United Nations (UN) General Assembly Special Session (UNGASS) on AIDS in June 2001, their declarations of global commitment and action are explicitly reframed by the comments of AIDS activists outside the UN building, which are inserted before and after their speeches. Such "book-ending" visualizes the argument offered by Alan Berkman of the Health GAP Coalition, who points out that the special session only came about because of activist pressure from below, that is to say, from inside the pandemic but outside the

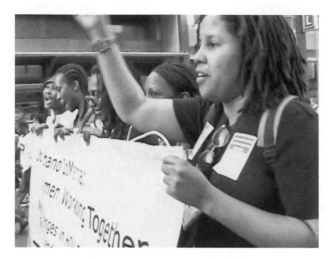

27. Frame capture from Pills, Profits, Protest: Chronicle of the Global
AIDS Movement (Anne-Christine d'Adesky, Shanti Avirgan, and
Ann T. Rossetti, 2005).

institutions of power. Moreover, in examining the place of AIDS on the global
agenda, the video repeatedly unpacks and contests the claims and justifica-
tions of the global elite through the swift dialogical insertion of countervail-
ing talking heads. However, Pills, Profits, Protest does not merely replicate the
strategies of earlier videos like Voices from the Front, for the makers understood
the specific new challenge for video activism in the global AIDS movement:
to construct a global discursive space within the video without obliterating
the specificity of the local. Although Pills, Profits, Protest introduces itself as a
"chronicle" of the movement, its organization functions more along spatial
lines than temporal ones. The pretitle montage of AIDS activists marching
in Durban, New York, and Washington generates a sensation of convergence
consolidated by the first scenes that depict the Thirteenth International AIDS
Conference in Durban in 2000, where global treatment activism first gained
substantial international media attention and important coalitions among
activists around the globe were forged. The video's repeated return to this
conference and the demonstrations it engendered points to what I would call
a logic of activist convergence (figure 27). Like the Durban conference, the
video's editing brings together activist talking heads from around the world
into a collective discussion situated in the politicized space of protest, which
the video visualizes through its numerous shots of AIDS activist demonstrations at sites of geopolitical power (the U.S. Congress, the UN building, the
Durban Conference Center).[54]

From Activist Memorials to the Memory of Activism

Pills, Profits, Protest is not only profoundly influenced by earlier AIDS activist videos, it also includes footage shot by Bordowitz and James Wentzy that originally appeared in their own videos. Sharing footage among video activists and reusing it in subsequent productions was in fact central to the collectivist ethos of direct-action video practices, which maintained a nonproprietary relation to the image, with the exception of requests for footage from local or network television channels, whom the collectives charged.[55] The reuse of footage by different video productions contributed to a sense of shared resources in the movement, even if images were often deployed for different ends. Arguably the most substantial reworking of activist footage in the movement occurred in the video memorials for deceased AIDS activists produced by friends and comrades for screening at memorial services, activist meetings, and on public-access television. To reuse would serve to recall.

The AIDS activist video collection at the New York Public Library includes the video memorials of a number of prominent ACT UP activists, including Ray Navarro, Katrina Haslip, David Feinberg, Aldyn McKean, Jon Greenberg, and Bob Rafsky. Sensing their historical value, Jim Hubbard made a concerted effort to track down as many video memorials as possible, but he suspects that many of them have become almost impossible to trace because their makers lost track of them once the master tapes were given to the activist's lover or family as a memento after the memorial service.[56] Ranging in length between eight to thirty minutes, the video memorials were produced even more quickly than other direct-action videos due to the limited time between the death of an activist and his or her memorial service. Since they frequently constituted a collaborative effort by several friends of the activist, their structure maintains the disjunctive, polyphonic collectivism characteristic of direct-action video. Footage excerpted from completed videos or mainstream media appearances is spliced together with interstitial moments of spontaneity, humor, or reflection retrieved from the archive of unedited protest footage. Jocelyn Taylor's and Wellington Love's 1993 memorial tape of Robert Garcia, their friend and fellow member of the video collective House of Color, displays a characteristically rich array of video sources, including Garcia's media appearances on *Donahue* and on gay cable-access television; clips and outtakes from other AIDS activists videos of interviews, speeches, and protest footage; step-printed video footage of personal photographs; and an essayistic monologue by Garcia spoken directly to the camera. In its diverse footage of varying discursive contexts, the tape testifies not only to

Garcia's tenacity and eloquence but also to the discursive multivalence necessary to effective acts of bearing witness to AIDS.[57]

Catherine Saalfield has described her collaboration with Bordowitz, John Greyson, and Jean Carlomusto in November 1990 on Navarro's video memorial as an opportunity to revitalize militancy in the process of mourning: "Faced with Ray's death, the four of us found ourselves conceptualizing a reservoir for our friend, a reservoir which turned out to be the power of collective action. For two days we were there, exorcising, purging, processing, crying, giggling, and longing for an image to last forever, or better, to come back to life."[58] These tapes refuse to follow the chronological structure of a life narration found in conventional memorials and obituaries (particularly on broadcast news), thus resisting the teleology from illness to death even in the event of death. Their circulation among memorial services, activist meetings, and public-access television constitutes one of the strongest examples of the imbrication of mourning and militancy in AIDS cultural activism. When screened at the memorial service, the tape brought activism into the space of mourning. Subsequent screenings in activist contexts — whether the ACT UP general meeting or at affinity groups — would then reverse the dynamic by bringing mourning into the space of activism.[59]

Wentzy's video memorial for Rafsky, which was broadcast on AIDS Community Television in March 1993, incorporates these dynamics of circulation in its formal structure. The tape opens with several activists at the ACT UP/New York general meeting expressing their utter shock at Rafsky's death and emphasizing both the imperative to speak of it and the impossibility to articulate its magnitude. Various footage of Rafsky's activism follows, including his widely reported confrontation with Bill Clinton during the 1992 presidential campaign. The tape repeatedly returns to the ACT UP meeting to hear other activists speak about Rafsky's loss and his inspiration to others, especially the younger generation of activists. Recalling the eloquence of Rafsky's speech at the memorial for a fellow activist, Tom Cunningham, one of the activists notes how Rafsky hated the way in which memorials immortalized the dead. The tape then presents the speech in which Rafsky articulated his quandary:

> To speak is a token of one's love and respect. Seeing Tom speak on that video, seeing him so young, before I knew him, and having to sit here and construct his past while he is no longer here is both excruciating and moving. I feel, on the other hand, that my speaking is also disrespectful because it flies in the face of the absoluteness of Tom's death and all the deaths, as if in the face of that my words could have some power, other

than to stroke my ego, or to those who hear them and are moved by them, to give a sense of closure, of significance, of comfort, when, in fact, another AIDS death signifies nothing and there isn't and shouldn't be any comfort, and in this room, I would only be preaching to the already converted.

Rafsky then vows to remain silent at all future memorial services out of respect for the dead and to prefigure "the absolute silence into which I will fall after my own death, which may come sooner, like Tom's, rather than later if our activism is not more successful." During these words, the video image becomes substantially grainier. After the final line of his speech in which he prays for the next generation of activists, the recording ends and video static fills the screen. As a hand appears over the static image, a slow zoom-out reveals a television monitor on which the speech has been played. The lights go up in the room, acknowledging the return to the space of the ACT UP meeting as a chant begins, "ACT UP! Fight Back! Fight AIDS!" The tape ends with the meeting's facilitator affirming the value of reflecting on the loss of Rafsky, but also of honoring his life by moving on with the work of planning future activism. Wentzy's zoom-out from the screen to the meeting literalizes the fluid movement of the video memorial between the material spaces of mourning and activism, which are then fused by the tape's broadcast in the mediated space of community television. The video memorial and its plural circulation demonstrate how the ability of direct-action video to reframe the relationship between mourning and militancy was not limited to the mediated space of its own discursive structure. It also proved to be an effective tool in actually linking the material spaces of AIDS cultural activism.

Wentzy's memorializing reuse of activist footage would take on a broader function in 2002 when he premiered his video chronicle, *Fight Back, Fight AIDS: Fifteen Years of ACT UP* at MIX: The New York Lesbian and Gay Experimental Film/Video Festival. Although *Fight Back, Fight AIDS* covers ACT UP activities from 1987 to 2002, the majority of the seventy-five-minute tape is dedicated to the early years of the group, with the first sixty minutes covering its first five years. In documenting the heyday of ACT UP in the late 1980s and early 1990s, Wentzy's video steadfastly refuses to engage in any explicit retrospective reflection or exposition about the group and its actions. The apparent absence of explicit discursive framing in Wentzy's *Fight Back, Fight AIDS* stands in sharp contrast to his sincere reflection in Ho Tam's *Books of James* (2006), a beautifully understated diary film that combines thirty years of Wentzy's own video footage (including his AIDS video activism), his voice-over reading from his own diaries, and shots of the intricate sketches in his notebooks. Although many of the diary entries in *Books of James* are historically concurrent with the footage they frame, the gap between recorded image and the voice-over spoken in the present by an older Wentzy provides a retrospective, reflective frame to the intimate portrait of this AIDS video activist.

In *Fight Back, Fight AIDS*, Wentzy employs footage of ACT UP actions, meetings, protest preparations, and speeches with a heightened sense of embodied immediacy, offering only the briefest of subtitles to historically identify the footage included. Moreover, the hand-held camerawork in the midst of the actions is even rougher than that used in *Stop the Church* or *Like a Prayer*. There are moments in the tape when all the viewer can feel is the momentum of activist bodies in the chaotic jostle of a demonstration. The rawness of the video's direct sound that has not been smoothed out in the editing process provides a persistent din of activist emotion and protest, enhancing the visceral effect of the video on the viewer. Speeches and actions play out in real time through single long takes, with *Fight Back, Fight AIDS* largely avoiding the frenetic editing techniques deployed by earlier direct-action videos.

Given the emphasis on earlier moments in ACT UP's history, one may read the tape's formal qualities in terms of a psychic attachment to the lost historical moment of ACT UP in its heyday. Lucas Hilderbrand argues along such lines when he calls the video "an affective archive" that allows access to the feeling of being an AIDS activist in the first decade of the epidemic, especially for his queer generation who just missed the radicalizing historical moment of ACT UP's zenith.[60] The intensified quality of the video's embodied immediacy can thus function as a psychic disavowal of the degraded present, allowing an "intergenerational nostalgia," in Hilderbrand's terms, for a past progressive social movement (307). However, these particular formal qualities also frame the scenes of the tape as pieces of raw historical documentation. Wentzy's holistic editing procedures preserve the historical integrity of the event recorded, whether it be a speech, a meeting, or an action. The degraded image quality of some of the early footage reminds us of the urgency to preserve such documentation. For example, the very first shots of the tape present ACT UP's inaugural protest on Wall Street in March 1987 in blurry, desaturated images. Due to the degradation of the VHS tape on which the footage was recorded, Wentzy letterboxes the image to mask the tracking marks at its top and bottom, thus creating an interplay between the local, contingent immediacy of the footage and the historical connotations of the pseudowidescreen format into which it has been placed (figure 28). In its doubleness, *Fight Back, Fight AIDS* oscillates between the visceral presence of

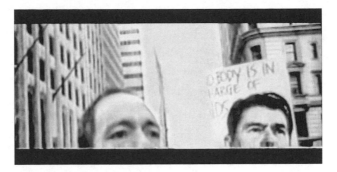

28. Frame capture from *Fight Back, Fight AIDS: Fifteen Years of*
ACT UP (James Wentzy, 2002).

its embodied immediacy and the blunt weight of its historical materiality. On
the one hand, the tape works to sustain a sense of ACT UP's continuity across
its fifteen year history of activism, while, on the other hand, it acknowledges
the historicity of the group and its greatest achievements. However, in its
drive to achieve both of these goals, *Fight Back, Fight AIDS* chooses to keep
out of the frame the growing emotional and political tensions within ACT
UP during the early 1990s and the subsequent decline of the movement by
the middle of the decade.[61]

Fight Back, Fight AIDS simultaneously embodies and documents the transformed discursive space that ACT UP was able to create, one in which AIDS
activists and people living with HIV/AIDS could bear witness to the AIDS
crisis in all its political, psychological, and medical complexity. Furthermore,
with its rawness and its lack of historical exposition, *Fight Back, Fight AIDS*
works to sustain a polyvalent memory of ACT UP among multiple constituencies: those who were most involved in the movement at its height, those who
recognize the faces of the now dead in the images before them, those who
recall the excitement of an ACT UP demonstration, those who were brought
into activism through the direct-action video, and those who draw intergenerational political inspiration from these sounds and images.

CHAPTER THREE

Related Bodies:

Resisting Confession

in Autobiographical

AIDS Video

The development of alternative AIDS media in the late 1980s and early 1990s coincided with a wider cultural trend in the global North toward what Jon Dovey has called "first person media."[1] These "subjective, autobiographical, and confessional modes of expression" have since become ubiquitous in print journalism (diary columns), popular literature (memoirs of personal trauma), nonfiction television programming (reality shows), and Internet culture (YouTube and blogging) (1). While this cultural turn to the politics of subjectivity has facilitated the growth of identity-based media production, including queer film and video, it has also allowed dominant media practices to increasingly privatize the understanding of historically and socially constructed experience. That is to say, just as social movements have fought for the political recognition of that which has been historically confined to the private sphere, particularly gender and sexuality, so has mass culture frequently worked to depoliticize the social as a realm of encounters between private individuals. With its contemporary abundance of confessional genres and its embrace of hand-held video technology, reality television has been a keen player in such transformations of the public sphere.

José Muñoz has argued that the participation of Pedro Zamora, a Cuban American gay AIDS educator, in the third season of MTV's The Real World in 1994 exemplifies this struggle to create queer counterpublicity in the midst of the majoritarian public sphere.[2] While the producers of the show saw the

presence of a young gay man of color living with AIDS as a significant catalyst to dramatic interaction among the young housemates, Zamora recognized activist opportunities in the show's dual reliance on the orchestration
of intensified social interactions and confessional talking heads to facilitate
the performance of an "authentic" self (or to use the discourse of the show,
when "people start getting real"). From the beginning of the show's taping,
Zamora responded to its continual coaxing of autobiographical acts as a
chance to expand his HIV/AIDS pedagogy to a national level. But, as Muñoz
points out, the producers persistently tried to contain the political impact
of Zamora's self-performance, especially the "new mode of sociality" enacted in his relationship with Sean Sasser, his HIV-positive African American
lover (159). The penultimate episode of the season infamously juxtaposed the
queer lovers' commitment ceremony in the Real World house with the bud-
ding heterosexual romance between Puck, the show's bad boy expelled from
the house, and his grunge girlfriend, Toni. Despite the producers' relativizing
edits, Zamora and Sean's relationship "forms a new space of self, identity and
relationality" in the face of its "tragically abbreviated temporality," which
was confirmed when Zamora died on 11 November 1994, less than two weeks
after the broadcast of the commitment ceremony (159).

In the year before Zamora's groundbreaking intervention in reality television, two independently produced AIDS videos, Tom Joslin and Peter Friedman's *Silverlake Life: The View from Here* (1993) and Gregg Bordowitz's *Fast Trip,
Long Drop* (1993), negotiated these idioms of first person media to bear witness to the modes of self, identity, and relationality available to gay men
living with AIDS at that particular historical moment, a time of waning hope
about the promise of political activism or of medical science to end the AIDS
crisis. This chapter examines how these videos turn to a similar strategy—
the doubling of the autobiographical subject—but do so to construct entirely different forms of testimonial address. Whereas *Silverlake Life* produces
an intimate address that draws from the video's construction of embodied
immediacy as the camera is passed back and forth between two lovers, *Fast
Trip, Long Drop* splits the autobiographical performance of its maker into two
characters, producing an ironic address that perpetually interrogates the
conditions and limitations of its own testimonial performance. I conclude
the chapter by turning attention to *Habit* (2001), Bordowitz's sequel to *Fast
Trip, Long Drop*, and Alexandra Juhasz's *Video Remains* (2005) to contemplate
the transformed imperatives of autobiography for queer AIDS since the development of combination therapies and the emergence of a global AIDS
activist movement.

In chapter 1, I discussed the prevalence and significance of the documentary portrait in queer AIDS media. However, the use of film or video to produce an explicit self-portrait or autobiography of a person with AIDS has proved much rarer. Whereas literary memoirs, diaries, and autobiographies by people with AIDS have been numerous and widely read, equivalent works in film and video have been less common.[3] Several experimental gay filmmakers living with AIDS have come to mix the autobiographical voice with other modes in their work. For example, blending poetry, fantasy, testimony, political commentary, and philosophical reflection, Derek Jarman's Blue, which I will discuss in chapter 6, arguably serves as the most prominent example of this tendency in queer AIDS media. The AIDS-themed films of Mike Hoolboom also demonstrate a similar heteroglossic quality that incorporates the autobiographical.

A small number of gay men living with AIDS have exploited the economy of home video technology by documenting their daily experience with a camcorder. For example, the French gay writer Hervé Guibert, who had already published several AIDS memoirs, picked up a camcorder on the encouragement of his publisher in 1990 and began to shoot a video diary. Serving as a record of his daily experiences of debilitating illness, reflections on his condition, and even a shocking suicide attempt, the footage was edited into an hour-long program and broadcast under the title La pudeur ou l'impudeur (Modesty or Immodesty) on public television in France and Switzerland after his death in 1991.[4] Serialized video diaries, such as Rubber Queen: An AIDS Docu-diary (Adam Gale, Chris Belcher, and Franklin Wassmer, 1992) and The Broadcast Tapes of Dr. Peter (David Paperny, 1992), similarly gained their television audiences by capitalizing on what Dovey has called the "camcorder cult" in television broadcasting.[5] Dovey argues that the low-grade video image has become "the privileged form of TV 'truth telling,' signifying authenticity and an indexical reproduction of the real world" (55; emphasis original). By performing "a localised, subjective and embodied account of experience," the first-person camcorder text—in contrast to the activist camcorder text—cooperates with the increasing privatization of the public sphere, in which individual subjective experience, framed within consumerism, becomes the emergent regime of truth (55). By focusing on their courageous individual videomakers, these autobiographical video diaries run similar risks as the documentary portrait, namely, the privatization of the AIDS crisis. If such autobiographical testimony remains framed as the intimate revelation of the private, it comes to bear witness only to universally identifiable human conditions, such as suffering, survival, or mortality. The social and political aspects that distinguish

HIV-related disease from other illnesses fall out and with them, so too does the imperative placed on the viewer to transform consciousness and to effect change.

Silverlake Life and *Fast Trip, Long Drop* constitute two quite different attempts to keep these imperatives in place in the practice of autobiographical video-making. Yet the two works do share a strategy of autobiographical doubling in their endeavor to keep their acts of bearing witness from turning into either the affirmation of a transcendental human consciousness or the commodified confessional discourse that saturates contemporary media. In *Silverlake Life*, the filmmaker Joslin's status as the autobiographical subject of the video is bisected by the copresence of his lover, Mark Massi. This doubling entails more than just the kind of multiplication of represented subjects that can be found in documentary group portraits like Marlon Riggs's *No Regret*. *Silverlake Life* is more than just an autoportrait of the couple, for it involves the continual transference of the camera between the video's two subjects. The unity of authorship, perspective, and embodiment to which the conventional autobiography aspires unravels in this exchange. Similarly, Bordowitz's introduction of an alter ego named "Alter Allesman" in *Fast Trip, Long Drop* destabilizes his already self-conscious and obviously rehearsed presence in the video. In the refusal to clearly demarcate the boundaries between "Gregg Bordowitz" and "Alter Allesman," *Fast Trip, Long Drop* constructs an autobiographical subject in quotes, allowing Bordowitz, the videomaker, the necessary distance to examine the social and political conditions under which people with AIDS can bear witness to their lives.

Autobiography and Textual Survival

As an autobiographical application of the video medium, *Silverlake Life* shares many of the characteristics and issues that define literary forms of AIDS autobiography. AIDS challenges the holistic ideal of autobiography as it was defined by literary criticism in the late 1960s and early 1970s when the form came to be academically recognized as a genre worthy of sustained theoretical attention. As a Western mode of self-production, autobiography is a concept that first emerges in the late eighteenth century, a discourse that Leigh Gilmore notes is "both a corollary to the Enlightenment and its legacy, and which features a rational and representative 'I' at its center."[6] By the nineteenth century, autobiography was increasingly recognized as a developmental narrative of the modern self, in which temporality and experience are organized according to a purpose or goal.[7] This ideal of the autobiographer as a self-identical, centered subject continues to be validated by many scholars of autobiography. For instance, John Sturrock argues that "autobiography represents an effort made by those who write it at the integration of their past lives and present selves: the autobiographer wishes to stand forth in print in the form of a whole."[8] Furthermore, the quest performed by the genre pursues, according to this model, what Philippe Lejeune calls "an identity between the author, the narrator, and the protagonist."[9] On the other hand, feminist scholars of autobiography, such as Nancy K. Miller, Susan Stanford Friedman, and Mary G. Mason, have argued that the autonomous, centered self is perhaps autobiography's deepest fiction of "masculine truth."[10] These critics have indicated how the textual production of such a holistic autobiographical subject as the defining feature of the genre ejects structurally looser forms of autobiographical discourse from the canon, including journals, diaries, and correspondence. In addition, it marginalizes works that focus on relationality rather than autonomy as the crucible in which the autobiographical subject is formed. Friedman thus contends that in writings by women and other minorities, the self is located not only in relation to a singular chosen other but also and simultaneously in that to the collective experience of the group.[11]

Such feminist readings of autobiography prove illuminating for the analysis of AIDS autobiography. Relationality, for instance, serves as a significant context for locating the production of subjectivity in AIDS autobiography. Writers frequently articulate their sense of self as a person with AIDS through their relation to significant others, who may be acting as caregivers, be also living with AIDS, or have died from AIDS-related illness. The cast of friends, family, ex-lovers, and community members may also embody any of these roles on the multiple occasions they appear in the social world of the text. Relating to the living or to the dead can in either case both support and disrupt the identity of the autobiographical self. But the relationality of AIDS autobiography must also be considered in terms of how it extends beyond the text itself. As an act of bearing witness, AIDS autobiography inscribes the relation to a listener or a reader into its textuality, constituting therein its address. Furthermore, in his study of AIDS diaries, Ross Chambers elaborates how the autobiographical forms chosen by gay writers living with AIDS prioritize a "witnessing impulse" over the "memorializing function" that defines conventional autobiography.[12] Less interested in the retrospective construction through memory of a coherent and meaningful life than in bearing witness to living with AIDS in the present, many gay writers with AIDS have turned to the temporally and narratively looser forms of the diary and the autobiographical essay.[13] Even those writers who employ the techniques of the novel in their autobiographical works manage, according to Jason Tougaw, "to give very clear indications of parallels between stages of the disease and narrative development, their fragmentation reflecting the authors' own ravaged communities and traumatized psyches."[14]

Time constitutes an important but problematic issue for AIDS autobiography. The person with AIDS endures a traumatic temporality in which there can be no after AIDS other than death. Citing Paul de Man's famous assertion that death in autobiography is primarily a "linguistic predicament," meaning that it is discursively unrepresentable, Tougaw argues that "an AIDS memoir, like life with AIDS, is haunted by death at every turn, constructed by and through the likelihood of early death" (251). Before the arrival of protease inhibitors and combination therapy, surviving AIDS could be nothing but a radically contingent concept. That contingency has not been resolved by the new therapies, merely deferred, since the hope they bring to people with HIV/AIDS is tinged with the real anxiety about how long they can remain medically effective. It is this temporal contingency of survival structuring the historical trauma of AIDS that most differentiates it from that of the Holocaust and other historical traumas in which the physiological persistence of trauma primarily constitutes a symptom of psychic repetition-compulsion. AIDS continues to be an ongoing medical crisis in which survivors living with AIDS are haunted not only by many others' deaths but also by the future threat of their own death, which marks the physical contingency of survival in the epidemic.

The discourse of survival, of living with AIDS, must be perpetually reconstituted under the encroaching shadow of dying from AIDS. This tension between living with and dying from AIDS can thus be seen as one of the defining features of AIDS autobiography. Tougaw suggests that writers living with AIDS evoke the well-known ACT UP slogan "Silence=Death" by persistently foregrounding their act of writing as a challenge to death-dealing silence. Yet in their work he also detects "an ambivalence about their own projects, a simultaneous devotion to and skepticism about the value of AIDS writing" (235). The trauma of AIDS, both on an individual and on a collective level, propels the writer to bear witness right here and right now. Such testimony bristles with immediacy and the feel of the live, for it is produced out of a sense of the near future of death. Yet imbued with the acknowledgment that, as discourse, it cannot alone sustain the life of its witness, AIDS testimony often propels its address into the future moment at which it will be read or heard. Realizing that he or she will not outlive the AIDS epidemic, the writer may invest the text itself with his or her desire to survive. Textual address as a form of survival becomes increasingly important to the writer with AIDS once he or she senses that his or her own physical survival is failing. It is at this point that autobiographical testimony takes on the function of an archive: to preserve in the hope of future use.

Joslin originally conceived *Silverlake Life* as a community portrait of the Los Angeles neighborhood where he and Massi lived, with Massi's AIDS as a structuring focus for the project. But as Joslin's own condition deteriorated faster than Massi's, Joslin, like many writers with AIDS, increasingly identified with the testimonial project as a form of survival. In one scene with their therapist, the conversation begins to illuminate a distinction between Joslin's desire to live for the project (as a form of survival) and Massi's determination to survive by whatever physical and medical means he can muster. This difference in attitude appears to be a source of tension in the relationship. By emphasizing it in this scene, *Silverlake Life* underscores the often contradictory structures of feeling lived by different people with AIDS at the time: to negotiate between survival against physical death and cultural survival after death. The forty hours of video footage shot over the short period from late 1989 until the following summer would become an archive of Joslin's own death, which occurred in July 1990.

Anticipating the "predicament" of the autobiographer's death, Joslin asked his friend (and former film student) Peter Friedman to complete the project in case of his physical incapacitation or his death. When Joslin's strength began to fail, Friedman helped Massi with the shooting and eventually took over the project. Friedman briefly returned to interview Massi several months after Joslin's death, which turned out to be only a few months before Massi's own death from AIDS-related illness in 1991. This interview with Massi provides the structuring frame for *Silverlake Life*, the feature-length documentary that Friedman edited over a period of fifteen months. *Silverlake Life* documents the final year of Joslin and Massi's twenty-two years together as they both struggle with AIDS-related illness. It shows the continual trips to the doctor, to energy healers, and to a therapist, but also moments of respite, which include a trip to Huntington Gardens, dancing to a new CD, and sunbathing on the balcony of their apartment. Friedman also incorporated two sections from Joslin's 1976 coming-out film *Blackstar: Autobiography of a Close Friend* into the video.[15] We see scenes from this earlier film in which Joslin interrogates his parents' attitudes to his homosexuality, describes his early sexual initiation by gay men, and films Massi reading a gay liberation manifesto from a rooftop. As Beverly Seckinger and Janet Jakobsen point out, the footage from *Blackstar* functions in *Silverlake Life* as a kind of flashback.[16] While the present crisis of AIDS reframes the earlier film as a now irrecoverable historical moment of liberational promise, the footage from *Blackstar* also places *Silverlake Life* in a long-standing queer politics of visibility.

The View from Here

The critical reception of *Silverlake Life* alternated between two terms to describe it, *documentary* and *video diary*, often in the same article. Yet neither term seems to really account for the complexity of its discursive construction. To label it a documentary certainly furnishes a sense of its status as a "record" of a particular "actuality" in the historical world, but it fails on the other hand to acknowledge how the autobiographical dynamics of *Silverlake Life* problematize the conventional power relations between maker and subject in documentary practice.[17] Similarly, to treat it as a video diary may aptly describe its principal medium and its mode of production, but the completed work is neither purely video nor completely a diary, since it incorporates film footage and its narrative structure breaks with the simple taxis of chronological "entries" that characterizes the diary form.[18] But like many video diaries, *Silverlake Life* does borrow heavily from the aesthetic and discursive vernacular of home movies in the video age. The camera is often hand-held and mobile, creating the sensation of embodied vision and presence. Subjects speak directly and with familiarity to the camera. If home movies, like domestic photography before them, are to be understood as a ritual practice now fully integrated into contemporary familial rites of passage such as births, birthdays, and weddings, then *Silverlake Life* signifies their perversion. I do not mean in the sense that it presents an alternative form of family organization, but rather because it documents the single rite of passage that both family photo albums and home movies never record — death. What appears so striking about *Silverlake Life* is not that it portrays the process of dying in such an unflinching manner, but rather that it does so using a visual vernacular that manifestly disavows such a process.

In its domestic focus, *Silverlake Life* demonstrates some of the important characteristics of what Michael Renov has coined "domestic ethnography."[19] As Renov and other critics have argued, autobiography acquires an ethnographic quality when the autobiographical subject situates his or her personal history within larger historical processes and cultural formations.[20] Far from being the transcendental, centered subject of the post-Enlightenment tradition, this subject is undeniably "in history" and thus produces what Bill

Nichols has called "embodied knowledge" and "a politics of location."[21] *Silverlake Life*'s subtitle, *The View from Here*, underscores this point. The video presents autobiographical discourse from a particular socially and historically determined perspective. Mary Louise Pratt employs the term *autoethnography* to describe such discourse: "If ethnographic texts are a means by which Europeans represent to themselves their (usually subjugated) others, auto-ethnographic texts are those the others construct in response or in dialogue with those metropolitan representations."[22] As a form of autoethnography, *Silverlake Life* delivers an oppositional "view from here" to counter the pathologizing gaze on the gay man with AIDS delivered by dominant media practices. But on closer inspection, the view from here in *Silverlake Life* is in fact bisected. Since Joslin and Massi exchange the camera throughout the work, the location of here as a position of embodied vision continually changes. This strategy remains crucial to the oppositionality of the project, for the doubling of the autobiographical subject works to stave off the containment of the video in the disciplinary frame of confession. Here is where Renov's notion of "domestic ethnography" proves valuable. Renov describes it as "a kind of supplementary autobiographical practice" that documents family members or people with whom the maker has maintained long-standing everyday relations.[23] It becomes autobiographical through what Renov calls "co(i)mplication": interconnected through communal and blood ties, the identities of maker and subject implicate one another in complicated ways. Renov writes, "With domestic ethnography, authorial subjectivity is explicitly in question or on display. There exists a reciprocity between subject and object, a play of mutual determination, a condition of consubstantiality" (143).

Exchanging the camera even performs a kind of "shared textual authority" between the two subjects (146). Neither Joslin's nor Massi's point of view (through the viewfinder) receives any discursive priority. Continually figured as an extension of their bodies, the camera becomes incorporated into their daily lives and their relationship. They often talk to each other through the camera: one is talking directly to the camera, while the other speaks from behind the camera's gaze with that kind of disembodied voice that ironically augments the sensation of embodied vision in the image (figures 29 and 30). As in the vernacular of home video, the one holding the camera persistently solicits engagement with the other being filmed by asking questions or merely requesting a gesture of acknowledgment in a wave or a smile. On a fundamental level, this interaction performs an act of bearing witness to survival, an insistence, supported by the immediacy and presence of the cam-

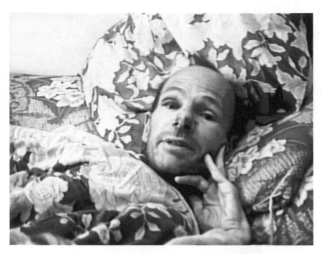

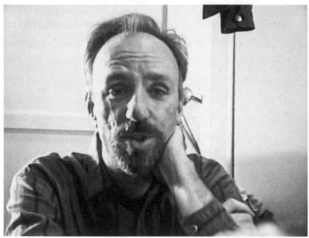

29–30. Frame captures from *Silverlake Life: The View from Here*
(Tom Joslin and Peter Friedman, 1993).

corder image, that "we are still here." There is often wit and irony in such declarations. In one particular scene, for instance, Massi is shooting Joslin as he sits in a pizza parlor eating lunch. It is a moment of respite, coming shortly after a scene in which Joslin taped himself in the middle of a sleepless night and expressing frustration at his lack of energy and the probable cancellation of the couple's trip to the Los Angeles Auto Show. Massi insistently prompts Joslin with the command: "You haven't told me where we are yet!" Joslin responds with a wry smile: "We're at Hard Times Pizza." Furthermore, the reciprocity of looks within and between scenes bears witness to the love between Joslin and Massi. At one point in the footage from *Blackstar*, Massi asks Joslin how he is going to "get the *we* in the picture." *Silverlake Life* answers Massi's question with its formal structure that reflects the reciprocity of love. Since their interaction is mediated through the look of the camera, the viewer of *Silverlake Life* quickly becomes sutured into the video's reciprocal rhythm, folded into its intimate exchange.

Joslin and Massi demonstrate a patent awareness that this intimacy is not "caught by the camera"; the video never generates the observational documentation of a private life together, despite their growing social isolation as their illnesses worsen. Nor are Joslin's confession-box moments, such as the rant he unleashes in the car as he waits for Massi to complete some basic errands, wholly spontaneous and candid. In the camera originals of *Silverlake Life* (now preserved and deposited in the AIDS Activist Video Collection at the New York Public Library) one can see how Joslin shot several takes for many of these scenes. The frustration he articulates in such scenes arises not only from the concern he is discussing but also from his repeated failure to record a satisfactory expression of his state of mind. He is frustrated at how his disease causes incapacities in both his everyday life and his attempts to record them in his videomaking. *Silverlake Life* can thus be considered a performative documentary in Stella Bruzzi's definition of the term: "The enactment of the notion that a documentary only comes into being as it is being performed, that although its factual basis (or document) can pre-date any recording or representation of it, the film itself is necessarily performative because it is given meaning by the interaction between performance and reality."[24] Bruzzi's definition helps explain a particular continuity between *Blackstar* and *Silverlake Life*. The latter enacts an extension of the former's use of a moving-image medium to serve as the public site for a performative politics of coming out.[25]

In addition to its production of reciprocal looks as an articulation of love, the camera's inscription in *Silverlake Life* also functions to emphasize the par-

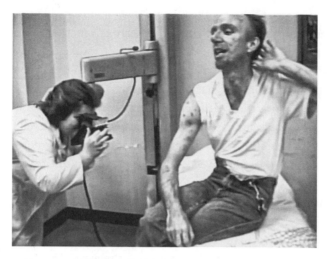

31. Frame capture from *Silverlake Life: The View from Here*
(Tom Joslin and Peter Friedman, 1993).

ticular internalization of the pathological gaze that people with AIDS, and especially gay men, are forced to experience. The video records numerous manifestations of the medical gaze: Joslin undergoes a brain scan; an emergency room doctor examines Joslin's body for symptoms of opportunistic infections; and Massi's doctors observe the progression of his Kaposi's sarcoma (KS) lesions on several occasions. One of these last scenes indicates how such surveillance of the body is mediated by both human and technological vision: Massi's doctor turns to a Polaroid of his KS-scarred back taken during his last consultation to monitor the progression of the cancer. Massi registers the objectification of this gaze with a camp, self-reflexive quip when a nurse prepares to take a new photograph: "I'm ready for my close-up now, Mr. DeMille!" (figure 31). Yet to maintain his own health as much as possible, Massi needs to internalize such objectification into a routine of self-scrutiny. But even this self-scrutiny is something that the two men inevitably come to share.

In a scene that brilliantly utilizes the feedback function of the video medium, Joslin and Massi tape themselves idly lying on their bed. The scene starts with a shot of a blank television screen sitting on a bedroom dresser. A tightly framed close-up of the two men's faces appears on the television screen (figure 32). It is clear that Joslin has just turned on the camera by pressing a button off-screen just below the frame line. Joslin and Massi turn and look intently off-screen to the upper left where we come to assume the monitor has been placed. The scene cuts to a full-screen version of the image that we have just seen on the television screen (figure 33). Massi turns to look directly into the camera, commenting, "I feel like I should be looking at the camera, but then if you look at the camera, you can't see yourself in the monitor." Joslin responds with the suggestion, "Let's look forward into the void instead." They turn their heads to look off-screen to the lower left. When the scene cuts back to their image framed in the television screen, Joslin and Massi are drawn back into looking again at the monitor off-screen in the upper left. They begin to play around with their own self-imaging, admiring the aesthetic arrangement of their bodies that they are contemplating in the monitor. In the midst of such harmless interplay, Joslin notices a red mark on Massi's eyelid, expressing concern that it may be another KS lesion of which Massi, it appears, has been unaware. This scene skillfully uses the video camera and the monitor to literalize the process of self-objectification arising from such self-scrutiny; Joslin and Massi literally see their bodies reflected back to them as objects of surveillance.[26] Similar to an earlier scene in which we see Joslin tape himself having the brain scan, this scene produces a certain *mise-en-abîme* effect in its camera setup. Such highly self-reflexive strategies qualify the camera's redemptive function (in mediating testimony) with the acknowledgment that this witnessing machine is similarly imbricated in the disciplinary structure of surveillance.

Another later scene concerning Massi's KS lesions demonstrates how quickly another person's phobic gaze can be internalized by a person with AIDS. Joslin and Massi are enjoying time at the swimming pool of a sympathetic acquaintance when she asks Massi to wear a T-shirt by the pool, inferring that his KS-marked torso is disturbing the other guests. Massi is subsequently interviewed curled up in a T-shirt beside the pool, acknowledging the shaming effect of the incident: "It feeds into a bad part of me, whereas normally I would be proud of it . . . of being alive for so long." The scene concludes with Massi returning to the pool without a shirt, an obvious attempt on his part to resist internalizing the phobic gaze. Asked by Joslin what he is doing, Massi responds obstinately, "Being political!" As the dramatic courtroom exposure of Andrew Beckett's lesion-marked torso in Jonathan Demme's *Philadelphia* (1993) illustrates, Kaposi's sarcoma lesions have a privileged relation in cultural representation to the signification of homosexuality as stigma. Massi's deliberate resistance to the phobic gaze in this scene is all the more noticeable since his attitude toward his KS lesions throughout the rest of the video entails a matter-of-fact practicality directed at treating them medically, which does much to weaken this stigmatizing function.

The couple's trip to the pool is the last time we see them together outside their apartment. As Joslin becomes increasingly sick and weak, the profilmic

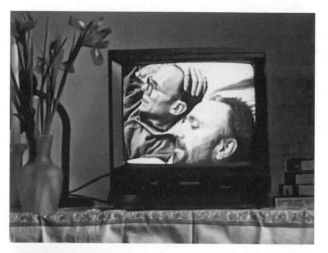

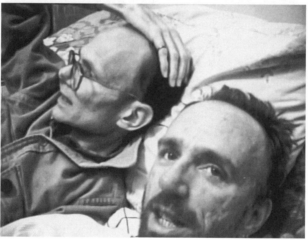

32–33. Frame captures from *Silverlake Life: The View from Here*
(Tom Joslin and Peter Friedman, 1993).

space shrinks to first their apartment and then almost exclusively to the bed-room in which Joslin eventually dies. With the video footage progressing in-exorably toward Joslin's death, Massi records time ever more emphatically. Scenes begin with Massi verbally inscribing the date from his position behind the camera, a reminder to Joslin that he has survived another day, that right now he is still here: "Good morning, Tom, it's June 1. You made it another month. We made it another month!" As these temporally marked scenes progress in Silverlake Life, we begin to experience the temporal inscriptions less as a sign of the present moment and more as an indication of the shrink-ing time before Joslin's death.

In her analysis of Silverlake Life, Peggy Phelan highlights its specific tem-poral structure, which, she argues, demonstrates more characteristics of cinema than of video.[27] Referencing Dziga Vertov's modernist application of hysteron proteron (the rhetorical placement of the last before the first), she indicates how the work exploits cinema's "giddy power" to manipulate time. Silverlake Life opens not with Joslin's death but rather with his absence after death. In the opening shot, Massi lies asleep on the sofa; Joslin's image, in-scribed with the words "Mark, I love you," fills a small television screen in the corner of the room. Massi explains in the following shot that "the thing I remember most about Tom is what he feels like, what his head, his forehead feels like, because I was so used to being able to just run in the other room and kiss him on the forehead. And I can't do that anymore." Following shots of Joslin's ashes magnify the absence of his living body, especially the initial shot of them, which is rendered in such an extreme close-up that they remain unrecognizable as a physical object. Then we see Massi holding a Polaroid of Joslin, followed by Friedman's hands picking up a box of videotapes. All these early shots in Silverlake Life can offer up only diminished signs that stand in for Joslin's human presence: a television image, his ashes, a photograph, and a collection of tapes. Even the title shot renders his body as a ghostly, skele-tal figure shrouded by the white gauze placed before it. What, then, is the effect of this hysteron proteron, of preempting the end at the beginning? While it breaks the initial narrative linearity of the work, this rhetorical structure fixes the temporal progression of the text toward its presumed teleological end in Joslin's death. The narrative suspense around what might happen has been displaced by the narrative anxiety about how much time may be left. As viewers, we are thus propelled into a structure of feeling shared by many people with AIDS in the era before antiretroviral combination therapy—an acute awareness of accelerated mortality that is nevertheless circumscribed by the uncertainty of its schedule.

Despite the gradual and highly visible mortification of Joslin's body and our knowledge that Joslin will die, Joslin's death still comes as an abrupt and surprising event in *Silverlake Life*. As viewers, we do not actually witness the moment of his death, only Massi's immediate reaction to it as he points the camera at his corpse: "It is the first of July and Tom has just died." The video renders Joslin's death through the space of a cut, splicing the image of his living but virtually inanimate body together with the image of his corpse. As Phelan points out, the viewer must rely on Massi's announcement for knowledge of Joslin's death, since the similarity between the shots is so close (169).

The event of death in documentary representation is, as Vivian Sobchack proposes, "an indexical sign of that which is always in excess of representation and beyond the limits of coding and culture."[28] The nonbeing of death can only be pointed to, it remains "over the threshold of visibility" and thus "perpetually off-screen." To represent the event of death in a moving image thus requires a perceptible contrast between two states of the physical body: "The body as lived-body, intentional and animated—and the body as corpse, as flesh unintended, inanimate, static" (287). *Silverlake Life* delivers such a contrast through the formal violence of a cut, a means of articulating the magnitude of Joslin's death, of refusing to naturalize or romanticize it. In forcing us to face the event of this shocking, unsimulated death, the video renders our very act of looking with an ethical charge, a responsibility produced by the documentary space of *Silverlake Life*. Sobchack indicates how such documentary space is constituted and inscribed as ethical space: "As much as documentary space points off-screen to the viewer's world, it is a space also 'pointed to' by the viewer who recognizes and grasps that space as, in some way, contiguous with his or her own. There is an existential—and thus particularly ethical—bond between documentary space and the space inhabited by the viewer" (294). That *Silverlake Life* involves such an intimate documentary space only compounds its constitution of an ethical space conjoining image and viewer. In the moment after Joslin's death, Massi's trembling camerawork (as embodied vision) provides the body through which the act of bearing witness is passed on to the viewer. As Sobchack reminds us, "whether by necessity, accident or design, the documentary filmmaker represents—and thus encodes—his or her act of vision as a sign of ethical stance toward the event of death s/he witnesses" (294). Standing before Joslin's corpse, Massi promises to finish the project for him, to complete the act of bearing witness that Joslin, in the nonbeing of his death, cannot now perform.

Massi and Friedman continue to tape the events following Joslin's death:

the arrangements with the undertaker, the memorial service, and the delivery of Joslin's ashes. Increasingly Massi relinquishes the camera to Friedman; the reciprocity of embodied vision found in the earlier scenes has gone. Friedman recedes behind the camera as Massi copes with his own contingent survival. Although Massi died in 1991 as Friedman was still reviewing the raw footage, Friedman decided not to incorporate Massi's death into the project: "I didn't want to trivialize it or reduce it to an appendage."[29] Furthermore, Friedman's decision to withhold Massi's death from viewers denies them the kind of cathartic ending that would risk closing down the video's ethical address.[30] *Silverlake Life* ends instead with a return to footage from *Blackstar*. Joslin and Massi dance, kiss, and then recount the famous deathbed exchange between Alice B. Toklas and Gertrude Stein, which is itself another instance of *hysteron proteron*: "Alice turned to Gertrude and asked, 'What's the answer?' And Gertrude replied, 'What's the question?'" This concluding return to the past should not be considered a gesture of melancholia on Friedman's part, for the anecdote inscribes *Silverlake Life* with an open-endedness that preserves the ethical considerations around witnessing and surviving the other's death.

Answering the Address

The question of whom *Silverlake Life* addresses as an audience became a major theme of the video's critical reception when it was screened at film festivals in the spring of 1993 and then broadcast nationally in the PBS series P.O.V. on 15 June 1993. While the critical response in the mainstream press proved overwhelmingly laudatory, the gay press exhibited a certain anxiety about address. Steve Warren, writing in the Philadelphia gay weekly newspaper *Au Courant*, typifies such concern:

> Who is the audience for *Silverlake Life*? People living with HIV, directly or indirectly, don't need to go to the movies to see more of it; and those whose lives have yet to be touched by AIDS won't be willing to sit down and watch it. As a recruiting film for caregivers it could backfire by scaring people off, even as it affirms others of the need for their services; and people with the disease may opt for suicide when they see what may be in store for them. It's certainly not for those who wish PWAs would stay indoors where they don't have to look at them, although I wouldn't go out of my way to cater to the tastes of those people.[31]

The critic feels caught between affirming a necessary cultural visibility and fearing the potentially depressive, resistive, or phobic responses to it. Even

Friedman himself admitted to doubts about recommending it to people with AIDS: "I don't actively encourage people with AIDS to see the film, but I don't discourage it either."[32] He noted, however, that a friend with AIDS, who had persistently requested a tape from the reluctant Friedman, acknowledged after seeing the video that it had helped him and his lover "validate their experiences with the ravages of AIDS."

Silverlake Life's intimate address frequently provided the focus for the critical discussion around it in reviews and in interviews with Friedman. A common question for Friedman became, "Are you sure this is a film that was meant to be shown publicly?"[33] In defense of the project Friedman reaffirmed the need for cultural visibility: "I suspect that the feeling of Silverlake Life's being too intimate is just a feeling that we're seeing something we shouldn't. It's a form of denial in a sense. It's a cultural taboo against death and also against seeing people with AIDS. Or seeing gay people, for that matter." While Friedman's mention of the cultural taboo around death may certainly partially explain the anxiety about the video, his argument that AIDS and gay people remain invisible in cultural representation elides the widespread conflation of AIDS and homosexuality in the dominant media during the first decade of the epidemic. What remains invisible in cultural representation is neither AIDS nor homosexuality, but the lived experience of gay sexuality, community, and intimacy in the midst of historical trauma.

To consider how the video's address actually functioned in its broadcast reception, it is necessary to turn now to the institutional and discursive framework shaping its broadcast and to the individual responses to the broadcast received by PBS. Through its broadcast on public television, Silverlake Life gained a far wider audience than most comparable works of independent queer film and video. The series producers of P.O.V. estimated in the early 1990s that the programs could attract an audience of several million nationwide, mostly in the coveted eighteen-to-forty-five age category.[34] The network initiated the P.O.V. series in 1988 with a stated mission to provide a platform for voices not present elsewhere in broadcasting or in the public sphere more generally. This mission appeared to finally provide independent producers with the opportunity to access a public television audience without having to abide by the ideological structures of "media balance" and "broadcast quality" regulating public television. By the time that Silverlake Life was broadcast, the P.O.V. series had gained a reputation for public controversy, built up around its broadcast of documentaries such as Robert Hilferty's Stop the Church (1990), Marlon T. Riggs's Tongues Untied (1989), and Michael Moore's Roger and Me (1989). As Patricia Aufderheide indicates, the series found its core identity "not in hard-hitting issue documentaries but in personal nar-ratives that push the envelope of American pluralism."[35] Yet these "personal narratives," such as *Tongues Untied*, continued to generate controversy, since they persistently engaged with subjectivity as a means to address wider social and political issues.

In a move that attempted both to manage the controversial aspect of its programming and to make the series more interactive, P.O.V. launched a "Talk Back" section at the beginning of its 1993 season, which can now be recognized as an important precursor to the Web-based discussion forums and blogs that permeate contemporary nonfiction media. After each broad-cast, viewers were encouraged to send in their responses to the show either as a written or a videotaped letter. As the season premiere, *Silverlake Life* was the first show to include this call for interactivity. Both PBS stations and P.O.V. received hundreds of letters after its 15 June broadcast.[36] Since the vast ma-jority of responses took the form of written letters, the series producers con-tacted a number of people who had written, asking them to tape a short video response using video equipment provided by their local PBS affiliate. Six of these "video letters" were subsequently broadcast in a "Talk Back" section after the next program in the season.[37] Chosen as a representative sample of responses, these video letters offered four positive responses and two nega-tive ones. An analysis of these video letters and the other letters received by P.O.V. reveals a number of significant tropes and patterns running through the public response to *Silverlake Life*.[38]

Many letters spoke of imperatives—the need to respond immediately after the broadcast, the necessity of sharing *Silverlake Life* with others, of making it required viewing. This imperative to respond and to pass on indicates the operation of an ethical address; the viewer bears witness to the witness, sharing the responsibility of trauma. Viewers also expressed an undeniable intimacy in their response to Joslin and Massi, particularly since almost all used their first names to describe and address them: "I wanted to tell Tom and Mark, I love you." Others articulated an intimate relation to them through the processes of identification and substitution. One woman wrote, "As I watched the film, I relived my son's death. He looked and sounded like my son. Ed's illness pretty much paralleled the death on the film. . . . I did not get to tape my son before he died. Having a copy of this film would help me." This woman wishes to privatize *Silverlake Life* as the home movie she failed to shoot, a substitute memento that can nevertheless assist her process of mourning. A young girl wrote of a similar resemblance between Joslin and her lost loved one: "Although my uncle was black, he looked so much like

Tom." One might be tempted to read this desire on the viewers' part to find physical resemblance between Joslin (or Massi) and their own lost beloved as a symptom of the ideology that reduces all gay male experience of AIDS to an identical descent into death through the process of corporeal emaciation. Yet in its desire to recognize shared experience, this identification appears, on the contrary, to function as a validation of the viewers' experience of traumatic loss. As a fundamentally relational act, bearing witness to trauma generates further testimonial acts of witness by the listener or viewer; the viewer has heard the witness, acknowledged his (or her) testimony, and reciprocated the act of bearing witness.

Of course many of the responses received were far from positive. One male viewer asked in his video letter, "How much longer are you going to try to wring out of your viewers what little sympathy we have for these gays who continue to live, flaunt, and kid about the self-inflicted, suicidal and immoral lifestyle which we are requested to approve?" Many of the religious viewers who objected to the coverage of Joslin's and Massi's "sinful" lifestyle and "self-inflicted" condition nevertheless felt compelled to acknowledge the emotional impact of the video. After expressing disdain for the homosexuality represented on the screen, one religious viewer admitted that the video had in fact been "real touching." Clearly the intimate address of *Silverlake Life* confounded many religious conservatives viewing the broadcast, pushing them to rely even more heavily than usual on biblical quotation as a rhetorical strategy. By incorporating virulently negative responses into the "Talk Back" section, the series producers not only managed the broadcast ideology of "media balance" but also employed the video camera, as Robert Hilferty had done in *Stop the Church*, as a witness to the very homophobia that contributes to the psychological trauma of AIDS.

A professed difficulty with watching *Silverlake Life* on television was not restricted to conservative viewers. Numerous positive letters stressed the difficulty of sitting through the whole program; one viewer noted that she was forced to tape the second half of the broadcast because she could not bear to see it all at once. But this avowal of difficulty was frequently situated within the expression of a set of polarities. One viewer wrote of being "devastated and comforted" by *Silverlake Life*, considering it simultaneously "agonizing and healing." Finding himself "shocked, saddened and elated by the program," another viewer recounted his own traumatized response: "I had some pretty amazing nightmares. I woke up agitated and it's 3pm and I'm still somewhat uneasy. I blame you and I thank you for it." The polarities in such responses are hard to read; they remain opaque, resisting any interpretative attempt to pin down a psychological or ideological explanation for them. While they presuppose a therapeutic function to the video, there remains also the implication of an unconscious pleasure in such horror, particularly in the latter response. It is ultimately not possible to evaluate how *Silverlake Life* affected these viewers beyond their immediate responses. Yet these letters are nevertheless profoundly useful in illuminating some of the complexity within the initial testimonial responses to *Silverlake Life*.

The Disaffiliation with Certainty

Fast Trip, Long Drop differs substantially from *Silverlake Life* in both form and tone. It lacks the latter's exploitation of the video medium's potential for immediacy and real-time coverage. Bordowitz demonstrates little interest in the kind of moment-to-moment documentation of life with AIDS that Joslin pursued. Similarly, in its montage structure and its radical open-endedness, *Fast Trip, Long Drop* refuses to construct a narrative trajectory for its autobiographical subject. Although *Silverlake Life* contains moments of wit and wry humor, it is essentially a deeply sincere work, striving to articulate the highest degree of expressive authenticity. *Fast Trip, Long Drop* distrusts such faith in the essential possibility of personal expression to empower the subject or foster social change. Drawing on the mordant optimism of Jewish humor, the video undercuts moments of personal expression with (self-)mockery, irony, and black humor.

In its formal fragmentation and dispersal of the authorial self, *Fast Trip, Long Drop* exemplifies what Renov calls "the essayistic in film and video."[39] Seeking to develop the critical vocabulary for the analysis of "new autobiography in film and video," Renov isolates the Barthesian model of the essay, with its triumphant plurality, as a powerful hermeneutic tool. He writes, "I privilege a writing practice that couples a documentary impulse—an outward gaze upon the world—with an equally forceful reflex of self-interrogation. This double or reciprocal focus effects an unceasing, even obsessive, exploration of subjectivity that situates itself within a matrix that is irreducibly material and of necessity historical" (105). Rather than attempt to articulate or discover a coherent identity as a person with AIDS, Bordowitz situates his subjectivity within a matrix of material and historical conditions that include sexuality, family, ethnicity, medicine, and political community. Through its inscription of Bordowitz in a montage of satirical sketches, rehearsed dialogues, interviews in the style of cinéma vérité, confessional performances, and archival footage, *Fast Trip, Long Drop* embodies the essayistic as a form that "*stages* subjectivity through a play of successive self-metaphorization" (105; emphasis original).

This Barthesian model of the essay is autobiographical in the sense that it strives to write autobiography against itself, to perform the self rather than to embody it. Roland Barthes borrows from the Brechtian formulation of the gestic when he announces, "I am speaking about myself in the manner of the Brechtian actor who must distance his character: 'show' rather than incarnate him."[40] Whereas Barthes's essayistic autobiography, *Roland Barthes by Roland Barthes*, disperses his subjectivity across multiple subject positions in language, namely, "he," "R. B.," "you," and "I," Bordowitz stages his subjectivity on the screen as two different characters, "Gregg Bordowitz" and "Alter Allesman."[41] Yet like Barthes, Bordowitz eschews the whole narrative for the fragment, turning to television spectatorship as a source for the video's aesthetic form.[42] As in Stuart Marshall's *Bright Eyes*, the seemingly arbitrary movement from one scene to another and the interruption of scenes by incongruous found images recall the experience of televisual flow, with its textually inscribed shifts in address and its spectatorially performed switches in channel. Bordowitz delights in the meaning produced by arbitrary conjunction. The video itself takes its title from a newspaper article in a local Idaho daily that mistakenly printed two paragraphs of an article concerning the death of Bordowitz's father in the middle of the lead report on Evel Knievel's failed attempt to fly across the Snake River Canyon in 1974. The relatively loose structure of the video demonstrates what Renov calls the essay's "disaffiliation with certainty."[43] *Fast Trip, Long Drop* refuses to locate a singular truth about either AIDS or Bordowitz; it disavows any claim to (self-)mastery. But the video is not without a structuring principle. Imbued with a Brechtian dialectical quality, the video plays conflicting assertions against each other. Bordowitz explains that "every time there is a positive assertion of identity, there is a counter made, a negation. I am Jewish, but I am queer, and I have AIDS, so what. There is always a negation made of the positive assertion—to bring it forward, displace it, and put it into another realm."[44]

Uncertainty perfectly defines the historical moment within the AIDS epidemic in which *Fast Trip, Long Drop* was produced. At the Ninth International AIDS Conference in Berlin in 1993, the results of the Concorde study seriously challenged the presumed effectiveness of the leading antiretroviral drug, AZT (azidothymidine), in slowing down the progression of AIDS.[45] Without any major alternative therapies on the horizon and with medical researchers' declaration that a cure was at best a decade away, one of the domi-

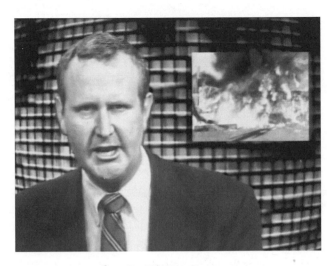

34. Frame capture from *Fast Trip, Long Drop*
(Gregg Bordowitz, 1993).

nant structures of feeling among people with AIDS in the global North—the
dogged commitment to outlive the epidemic—began to be displaced by an
emergent despondency at the lack of material and psychological prospects.

Fast Trip, Long Drop opens with the public announcement of this state of
uncertainty (figure 34). Reporting that there are now 40 million people infected with HIV, a fictional newscaster (Bob Huff) comments, "If you are
one of them, panic! That's right, panic! There's not a thing to be done for you.
Yeah, I know I'm supposed to be the news guy. I'm supposed to bring you
to the edge of worry and not beyond. Give you just enough anxiety to keep
coming back for more. . . . If you don't have AIDS, don't worry about it. I'm
not going to discuss it. I'm reporting on behalf of the uninfected. And we
know who we are." This opening scene establishes two significant and related
issues in *Fast Trip, Long Drop*. First, it articulates what Douglas Crimp calls
"the incommensurability of experiences," which occurs when the physical
and psychological trauma produced in the communities most affected by the
epidemic is unacknowledged, ignored, and, at worst, condoned by society
at large and by the mass media in particular.[46] The second emphasis of this
opening scene is the question of media address. As the previous chapter elucidated, the person with AIDS remains excluded from the address of mass
culture, particularly of news media. Rather than refuse any form of address
to people with AIDS in the manner of dominant media discourse, this scene,
like Huff's own video *Rockville Is Burning* (1989), openly addresses people with

AIDS, but with a caustic attitude that reveals the phobic message behind that refusal to address performed by mass culture.

Exemplifying the practice of alternative AIDS media, Bordowitz's video-making has long been concerned with the question of address. Dropping out of art school in the mid-1980s to join the emergent AIDS video activist scene in New York City, Bordowitz soon became a founding member of Testing the Limits. His opportunities to produce community media increased when he joined Jean Carlomusto at Gay Men's Health Crisis (GMHC) in its Audio-Visual Department in 1988. Over the next five years, Carlomusto and Bordowitz collaborated on a variety of projects, including group-specific safer-sex videos and Living with AIDS, the weekly cable access show designed for people with AIDS. The show broadcast a variety of material in different formats, including studio interviews, roundtable discussions, independently produced tapes, and video coverage of recent activist actions.[47] When the original Testing the Limits collective split over the ambition of some members to institutionalize the group as a grant-funded nonprofit organization producing for a public television audience, Bordowitz switched his energies to the newly formed DIVA TV collective, of which he was also a founding member.

The exigency of producing alternative media for specific community needs in the context of governmental repression and censorship often forced Bordowitz and his colleagues to bracket certain issues for the sake of producing materials that would be most accessible to those communities in urgent need. For example, the GMHC-produced Safer Sex Shorts, made to fill the gap in community-specific safer-sex information, often elided the complexity of sexual identities and practices for the sake of a clearly articulated community address. Bordowitz recalls that by the early 1990s, "we could no longer produce work that was satisfying and relevant to our situation as people with AIDS without overturning the limits we had established earlier on."[48] In producing Fast Trip, Long Drop, Bordowitz turned to his own experience to explore the complexity and uncertainty of that particular moment in the epidemic: "I no longer impose fetters on the work for the sake of what I envisioned to be the good of the community it was intended for. Rather, I've tried to overturn any limits placed on the work for particular uses (89). It is in this sense that Juhasz has dubbed Fast Trip, Long Drop "the first meta-AIDS video."[49] The video interrogates the conventions of a wide array of subgenres in alternative AIDS media, many of which Bordowitz has produced himself—the experimental media critique, the activist tape, the PWA cable-access show, the HIV prevention tape, the documentary portrait, and the support group video.[50]

The Political Problem of Despair

In classic expository fashion, *Fast Trip, Long Drop* locates the time and place it is documenting through establishing shots of the New York City skyline and providing intertitles that give the year as 1993. But this conventional documentary code is interrupted by postwar archival footage of city buildings under demolition. The anonymous and anachronistic quality of such found images pushes their meaning away from indexical reference and toward metaphor — a community under threat, collapsing physical bodies, or the embodiment of despair. The camera pans across a cramped apartment to find "Bordowitz" in a "Silence=Death" T-shirt lying on the bed. In a gesture suggesting perhaps a deliberate citation of the intimate yet self-reflexive discourse of *Silverlake Life*, a video monitor faces "Bordowitz," supplying him with a feedback image. He speaks wearily to the camera of his present predicament — he is feeling ill, but he remains uncertain as to what it might be. He lists a number of serious opportunistic infections as possible candidates: Lyme disease, tuberculosis, hepatitis, or mononucleosis. This potentially confessional moment is punctured by several archival images of daredevilry: a tightrope walker and a flaming stuntman jumping into a pool. The scene shifts to a television producer's control room as a fictional cable-access show, *Thriving with* AIDS, goes on the air. Henry Roth (Bob Huff), its ponderous host, attempts to wake up his dozing guest, Alter Allesman (performed by Bordowitz), with a question. Roth enunciates the final three words with a slow, obnoxious deference: "How long have you been *living with* AIDS?" Responding with obvious resistance to Roth's almost pitiful tone, Allesman proclaims to identify with his own illness and sarcastically acknowledges his mortality: "I will die. Of course, I may not. Like everyone else, I could get hit by a bus, get murdered, kill myself." Bemused, Roth can only offer the absurd reply: "OK, we can always hope."

These two scenes set up the structure of alternation between "Bordowitz" and Allesman that continues throughout the video. "Bordowitz" appears in a number of different contexts: discussing his outlook with an HIV support group of gay male friends; recalling his coming out with his mother and stepfather in their Long Island kitchen and talking about its relation to his subsequent HIV disclosure; sharing his feelings about mortality with his friend and fellow artist Yvonne Rainer; and contemplating the death of his estranged father in a bizarre traffic accident. The video regularly returns to the studio of *Thriving with* AIDS, an obvious parody of the affirmative *Living with* AIDS show Bordowitz coproduced, to find an increasingly embittered and uncooperative Allesman. When Roth at one point fails to engage Allesman in conversation, he asks the producer to roll a documentary segment on Allesman's daily life. The character who appears in the segment seems to demonstrate more the contemplative weariness of "Bordowitz" than the virulent contempt of Allesman. Yet we cannot be sure. There are no subtitles to differentiate the characters at this point. In several scenes, in fact, Bordowitz subtitles the names of everyone except the character whose presence his body signifies, leaving us unsure as to who is speaking, "Bordowitz" or Allesman. The mounting slippage between these character doubles blocks any attempt on the viewer's part to locate a singular and authentic autobiographical self behind such testimony.

Clearly Bordowitz wished to do damage to the concept of autobiography in its conventional sense. He originally scripted Allesman's lines as platforms for serious monologues: "Splitting myself into two characters enabled me to act out versions of myself that I was afraid to show."[51] But working in rehearsal with Huff, Bordowitz began to change his relationship to his own testimony. Tapping into Huff's experience in the New York downtown theater scene, the two developed a darkly comic undercurrent to their performances. In fact, the video's investment in paradox, ridicule, and black humor demonstrates a noticeable affinity with the aesthetic strategies of ridiculous theater. Bordowitz has indeed argued for the connection between AIDS activist video practices and ridiculous theater as epitomized by the dramaturgy of Charles Ludlam.[52] In its rigorous challenge to the orthodoxies and idioms of AIDS video activism and the AIDS activist movement more generally, *Fast Trip, Long Drop* engenders the spirit of Ludlam's manifesto for ridiculous theater: "Test out a dangerous idea, a theme that threatens one's whole value system. Treat the material in a madly farcical manner without losing the seriousness of the theme. Show how paradoxes arrest the mind."[53] The simultaneous maintenance of farce and seriousness provides the constitutive tension—the double voicing—at the heart of *Fast Trip, Long Drop*. It is driven by the urge to bear witness, yet it remains steadfastly skeptical of the conditions under which it can be enacted. Furthermore, the video questions for whom and in whose interest the act of bearing witness is performed.

Fast Trip, Long Drop bears out this uncertainty around testimony's ethical and political valence through its deployment of montage and its doubling strategy. If testimony is the discourse of the survivor, then *Fast Trip, Long Drop* illuminates what happens when the survivor begins to doubt the possibility of survival. This becomes very apparent in the conversation among members of the HIV support group. In the face of increasing loss and despair, "Bordowitz" recalls his former conviction that he would outlive the epidemic through the power of collective action, a belief he now finds difficult to hold. Another member of the group, Derek, admits that "there's a part of me that's willing to give myself to death." Once again, images of daredevilry punctuate the conversation, this time from demolition derbies and automobile stunts. These found images of the body at risk interrupt a number of testimonial scenes throughout the video, each time nudging us to contemplate our spectatorial relation to the testimony before us. The daredevil's body in these found images is endangered solely for the purpose of spectacle, to produce thrilling pleasures for the audience. Cut into the testimonial scenes, these images suggest an altogether different risk—that the experience of risk and mortality in AIDS testimony may produce forms of unconscious pleasure for its audience. Testimony subsequently loses its ethical address in becoming a spectacle of transgression and suffering; it slips into the kind of commodified confession that has become a pervasive aspect of contemporary first person media.

While the persistent insertion of archival images into scenes with "Bordowitz" works to interrupt the passive consumption of his testimony by a voyeuristic general public, the character of Allesman vociferously resists a related form of appropriation enacted in the AIDS activist movement itself, and in lesbian and gay communities more generally. When asked by Roth if he is "a powerful model of someone surviving and thriving with AIDS," Allesman loses his temper. He declines to be a model of any sort and blatantly rejects the notion that, as a person with AIDS, he is either "a revolutionary body" or "an angel." He turns the table on Roth, asking him, "How do you live with AIDS?" In this outburst Allesman spotlights a major critical target of Fast Trip, Long Drop: the burdens that people with AIDS bear on behalf of those around them who are neither sick nor infected. What is being articulated in this scene is the complete frustration with the "truths" projected onto people with AIDS from within as well from outside their own communities, namely, that people with AIDS may enjoy a closer relationship to a transcendental truth due to their proximity to death or that their survival offers the promise of collective redemption for either the movement or the community.

At this crucial moment Allesman turns to look right into the camera and addresses people with AIDS directly (figure 35): "I want to speak to people with AIDS. Aren't you sick of all this shit? . . . Why is it my burden to survive and thrive with AIDS? No one can take my place for me. No one can die for me. Aren't we all living with AIDS? Isn't this a crisis for all of us? I used to

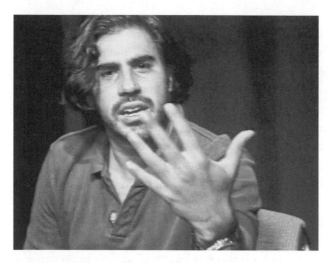

35. Frame capture from *Fast Trip, Long Drop*
(Gregg Bordowitz, 1993).

think so once. Now I think that some of us are living with AIDS and some of us are dying from AIDS." The ultimate irony of Alter Allesman's name now becomes apparent; it translates from Yiddish as "old everyman," the qualifying adjective suggesting the "old trope" of the everyman. But *alter* also carries the Latinate sense of otherness. Trapped in the paradox of being a person with AIDS, Allesman bears the burdens of both pathological otherness and transcendental representativeness, which have been projected onto him from different quarters.

Alisa Lebow argues that this tension lies at the heart of the video's engagement with Jewish identity and its relationship to AIDS. This "Jewification of suffering and resistance," which simultaneously particularizes the suffering Jew and universalizes the Jew as suffering, furnishes the video with a historical optic through which to understand the paradoxes inherent in the representation of people with AIDS. Moreover, Lebow reads Allesman as a self-conscious citation of the figure of Jew as "conscious pariah," who was "by nature difficult, ornery, prepared to be reviled, yet . . . spoke his conscience and took a stand wherever hypocrisy or complacency lurked."[54] Through Allesman, Lebow links the "unmanly conduct" of the cultural figure to the "sedentary, serious, studious sissy" at the heart of the rabbinical model of Jewish masculinity, which the historian Daniel Boyarin has traced (144). Not only does this trope provide Bordowitz with an alternative image of Jewishness to the militarized masculinity of contemporary Zionism but it also offers an opportunity to articulate all that has been repressed by the heroic discourse of AIDS militancy, the masculinism of which became increasingly detrimental to AIDS activism, according to Crimp, as queer structures of feeling in the early 1990s began to question the activist optimism of the late 1980s.[55]

Fast Trip, Long Drop further probes the questions of representation and address through several parodic sketches that target public figures living with AIDS. In each of them, parody performs a revelatory function in that it uncovers the subtext underlying each particular act of testimony. Recalling Mary Fischer, the woman with AIDS who addressed the 1992 Republican Convention, "Charity Hope-Tolerance" (played by the artist Andrea Fraser) appears in a public service announcement against AIDS discrimination. Pausing briefly after each assertion she makes, this mild-mannered WASP declares directly to the camera, "I have AIDS. That's supposed to shock you. Feel sorry for me. See, if I'm not so bad, then those other people with AIDS—you know who I mean—we can live with them, can't we? I am brave. And I have resources. Feel bad for a few more seconds. OK, that's enough." Filled with an imperative call for pity, which is usually disguised as compassion, her speech functions to maintain the otherness of people with AIDS rather than to challenge it. Her self-identification as a person with AIDS produces her demand for pity, while her disidentification with other people with AIDS reassures her privileged white audience that survival is possible, but only if one has what she and her audience share—resources and privilege.

In another parody of AIDS public service announcements, the black basketball star "Hex Larson" (Maszaba Carter) delivers an HIV prevention message: "I'm talking directly to the uninfected. People with AIDS, this isn't for you. Use a condom. Don't worry about me. I still get mine. I'm going to beat this thing. It's just another game in which there are winners, losers, and spectators." Obviously modeled on Earvin "Magic" Johnson, Larson offers a similarly privatized message of survival, reassuring his audience that he will survive even if others may not. Both Larson and Hope-Tolerance speak neither to nor on behalf of other people with AIDS. Paradoxically, their address to the uninfected is premised on a disidentification with the very group of people they are assumed to represent. Fast Trip, Long Drop includes a third parodic sketch involving a public figure with AIDS. Based on the outspoken writer and activist Larry Kramer, "Harry Blamer" (Bob Huff) does in fact speak to fellow activists (as well as researchers), but he only offers the same kind of self-interested, disidentificatory discourse as Larson and Hope-Tolerance: "What about my needs? You're all wastes of human flesh if you can't find a cure for me."

Conversely, "Bordowitz" does venture to speak to and for a particular community by the end of the video, albeit ironically. As an incisive parody of the political stump speech, the scene shows him running for political office in "this nation of the ill and dying." He offers his candidacy for "a constituency of the burnt out, the broken hearted, and you, all of you, the profoundly confused." His speech is edited into real footage of an earlier demonstration from 1988 in which we have already heard him speak; he even wears the same clothes. In the earlier speech, Bordowitz had insisted on the imperative to come out as a member of "the AIDS community," to embrace one's medical status as an identity around which to organize and survive collectively. With that community physically and psychologically decimated, his new speech explicitly poses the question of despair as a political problem. What are the possibilities for empowerment and organization in the context of despair and uncertainty as pervasive structures of feeling?

Fast Trip, Long Drop struggles to answer this question throughout its fifty-four minutes by investigating the historical conditions that determine Bordowitz's subjectivity: his coming out as an HIV-positive gay man; the early loss of his father; his Jewishness; and his media activism. His investigations do not resolve the problem, but they do compel him to acknowledge the category of the limit or the unknown as a necessary precondition for tackling the problem. Yet as a contemplation of mortality in the midst of an epidemic, Fast Trip, Long Drop refuses through its dogged historical materialism to understand this limit in the transcendental sense that some AIDS art and media have assumed.[56] To accept the limit within a transcendental frame would facilitate resolution and thus foreclose the articulation of the epidemic's magnitude, which Bordowitz refuses to grant a transcendental dimension. Fast Trip, Long Drop literally refuses such closure. As Cynthia Chris has pointed out, the video includes three consecutive attempts to end: Bordowitz ambles through a shopping mall reflecting on his desire to "go from being to extinction without dying . . . to disperse"; Bordowitz steps off the curb in front of an oncoming bus (a mordant joke that runs through the video); and finally, after the credits, Bordowitz is once again seen on his bed as he remarks, "Death is the death of consciousness, and I hope there's nothing after this," and then he breaks into laughter, drops his cigarette, and mutters, "Oh shit, cut," and the video finally concludes.[57] The video thus ends without closure, terminating in rhetorical terms merely by the instruction to cease shooting. Similar to Silverlake Life, Fast Trip, Long Drop thus ends in open-endedness, and in doing so, it preserves the structural condition necessary to the act of bearing witness. For all its critical interrogation of such an act and its conditions of possibility, the video stubbornly refuses to surrender its redemptive promise. The double voicing of the video's ironic address always brings it back to the original imperative to bear witness. If anything at all, it bears witness to the fundamental problems of bearing witness to the AIDS epidemic.

Silverlake Life and Fast Trip, Long Drop both clearly exploited the video medium's ability to complicate the first person in AIDS autobiography. In pluralizing the autobiographical subject, they do not take on the linguistic position of first-person plural as in the pronoun we; rather, their plural performance of the first person involves the inscription of a relationality that is crucial to both the constitution of the subjectivities represented and to the act of bearing witness. In Silverlake Life, that relationality is embodied in the structure of camera exchange between Joslin and Massi, which not only elucidates the coimplication of their subjectivities but also folds the viewer into the reciprocal address of their love. While the intimate address of the video largely elides the issue of community response to the epidemic, it arduously bears witness to the way in which dying from AIDS involves a gradual and oppressive reduction of one's worlds, both individual and social, private and public. Joslin's bearing witness through the video camera became for him a means to resist such obliterating reduction by creating a public address that would survive him. The relationality posited by Fast Trip, Long Drop is substantially more social and historical in scope. Bordowitz struggles to understand his subjectivity as a person with AIDS at a particular historical moment through a complex matrix of relations. But the video also profoundly questions whether film and video media can engender relationality at that historical moment and not merely reinforce the othering of people with AIDS. The video's ironic address thus bears witness to the problem of despair as a pervasive structure of feeling among people with AIDS, particularly activists, during the early 1990s.

Redemptive Habit and Recovered Remains

In concluding this chapter, I want to turn to the question of how queer makers have used autobiographical video practices to address the challenges posed by the normalization of AIDS in the global North since the late 1990s. A number of queer makers with a long history of AIDS video activism have taken up this question, including Bordowitz in Habit, Juhasz in Video Remains, Jean Carlomusto in Shatzi Is Dying (2000), and Richard Fung in Sea in the Blood (2000).[58] While all these videos appropriate and reframe earlier images of the AIDS crisis in the service of working through its transformation in the

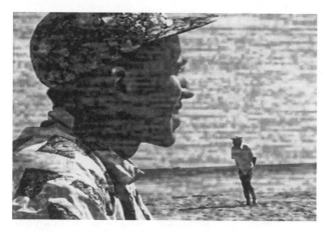

36. Frame capture from *Video Remains* (Alexandra Juhasz, 2005).
Courtesy of the artist.

present, I have chosen to focus on *Video Remains* and *Habit* since these two
videos demonstrate the most sustained and explicit attempts of this group
to revisit the witnessing dynamics of earlier AIDS video. Although neither
video uses the doubling strategy of *Silverlake Life* and *Fast Trip, Long Drop*, they
do retain, and in fact intensify, the focus on the autobiographical subject's
relations to intimate others that is found in the earlier videos. It is through
these relationships that *Habit* and *Video Remains* examine the relationship of
the normalized here and now to their others: the traumatic there of the worsening global pandemic and the traumatic then of the era before combination
therapy.

The basis for *Video Remains* is a tape Juhasz recorded in 1992 of her best
friend, James (Jim) Lamb, who was dying from AIDS. An off-Broadway actor
and performer, Lamb asked Juhasz to record a fitting testimonial account of
his life story before it was too late. Thus during a short vacation they spent
together in Florida, Juhasz videotaped a fifty-five-minute conversation with
Lamb on the beach as he recounted stories of his life, his family history,
and his friendship with Juhasz (figure 36). Since recording it, Juhasz had
always felt profoundly ambivalent about the original tape, particularly after
Lamb's death less than a year later, for it seemed radically unable to capture
her beloved friend: "There is little to nothing of his amazing, vital presence
in those pixels and yet, there he speaks, and smiles, and suffers, more tangible although somehow less flexible than a memory."[59] Her ambivalence
toward the tape, "a haunted and hated object," was exacerbated by her suspicion that Lamb was suffering from AIDS-related dementia when it was shot,

which rendered much of his testimony meandering and confusing.[60] Juhasz employs the whole of the original interview tape as the literal foundation of Video Remains, overlaying the original footage with an array of recently recorded conversations about the nature of memory in the third decade of the AIDS pandemic, including telephone calls with lesbian AIDS activist friends about why they do not talk about AIDS anymore, an unanticipated conversation with a hairstylist recalling the memory of a long-dead friend and a lost age, and observational footage of gay teens in an HIV prevention workshop in Los Angeles discussing their relationship to AIDS. Juhasz uses very slow dissolves and sound bridges to render the quality of a palimpsest to Video Remains, thus allowing the video's formal structure to mirror the meandering drift of Lamb's testimony. Since Juhasz refuses to let the original tape stand as a fitting tribute to her beloved friend, her engagement with it continually shifts between the external witnessing of Lamb as a dying intimate other and the internal witnessing of her intimate relationship to him and to the AIDS activist movement of which they were both part.

Video Remains reframes Lamb's witnessing body at the same time that it questions the very possibility of such reframing. The traumatic past stubbornly remains below the surface of the normalized present, yet resistant to any present attempt to frame it, as it consistently fades back into picture. The ambivalent duality of the video's title thus becomes clear. The original video remains in existence with little material degradation; it is testimony that has survived its speaker, an archival preservation of the past that now registers the difference of the present. As Juhasz notes, "The tape stays the same, even as I change" (323). But the material remains of the video are also like the physical remains of the dead, all too evident embodiments of loss. Such loss is doubly inscribed in the image of Lamb. His AIDS-related dementia had first deprived him of the sagacity and eloquence he so desired for his final testimonial performance; second, his death had robbed Juhasz of her best friend. Video Remains struggles with the specter of a third potential loss—the individual and collective forgetting of the epidemic, even among those who had demonstrated the highest level of commitment during the 1980s and 1990s to ending the AIDS crisis in the United States. Juhasz describes Video Remains in terms of a "queer archive activism" that relies "upon the recorded personal stories of regular people played out largely in respectful real time" (326). But to wrench the original tape from a "debilitating, private melancholic remembrance of AIDS in the 1980s," Juhasz must also subject it to the often oblivious present (327). Memory wrought from an interrogation of our forgetting, whether individual or collective, is more than a straightforward act of remembrance, for it revitalizes the past by forcing us to simultaneously recognize both its resonance with *and* its difference from the present.

Whereas the structural basis for *Video Remains* lies in the real-time duration of a conversation recorded well over a decade earlier, the temporal structure of *Habit* takes a different, if equally simple form: the habitual actions of the everyday in Bordowitz's present life. *Habit* serves as a sequel to *Fast Trip, Long Drop*, which, in light of Bordowitz's worsening health in the early 1990s, was conceived as his last work. Made almost a decade later as Bordowitz lived a more stable life on antiretroviral drug therapy, *Habit* reworks many of the scenes and strategies from the earlier video through the optic of his supposedly normalized existence. However, it becomes clear from the very opening scenes of the video that *Habit* contests the notion that the supposed normalization of AIDS from antiretroviral therapy has ended the AIDS crisis at the same time that the video attests to the substantial political, psychological, and medical changes brought about by this new historical period of the AIDS pandemic. But Bordowitz is also well aware of the redemptive aspect of habit. In writing about the video, he comments, "I embrace the notion of habit. I do not reject it as deadening or stultifying. Habit is understood as the backdrop against which epiphany rises."[61]

The video opens on an image of serenity: a woman, who we later learn is Bordowitz's partner, Claire Pentecost, sits in a living room in the lotus position. The subsequent shots depict the everyday rhythms of domestic routine: Bordowitz waking up, Pentecost doing yoga, Bordowitz making coffee. It is the voice-over conversation between Pentecost and Bordowitz that radically qualifies this image of domestic normality since they discuss the ramifications of his until recently imminent sense of mortality. Pentecost ruminates about the changes brought about by her partner's antiretroviral drugs: "I guess I've started to think differently. I've started to fall into that normalcy—like our life will just go on and on. But sometimes I get into a panic." Bordowitz asks, "When?" Pentecost calmly replies, "Every day." Uncertainty, anxiety, and the awareness of mortality remain, albeit in different manifestations. Reworking a scene from *Fast Trip, Long Drop* in which Bordowitz's subjectivity in crisis is visualized in the split image of his face in the doors of a medicine cabinet while he is shaving, *Habit* returns Bordowitz to the bathroom, but this time he looks pensively in the mirror, scrutinizing his face as he smiles broadly, almost sarcastically. He pulls back the skin on his slightly gaunt face in a mock face-lift (figure 37). The new scene offers both literal and metaphorical interpretations. Bordowitz's self-scrutiny and his attempt to momentarily recapture an earlier shape of his face admit a concern

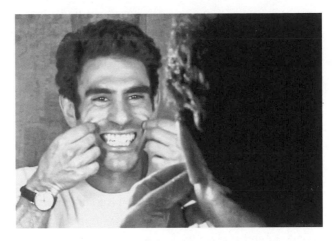

37. Frame capture from *Habit* (Gregg Bordowitz, 2001).

about the physical side effects of the combination therapy on his body. But the self-conscious performance of the smile in this context also implies an underlying anxiety about his normalized present state.

Not only does Bordowitz problematize the discourse of normalization "after" the AIDS crisis in the global North but he also situates his current everyday life on antiretroviral therapy alongside the contemporary struggle for treatment access by South Africans living with HIV/AIDS. *Habit* shifts between Bordowitz's life in Chicago and footage he shot in South Africa during the Thirteenth International AIDS Conference in Durban in 2000, which includes interviews with AIDS activists Zackie Achmat and Promise Mthembu from the Treatment Action Campaign (TAC), South Africa's most effective AIDS activist organization. Combining tactics and organizing strategies drawn both from ACT UP and the antiapartheid struggle, TAC has been at the forefront of the struggle against both the AIDS profiteering of the international pharmaceutical industry and the AIDS denialism of Thabo Mbeki's government. Invoking the memory of ACT UP in its heyday, *Habit* also contains several scenes of the group's vigorous protests during the conference.

While the video is emphatically structured around both spatial and temporal difference, it refuses to frame those dynamics around the ideological assumption that South African AIDS activists are now where ACT UP was in the late 1980s. *Habit* never tries to resolve the gaping difference between Bordowitz's experience of AIDS in Chicago and that of Achmat or Mthembu in South Africa. Rather than posit this relationship in terms of the discourse of a shared humanity, which has been deployed in contemporary AIDS documentaries like the HBO-funded series *Pandemic* (Rory Kennedy, 2002), Bordowitz leaves open that glaring discontinuity as an implied ethical question: What historical conditions are responsible for this inequity?[62] In its presentation of activist arguments from South Africa and other parts of the world about the political and economic determinants of treatment access, *Habit* provides its viewers with the knowledge to begin facing that question. *Habit* demonstrates that the ethical imperative to fight the global AIDS pandemic cannot be pursued from an omniscient, humanist position outside history, outside a consideration of the structural violence wrought by global capitalism. One of the most important aspects of *Habit* is therefore how situated its autobiographical performance is, both historically and culturally. It speaks from a very specific subject position, often detailed in the most mundane daily habits. It both reflects on that position and provides a space in which it both listens to and allows us to listen to testimony from subject positions radically different from its own. Bordowitz has expressly described the video in terms of its commitment to listening: "I went somewhere, I had a profound experience, and I realized that the thing that I could, the only thing that made sense to me to do, was to bear witness. And so, *Habit* is organized around the notion of Silent Witness. Just listening, but being active. Being active through listening."[63] In its commitment to listening, *Habit* stands in sharp contrast to *Fast Trip, Long Drop* with its biting loquacity.

Arguably the most influential voice to which *Habit* listens is that of Achmat, the chairman of TAC. Although Bordowitz does not explicitly structure the South African sections of *Habit* around Achmat's interview, the pledge that Achmat made in 1998, and which he repeats in *Habit*, remains key to the ethical project of the video. In a Gandhian act of embodied witnessing, Achmat refused to partake in antiretroviral drug therapy until all South Africans who needed the medication could get them through the public healthcare system. He could have gotten access to such treatment due to the generosity of friends willing to pay for the medications that he could not himself afford. But as the chairman of TAC, he argued that he could not in good conscience lead the treatment-access movement if he was benefiting from an economic privilege denied those he was leading. In its ethical clarity, *Habit* acknowledges that to effectively build a global AIDS activist movement, Bordowitz and Achmat must adopt fundamentally different witnessing practices. Moreover, it makes clear that part of Bordowitz's responsibilities lie precisely in articulating that difference. The video thus consistently cuts abruptly between U.S. and South African contexts to posit the radical discontinuity of their AIDS crises as the central, unresolved issue of global AIDS (figures 38 and 39).

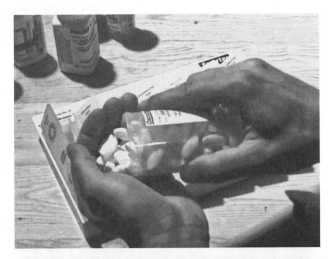

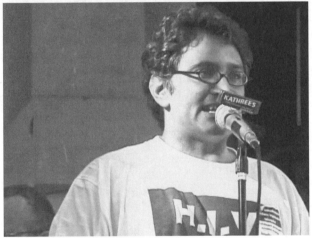

38–39. Frame captures from *Habit* (Gregg Bordowitz, 2001).

In writing about the video, Bordowitz insists that he aspired to make a political work of art, "one that embodies in its form the ethical demands faced in our encounters with others as they arise out of current conditions of existence."[64] For Bordowitz, such political media making functions through the production of blunt irresolution as the most effective catalyst for the active engagement of his audience. In its specific address to an audience in the global North, *Habit* recognizes that the ethical demand of Achmat's pledge can only be grasped within the historical conditions that have necessitated it. Those conditions are simultaneously local and global, but each sphere requires a different form of political engagement. Bordowitz's autobiographical exploration of the psychological ambivalence that he experiences in living with AIDS on antiretroviral treatment would seem to be a luxury that South African audiences can hardly afford to entertain. But for North American audiences, it is absolutely necessary if they are to fully recognize the ethical address of Achmat's pledge and not merely treat it in a typically liberal humanist way, that is to say, as the courageous gesture of a heroic individual. I will continue to consider these issues in the next chapter as I examine the testimonial space of song in John Greyson and David Wall's *Fig Trees* (2003), a video opera installation centered on the ethical complexity of Achmat's pledge.

□

Queer Anachronism and
the Testimonial Space
of Song

No scene in Jonathan Demme's *Philadelphia* (1993) has generated more critical attention and disagreement than the "Mamma Morta" scene in which Andy Beckett (Tom Hanks) breaks off trial preparation with his lawyer Joe Miller (Denzel Washington) to listen in rapture to a recording of Maria Callas singing the "Mamma Morta" aria from Umberto Giordano's *Andrea Chénier* (1896). Some scholars have approached it in terms of the intersubjective dynamics of its sentimental pedagogy, what Charles I. Nero dubs its "operatic tutelage," in which the straight African American man learns how to feel from the gay white man.[1] Others have focused on the scene as a privileged moment of sublimity for Andy. Thus, while Brett Farmer reads this affirmatively as "a delirious transcendence of embodied identity," Dennis Allen argues that the scene merely subtends heteronormativity by pathologizing Andy's homosexuality as an irrational, unstable, and incoherent identity.[2]

Regardless of their ultimate ideological assessment of the scene, most scholars agree that its formal qualities render it a privileged moment in the film. As Andy becomes ever more transfixed by Callas's singing and moves around the empty floor in ecstatic gestures, the camera shifts to a high-angle position, framing his body tightly in an increasingly abstracted space. Expressionist red lighting enhances the unreality of the moment, as Andy asks, "Can you feel it, Joe?" A more naturalistically illuminated Joe merely looks on, appearing utterly bewildered. After the aria is over, he excuses himself and makes a hasty exit from Andy's apartment. In the hallway, Joe equivocates momentarily about returning to Andy, but then continues his exit. This brief gesture of indecision subtly registers the emotional impact that the shared experience of hearing the aria has had on Joe. The film also distinguishes this encounter through other formal means that contrast it to an earlier exchange between Andy and Joe in the law library. In that scene, Joe witnesses the discrimination that Andy suffers at the hands of the law librarian and comes to bond with him over the law, a connection that will prove the turning point for Joe's commitment to Andy's case. In contrast to the aria scene, their conversation in the library is filmed from a noticeable low-angle position on the desk, as if the camera was occupying the position of the legal texts that draw the two men together. *Philadelphia* marks its aria scene as a particularly special moment of witnessing, one that exceeds the legal and political discourses that constitute the dominant testimonial frame of the film.

Does song, then, offer a discrete and privileged mode of enunciation for bearing witness? Can song provide unique opportunities to reframe the mediated body of the witness and his or her utterance? In her analysis of Claude Lanzmann's landmark Holocaust film *Shoah* (1985), Shoshana Felman argues that song is central to both its structure and its address.[3] *Shoah* opens and closes with the performance of songs by Simon Srebnik, one of the only two survivors of the Chelmno concentration camp in Poland. Having persuaded Srebnik to return to the site of trauma, Lanzmann opens the film with Srebnik sitting in a boat on the river in Chelmno as he sings once again the Polish and German folk songs that the camp guards forced him to sing. At the end of the scene we hear an elderly Polish woman declare in voice-over, "When I heard him again, my heart beat faster, because what happened here . . . was a murder." Her comment acknowledges how the song of the witness-survivor (*superstes*) can enter the body of the witness-observer (*testis*). "Opened by the song, the film does not simply show itself, it calls us," notes Felman. "It calls us through the singing it enacts. It is asking us to listen to, and hear, not just the meaning of the words, but the complex significance of their return, and the clashing echoes of their melody and of their context" (271). Felman's analysis indicates how the testimonial potential of song is realized not through the Romantic conception of vocal music as a transcendental experience but through its historical specificities and the contrapuntal dynamics they produce.

In the context of queer AIDS media, no one has been more attuned to this than John Greyson, whose film musical *Zero Patience* (1993), scored by Glenn Schellenberg, and video opera installation *Fig Trees* (2003), a collaborative project with the composer David Wall, serve as the focus of this chapter.[4] I have chosen to analyze Greyson's works here less for the auteurist coherence they might offer than for the historical and aesthetic range that they permit me in addressing these questions around the testimonial space of song. Whereas Zero Patience appropriates the popular cultural form of the film musical to bear witness to both the structures of feelings and the politics of AIDS activists in the late 1980s, Fig Trees turns to the high art realms of opera and gallery installation to bear witness to the resurgence of radical AIDS activism at the turn of the millennium in South Africa. I am also interested in these works for their queer anachronism, that is to say, their fanciful retrieval of queer figures and their works from the cultural archive (Richard Burton, Gertrude Stein, and Virgil Thomson), whose encounters with the present play a considerable role in the witnessing dynamics performed by these works.

A key figure in queer Canadian cinema, Greyson has produced an audacious body of work that finds its structuring principle in the dialectics of queer cultural production in the era of AIDS. In addition to Zero Patience and Fig Trees, Greyson produced several short AIDS activist videos in the late 1980s, including The ADS Epidemic (1987), a public service announcement/music video; The World is Sick (sic) (1989), a documentary about AIDS activism at the Fifth International Conference on AIDS in Montreal in 1989; and The Pink Pimpernel (1989), a chronicle of AIDS activism in Toronto that includes a queer remaking of The Scarlet Pimpernel (Harold Young, 1934) and safer-sex shorts modeled on queer avant-garde classics such as Andy Warhol's Blow Job (1963) and Jean Genet's Un chant d'amour (A Love Song) (1950). Greyson's films and videos use passion, intellect, and cheek to play on the dialectical tensions between aesthetics and activism, grief and anger, entertainment and pedagogy. Whether feature films, activist videos, or public service announcements, Greyson's works are marked by a rigorously self-reflexive play with form (especially genre), a deeply political engagement with representation, a dense historical and cinematic intertextuality, a camp sensibility, and, above all, an erotic impudicity. For example, his irreverent short film The Making of Monsters (1991) brings back to life Georg Lukács and Bertolt Brecht (played by a fish in a tank) in contemporary Toronto to argue how best to produce a film about queer bashing based on the actual murder of a gay schoolteacher in 1985. Presented as a "making of" documentary about a fictionalized television movie about the murder, The Making of Monsters pits Lukács, the social realist who embraces dramatic narrative and empathetic identification, against Brecht, the modernist who prefers the antirealism of song-and-dance numbers for their potential to produce more politically engaged and critically aware audiences. Refusing to champion one strategy over the other, the film shifts vertiginously between powerful scenes of personal testimony, such as the victim's mother lamenting the normality of homophobic violence, and rambunctious spectacles of political didacticism, such as the pop-choreographed musical number about homophobic violence and the male homosociality of sport performed by four young men clad only in hockey masks, socks, and jockstraps.

In his history of Canadian queer cinema, Thomas Waugh indicates the salience of music in Greyson's work, tracing its development from the appropriation of pop music in his Kipling Trilogy (1984–85) through the witty adaptation of Brecht and Kurt Weill songs in The Making of Monsters to the original musical compositions of The ADS Epidemic, Zero Patience, and Fig Trees.[5] Furthermore, in a lecture he gave at Concordia University in 2006, Greyson himself acknowledged the two principal threads running through his work: "First, AIDS: an engagement that now spans two decades, with the meanings and material experiences of the pandemic. Second, an ongoing interest in song: song as narrative, polemic, eulogy."[6] Just as Greyson has maintained a radically heterogeneous visual aesthetic that incorporates narrative, performance, appropriated images, interviews, and documentary footage (what Waugh dubs his "narrative essay-mosaic"), so too has his engagement with song been similarly diverse and disjunctive: "Song as dialogue between cultures, across continents, through centuries. Song as disruption of realist conventions and complacent representations. Song as humour. Song as counter-point and catharsis. Song as Trojan horse, a double agent infiltrating the cold-war worlds of high and low art, betraying both sides, taking no prisoners." For Greyson, song is thus, like the act of bearing witness, both communicative and interruptive. It harbors the ability to simultaneously attest and contest, which he sees rooted in its dialectical treatment of affect: "Sung words simultaneously distance us and draw us closer, making the emotions both more stylized and more heartfelt, appealing to a sensuality transcendent of naturalism."[7] Greyson's conception of song's dialectical capacities here clearly invokes the dynamics of camp, which Steven Cohan has argued can be understood, among other things, as "the formation of a queer affect: of taking queer pleasure in perceiving, if not causing category dissonance."[8] Moreover, Greyson's camp embrace of song is deeply embedded in his critique of representational practices and institutions. Made a decade apart, Zero Patience and Fig Trees each focus on a historical figure, in both cases a gay man who has played a significant role in the cultural representation of the AIDS pandemic at specific moments in its history: Gaetan Dugas and Zackie Achmat. Both have become mythologized historical figures, but each at different ends of the shadow archive: Dugas as the repressive portrait of the disease-spreading deviant and Achmat as the honorific portrait of the disease-defying hero.

Zero Patience attempts to untangle and debunk the mythology around Dugas as the so-called Patient Zero. Dugas was a French-Canadian flight attendant who participated in one of the earliest cluster studies in the early 1980s that determined that the (as then unnamed) virus could be sexually transmitted.[9] It was in Randy Shilts's 1987 bestseller And the Band Played On: Politics, People, and the AIDS Epidemic that he was publicly given the moniker Patient Zero. Shilts painted a lurid characterization of an arrogant man who seemed to use his sexual promiscuity to willfully infect others. Zero Patience figures Dugas in the character of Zero (Normand Fauteux), who returns to Toronto in the early 1990s as a ghost, unable to be seen by others save by Sir Richard Francis Burton (John Robinson), the famous nineteenth-century British explorer and scientist, a second historical figure fantastically resituated in the present of the film. The voice-over narration informs us that Burton has had "an unfortunate accident with the fountain of youth" and is still alive today, working as the chief taxidermist and diorama artist at the Natural History Museum in Toronto. The narrative concerns Burton's attempt to assemble a new exhibition, The Hall of Contagion, in which the sensationalist depiction of Zero as "the Man Who Brought AIDS to North America" will become the main attraction, the spatial and historical culmination for an exhibition covering centuries of epidemic disease.[10] Burton tracks down many of Zero's old friends, including the ex-junkie Mary (Dianne Hetherington) and the schoolteacher George (Richardo Keens-Douglas), who is struggling against blindness from cytomegalovirus. Now all AIDS activists in a group resembling ACT UP or AIDS Action Now (its Toronto counterpart), they resist Burton's sensationalist agenda and plot a protest zap against the museum. Burton's investigations cause him to eventually encounter Zero's ghost, who also contests Burton's project but gradually develops a more complicated relationship with the older man. Although the ethical and erotic encounter between these two men forms the principal narrative structure of the film, I concur with Waugh when he argues that the nine song numbers provide the essential coherence to the film with its "typically centrifugal narrative/expository structure that dashes off self-reflexively in all directions."[11] Songs become the principal vehicle to tell Zero's story, to bear witness to Dugas.[12]

Fig Trees centers around Achmat, who cofounded the Treatment Action Campaign (TAC) in 1998.[13] Achmat's pledge not to take antiretrovirals until they were universally available in South Africa brought unprecedented national and international media attention to TAC and its fight for universal

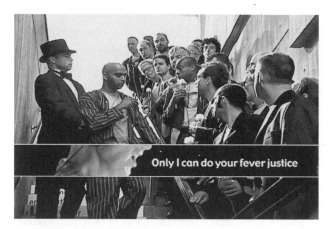

Only I can do your fever justice

40. Still from the video installation *Fig Trees* (John Greyson and David Wall, 2003). Courtesy of the artists.

access. But it also fostered an image of Achmat as the quintessential hero of the global AIDS pandemic, earning him numerous awards and a Nobel Prize nomination in 2004.[14] In an act of fantastical historical anachronism similar to that of *Zero Patience*, *Fig Trees* brings Achmat together with Stein and Thomson, the queer modernist poet and composer who had collaborated on the 1934 experimental opera *Four Saints in Three Acts* (based on the lives of Saint Theresa and Saint Ignatius, as well as several invented saints). Stein and Thomson appear in *Fig Trees* in search of new subjects for a follow-up to *Four Saints*. They try to persuade Achmat to let them write an opera about what they see as his act of martyrdom worthy of canonization. Along the way, Thomson must compete in a "Staircase Motet" with twenty other queer modernist composers for the rights to Zackie's story (figure 40). But in the final scene of the opera, "Fig Orchard," Zackie decides that it is time to start taking his medications, thus denying Stein and Thomson of their operatic martyr. In August 2003, three months before the premiere of *Fig Trees*, the TAC membership appealed to Achmat to end his strike, arguing that they needed a living leader, not a dead martyr. In agreement, Achmat announced on national television that he would start taking antiretroviral drug therapy because he would not let the AIDS denialists in the African National Congress (ANC) government kill him.

Zero Patience and Fig Trees both focus their narratives self-reflexively on the project and process of cultural representation, notably situated in powerful institutions — the museum and the opera. Through the anachronistic encounter with queer historical figures the two works interrogate the contemporary discursive production of villains and heroes in the cultural narratives of the pandemic. But neither work serves merely as an ideological critique of cultural representation. For in each case, the performance of songs provides the space in which the subject of the representational project not only contests the image and the enunciative position that have been constructed for him but also attests to the structures of feeling shaping his subjective experience of AIDS. Songs have discrete communicative and performative characteristics that make them an apt medium for acts of bearing witness. Songs exceed the bounds of regular speech. We listen to songs as an experience that can be at once intensely subjective and highly social, regardless of whether they are solo performances or a chorus. Although other performing and literary arts may also engender an address that is simultaneously singular and collective, the musical performance of the voice in song intensifies this tension. Songs create a permeable space. Like other forms of music, song has the propensity to fill a room, but it also has a capacity to fill us. According to the literary scholar Mark Booth, "the singer's words are sung for us in that he says something that is also said somehow in extension by us, and we are drawn into the state, the pose, the attitude, the self offered by the song."[15] Moreover, the prominence of voice as a signifier of embodiment is heightened when a person breaks into song, even if the song is experienced through the mediation of a recording. Wayne Kostenbaum describes these dynamics in a particularly eloquent passage in his book on opera:

> A singer's voice sets up vibrations and resonances in the listener's body. First, there are the physiological sensations we call "hearing." Second, there are gestures of response with which the listener mimics the singer, expresses physical sympathy, appreciation, or exultation: shudder, gasp, sigh; holding the body motionless, relaxing the shoulders, stiffening the spine. Third, the singer has presence, an expressive relation to her body— and presence is contagious. I catch it. The dance of sound waves on the tympanum and the sigh I exhale in sympathy with the singer persuade me that I have a body—if only, by analogy, if only a second-best copy of the singer's body.[16]

As Kostenbaum here contends, the listener may in fact experience the song as a moment of corporeal mimesis.

In both *Zero Patience* and *Fig Trees*, the space of songs becomes central to their testimonial dynamics, which emerge from their specific generic forms. *Zero*

Patience thus exploits the privileged functions of direct address and mise-en-scène in the film musical, while *Fig Trees*, as a gallery installation, constructs a distinct material space for each song. The song number in a film musical disrupts the narrative flow, creating a discursively differentiated space.[17] The song number reconfigures space because it avows its status as a performance. Unlike the spectatorial relations of classical narrative cinema, the song number acknowledges its audience on the other side of the screen, that is to say, in the auditorium. Song numbers often inscribe a diegetic audience whom the singer addresses, yet this usually functions as a suturing device to bridge the shift to a direct address of the film's audience. The film musical is one of the few genres of popular narrative cinema that permit such shifts to a direct address.[18] Furthermore, the performer's placement within, and movement around, the profilmic space foregrounds the mise-en-scène of the song number, transferring the dominant signifying function from narrative to spectacle. And finally, the prerecorded singing that characterizes the numbers of a film musical differentiates them as privileged spaces discursively demarcated from the rest of the film. They are always louder in volume and, due to postsynchronization, the singers' voices literally come from another time and space than the one seen on the screen.[19] Although such film technology further mediates the communicative act performed by the song, it does not disqualify or mitigate its status as direct address. On the contrary, it enhances the recognition of its paradiegetic qualities.

Gallery installations (as a form of installation art) considerably complicate questions of address and mise-en-scène. The viewer becomes a visitor to the work, entering it as a physical space that both addresses the visitor by its material design and renders the visitor an element of the work's mise-en-scène.[20] Installation art simultaneously liberates and disciplines visitors in their engagement with it by allowing degrees of choice in movement and attention, but only ever degrees. Nevertheless, such generally freer engagement usually permits installation visitors some agency in determining their temporal and spatial experience of the work. Works of installation art tend not to posit a fixed, stable, or ideal position for visitors, and those that do usually encourage them to recognize the construction of their position and may intimate means to resist it. Visitors' bodily movements within and in response to the physical space and design of the work render installation art an aesthetic mode in which the viewer's embodied experience becomes paramount. In their giving formal privilege to space, both the film musical and the gallery installation offered Greyson apposite means to interrupt the cultural narratives constructed around Dugas and Achmat.

Redeeming the Ghost in the Machine

Zero Patience constitutes at once a challenge to the specific claims of Shilts's *And the Band Played On* and a critique of the historiography on which it is grounded. For all its interweaving narrative strands as the book moves among key individuals involved in the early years of the epidemic, *And the Band Played On* engenders a historiography grounded in clearly articulated linear causality. Through his self-identification as a hard-hitting investigative journalist, Shilts understood epidemiology to be first and foremost a matter of etiology, requiring the need to uncover the linear causality of the epidemic, to track down its source. Greyson's film seeks to not only redeem the memory of a fellow gay Canadian but also to constitute a form of genealogical critique (in the Foucauldian sense) of the very discourses that made a figure such as Patient Zero imaginable in both cultural fantasy and historical narrative.[21]

Published to great critical acclaim in the mainstream press, *And the Band Played On* offered the first popular chronicle of the AIDS epidemic and quickly became the most widely read book on the subject in the United States. A gay journalist writing for the *San Francisco Chronicle*, Shilts conceived of the book as a work of committed nonfiction: "A tale that bears telling, so that it will never happen again, to any people, anywhere."[22] The language Shilts uses here to frame his project indicates that he envisioned his own work as a form of journalistic witnessing—testimony to the past as prophylaxis to secure the future. In his "Notes on Sources" at the end of the book, he lays claim to its objectivity: "This book is a work of journalism. There has been no fictionalization. For purposes of narrative flow, I reconstruct scenes, recount conversations, and occasionally attribute observations to people with such phrases as 'he thought' or 'she felt'" (607). However, in addition to its prologue, epilogue, epigraphs from Albert Camus's *La peste* (*The Plague*), and a printed roster of dramatis personae, the book is also organized and phrased precisely in the fashion of a Victorian serialized novel, with very short episodic chapters.[23] Citing Roland Barthes's concept of "zero degree writing," Douglas Crimp has characterized Shilts's writing style as the arcane articulation of a universal point of view typical of nineteenth-century bourgeois writing: "The bourgeois writer [is] sole judge of other people's woes and without anyone else to gaze on him."[24] Erasing his own presence as a witness from the text, Shilts narrates the early years of the epidemic through his fictionally reconstructed witnesses, all the while laying claim to his cherished sense of committed journalism and its ethos of bearing witness.

Abiding by the melodramatic structures of such zero degree writing, Shilts divides the dramatis personae into clearly defined heroes and villains: "The AIDS epidemic is, ultimately, a tale of courage as well as cowardice, compassion as well as bigotry, inspiration as well as venality, and redemption as well as despair."[25] Despite all its vilification of bureaucratic indifference and scientific arrogance, the book renders as its principal villain Patient Zero. For Shilts, he is a one-dimensional scoundrel from a gothic novel and an emblem of gay lifestyle in the postliberation era, obsessed with his own pleasure and vanity, continually looking into mirrors, and uttering vanities worthy of the Evil Queen in Snow White: "I'm still the prettiest one" (47). Shilts never interviewed or even met Dugas, so he depended on other testimonies to construct his characterization, principally that of the Centers for Disease Control and Prevention (CDC) sociologist William Darrow, who publicly repudiated Shilts's character assassination of Dugas in the book, arguing that Dugas had in fact eagerly cooperated with the epidemiological investigation. In an earlier historical account of the epidemic, Darrow's description of Dugas's character differs markedly: "He felt terrible about having made other people sick. He had come down with Kaposi's but no one ever told him it might be infectious."[26] In promoting And the Band Played On by focusing on the Patient Zero theory, Shilts's publisher, St. Martin's Press, made immediate media stars of both Shilts and Dugas. Yet Crimp has argued that the bigger problem behind Shilts's and his publisher's blatant exploitation of Dugas lies in Patient Zero's prior existence "as a phobic fantasy in the minds of Shilts's readers before Shilts ever wrote the story."[27] Fittingly, Greyson's film pulls Zero from the shadow archive of AIDS representation in the form of a ghost—a figure haunting the cultural imagination, but also an ordinary gay life in the end unseen and unrecognized by public culture, and thus a loss still waiting to be mourned. While the figure of Patient Zero stands center stage in the spectacle of AIDS, the actual life and death of Dugas remains wholly unimaginable and unrepresentable. He is one of the epidemic's "Drowned," to borrow Primo Levi's term, a "true witness" because he had no opportunity to bear witness to his own dying.[28]

The film's redemptive project for bearing witness to the life and death of Dugas thus necessarily takes place within a complex historical analysis of dominant media discourses and the visual technologies through which they are communicated. In the following pages, I examine how Greyson constructed specific song numbers in the film as witnessing spaces in which such dual labor could be enacted. The film's credit sequence posits Zero first and foremost as a trope of media representation: the opening title shot reads, "In 1987 newspapers around the world accused a canadian flight attendant of bringing AIDS to north america. They called him patient zero."[29] Credit shots subsequently present pixelated fragments of monochrome photographs showing Zero's naked torso. A similar photograph then appears on a flyer explaining the Patient Zero theory, anonymously thrown at Burton as a paper airplane (presumably by the self-conscious hand of the author). Just as Burton begins to realize how he can use the figure of Patient Zero to replace the cancelled "Düsseldorf plague rat" in his Hall of Contagion exhibit, an intertitle shifts the scene to "meanwhile somewhere between existential limbo and the primordial void," where Zero appears to languish. So begins the film's first song number, "Just Like Scheherazade," a pop ballad visualized in a music-video montage that includes long shots of Zero dancing with a glitter ball in a deserted swimming pool, tightly framed close-ups of Zero singing, and overhead and underwater shots of water ballet dancers: 1980s music video meets 1940s Metro-Goldwyn-Mayer (MGM) Esther Williams vehicle.[30] Frequent dissolves between Zero's facial close-ups and the water ballet shots imply his spectral state (figure 41). But they also align the interlocking movements of the water ballet with the erotic and utopian desires of his lyrics:

Tell the story of my life
From zero hour to 12 a.m.
From the good to the bad
Tell the tale, save my life
A life I could have had
Just like Scheherazade
I've been dead for years and years
Sick with loneliness
No one sees or hears me
I'm dying for a kiss

The Scheherazade motif has appeared beforehand during the credit sequence in shots of a classroom in which George is teaching French to his pupils with the use of *Arabian Nights*. Holding a copy of the book with a photograph of Burton (its English translator) on the dust jacket, a young boy translates the story of Scheherazade from George's French transcription on the blackboard (figure 42). Storytelling in *Arabian Nights* is nothing less than a matter of life and death. The collection of fairy tales is filled with individuals whose lives depend on the responses of their listeners to their tales. "If all the characters incessantly tell stories," notes Tzvetan Todorov, "it is because this action has received a supreme consecration: narrating equals living."[31]

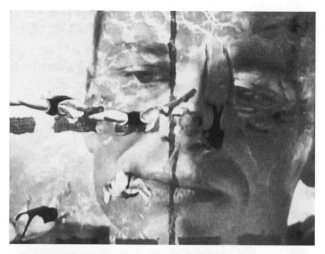

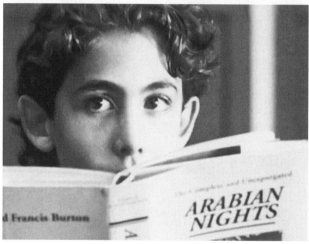

41–42. Frame captures from *Zero Patience* (John Greyson, 1993).

In his characterization of the book, Todorov here unwittingly proposes *Arabian Nights* as a promising counterpoint to the logic of "Silence=Death." As the character at the heart of the frame story of the collection, Scheherazade is clearly the most significant of the book's storytellers. She is able to stave off King Shahryar's threat of execution only by continuing to tell him stories. Her survival strategy of narration is ultimately underpinned, according to Jack Zipes, by a larger moral pedagogy both in her motives and in the social function of the book itself.[32] Her storytelling serves three principal functions. She wishes to morally reeducate Shahryar, to reinstall his humanity through narrative, which she achieves by the end of the book. She also teaches her younger sister, Dunazade, who is the other listener to her tales, how to narrate her own destiny and achieve a level of autonomy in a patriarchal social world. Finally, Scheherazade's storytelling serves to socialize contemporary Muslim readers: "Without disregarding the entertaining and humorous aspects of these stories, they are primarily *lessons* in etiquette, aesthetics, decorum, religion, government, history, and sex" (588; emphasis original). In its use of Scheherazade as a major motif, *Zero Patience* takes up this pedagogic imperative behind her storytelling function in *Arabian Nights*. The lessons to be learned are in the same areas mentioned by Zipes, but they come not from the medieval Muslim world, but from contemporary gay culture in the midst of an epidemic.

Pedagogy continues as a principal motif in the second song number in the film, "Culture of Certainty," a raucously didactic song in the vein of Brecht and Weill, in which Burton presents a slide show to the museum director, Dr. Placebo (Bernard Behrens), in an attempt to convince him that Patient Zero should be the centerpiece of the exhibition. Although Placebo functions as the diegetically inscribed audience for Burton's song/illustrated lecture, the frontal staging of the number allows Burton to address us directly with his exuberant faith in empiricism. Both the lyrics and the images of the slide show parallel the moralizing pathology of AIDS science in the context of Victorian empiricism, highlighting Burton's own idiosyncratic interventions in Victorian sexology, which included translations of the Kama Sutra and empirical studies of penis size. Burton is a curiously contradictory figure in Victorian culture whom Edward Said sees "both as a rebel against authority (hence his identification with the East as a place of freedom from Victorian moral authority) and as a potential agent of authority in the East."[33]

In a later scene in which Burton tries to capture Zero's image on videotape, he asks him to read something, and Zero chooses Burton's "Terminal Essay," a piece on homosexuality from 1885, in which Burton articulated his

"Sodatic" theory of pederasty. In the essay, Burton posited that homosexuality was only indigenous to tropical climates, thus assuring his English audience that sexual inversion was safely contained in a geographically located other. Greyson seems to concur with Said's ambivalence toward Burton when he has the character defend his theory as the strategic avoidance of censorship. Nevertheless, by having Zero confront Burton on this issue, the film suggests that Burton's theory forms a part of the discursive genealogy that permitted Shilts and the U.S. media to construct Dugas as an alien sexual other—a French-Canadian homosexual. Right before Burton sings "Culture of Certainty," his mention of Zero's French-Canadian identity to Placebo appears to finally mitigate the museum director's reluctance to highlight "a promiscuous, irresponsible homosexual Canadian" in a national cultural institution. Stuffy Anglo-Canadian hegemony in the end allows Zero to function as a contaminating other on both sides of the border.

Despite its simplicity, the mise-en-scène of "Culture of Certainty" holds a larger thematic significance. Burton's use of a slide projector invokes the nineteenth-century practice of the illustrated lecture, which, as I discussed in chapter 1, constituted one of the precursors to documentary film, itself a representational form key to the spectacle of AIDS and one that Burton subsequently deploys in the video about Zero for the exhibition. As a prominent visual practice of nineteenth-century public culture, the illustrated lecture contributed to the development of modern structures of surveillance and spectacle. It was a site at which popular science and entertainment met. The mise-en-scène of two other song numbers in the film highlight other visual technologies key to the popular visualization of modern science: "Contagious" is staged in a habitat diorama at the museum and "Scheherazade (Miss HIV)" plays out in Zero's blood, which Burton and Zero view through a microscope.

The diorama plays a substantial role in the film's museological mise-en-scène. This visual technology common to the late nineteenth-century museum combined spectacle and narrative in its spatial serialization of tableau displays and thus served as a precursor to cinema.[34] The film stresses the genealogical significance of this particular visual technology through Burton's insistence to Placebo that the exhibition culminate with the Patient Zero display using the latest multimedia technology. Zero is to constitute the contemporary end point for a history of epidemics depicted in earlier moments with waxwork dioramas (of Typhoid Mary and the Tuskegee Experiment) and a taxidermic diorama of the African green monkey. The Hall of Contagion thus conjoins two historical narratives in its spatial organization—the historical progression of human epidemics and the historical development of modern visual technologies.[35] Despondent in his continued failure to materialize, Zero engages in an imaginary conversation with the stuffed African green monkey in Burton's Hall of Contagion, pitying himself in comparison to the animal's ignorance of the politics of blame, which position them both as "causes" of the AIDS pandemic. Suddenly the green monkey comes to life, anthropomorphizing into the figure of a butch lesbian activist (Marla Lukofsky) who angrily repudiates Zero's self-pity with the song "Contagious":

> This pack of pariahs is feeling outrageous
> The plague we've got is one called rage
> Skin us and stuff us, we're snapping and snarling
> The law of the jungle, break out of the cage

Several other taxidermy animals also break out of the diorama display, anthropomorphizing into a multicultural group of dancers whose exuberant movements embody the utopian desire to break the institutional and discursive structures of representation.[36] The film's consistent return to Burton's taxidermy for the museum dioramas (often in slow panning shots) provides an apt metaphor for the violence performed by modern systems of visual representation: the body is eviscerated, stuffed, and rendered inert or animatronic.

The microscope, another modern visual technology deeply implicated in the scientific objectification of the body, plays a central role in the song number "Scheherazade (Miss HIV)." After Burton has stolen Zero's blood samples from the original epidemiological study, Zero inquisitively places them under Burton's microscope (figure 43). What he sees is quite spectacular: sitting on a float holding a large parasol emblazoned with the letters "HIV" and surrounded by other smaller anthropomorphized viruses swimming around her, is Miss HIV, played by Michael Callen, the AIDS activist, long-term survivor, and performer (who had also appeared at the end of Bright Eyes) (figure 44). This scene presents the retrovirus as an acerbic drag queen who not only questions the dominant scientific theory that HIV causes AIDS but also vindicates Zero as an innocent victim of the politics of blame by pointing out the inconsistencies of the Patient Zero theory (particularly as it relates to the latency of AIDS). The scene provides a pedagogic spectacle on the scientific debate about the relationship between HIV and AIDS, which was still an important political and therapeutic issue for PWAs in the early 1990s, not the pernicious, conspiracy-laden denialism it became over the following decade. But the song that Miss HIV sings is unlike the earlier didactic

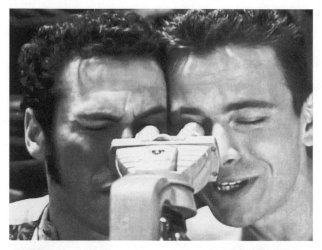

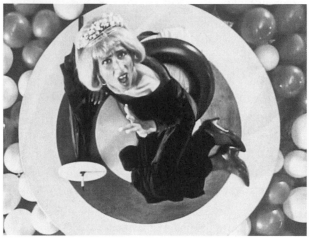

43–44. Frame captures from *Zero Patience* (John Greyson, 1993).

numbers. Rather, it articulates the dialectics of politics and pathos in the epidemic through the thematic symmetry of its mere six lines:

Tell a story of a virus
Of greed and ambition and fraud
A case of science gone bad
Tell a tale of friends we miss
A tale that's cruel and sad
Weep for me, Scheherazade

Callen's defiant insistence on holding the final high note of the song longer on screen than Barbra Streisand, while clearly the ruse of a gay diva, heightens its expression of emotional authenticity. The testimonial aspect of the song momentarily ruptures the diegetic world of the film, for the song's voice is clearly that of a PWA rather than that of a drag queen retrovirus. It is the performer Callen singing of "friends we miss," not the character Miss HIV.[37] This number plays on the prevalent cultural slippage between the virus/syndrome and the person with the virus/syndrome, but it does it through the ironic performativity of camp and drag.[38] The number connects formally and thematically to others in the film that convey the structures of feeling of gay men with AIDS, namely, Zero's plaintive "Just Like Scheherazade" (of which it is a reprise) and "Positive," George's poignant expression of the emotional seesaw between courage and doubt that marked the lives of PWAs at the time (the number plays off the ambiguities of the term positive in the era of HIV).[39] Although Greyson often described the film as a celebration of the international AIDS activist movement, inspired by the camp, wit, and humor of ACT UP, musical numbers such as "Positive" and "Scheherazade (Miss HIV)" bear a distinctly Brechtian imprint with their dialectical approach that refuses to merely preach the "right position."

This spectacle seen through the lens of a microscope in the Miss HIV number constitutes an additional imbrication of science and entertainment. Callen's performance is shot from an overhead position to suggest Zero's point of view as he looks into the microscope. The overhead shot is in fact a privileged device in the film, occurring in many of its spectacular numbers. Greyson suggested in an interview that we regard these perspectives as the visualization of scientific discourses of "objectivity" that posit an enunciative position outside and above the object of study.[40] Although this overhead shot of Zero's blood invokes a scientific gaze, its performative spectacle of song and dance seen from above also implies the popular cultural gaze associated with Busby Berkeley musicals. When the film cuts from Zero looking into the microscope to the spectacle in his own blood, it replicates the shift to the "impossible space" of spectacular performance so common in Berkeley musicals.[41] The abstraction of bodies accomplished in Berkeley musicals, where women's body parts are fetishized as a kaleidoscopic pattern, is reversed in Zero Patience. Zero's body, which has been fragmented into the microscopic image of his blood cells, recorporealizes in the embodied form of Miss HIV. Zero's viewing of such a spectacle through a binocular eyepiece bears traces of the spectatorial dynamics found in a visual technology with a radically different function than the microscope—Thomas Edison's kinetoscope. Edison's early cinematic technology involved an individualized spectatorship in which the viewer peered down into a binocular eyepiece, to be gratified with short spectacular entertainments such as dancers and other performers. This genealogical trace of yet another apparatus of modern visuality points to the complex interrelationship between the visual technologies of science and of entertainment that construct AIDS in the public sphere.[42]

Arguably the most significant visual apparatus in Zero Patience is the film's museum setting, which features in several song numbers, most prominently in the final number, "Zero Patience," when the AIDS activists break into the Hall of Contagion to radically retool it, and Burton helps Zero disappear again into the primordial void. The film's museum setting draws on two specific museum controversies that directly preceded Greyson's writing of the script. His fictional Museum of Natural History invokes the Royal Ontario Museum, which had prompted vociferous protests against the alleged neocolonial ideology of its 1989 exhibition Into the Heart of Africa, while the AIDS activist protests against Burton's Hall of Contagion recall ACT UP's picketing of the Museum of Modern Art in 1988, protesting the alleged pathological gaze of Nicholas Nixon's documentary portraits of PWAs.[43]

But the significance of the museum setting extends beyond these specific historical intertexts, for the film treats the museum as a modern apparatus of disciplinary power that forms part of the discursive genealogy of the spectacle of AIDS. Tony Bennett reads the birth of the modern museum in the nineteenth century in terms of the period's "exhibitionary complex," which included the widespread popularity of expositions, world fairs, and nascent public museums and permitted the construction of a temporally organized order of things and peoples, "an order which organized the implied public—the white citizenries of the imperialist powers—into a unity, representationally effacing divisions within the body politic in constructing a 'we' conceived as the realization, and therefore just beneficiaries, of the processes of evolution and identified as a unity in opposition to the primitive otherness of conquered peoples."[44] The construction of a "general population" and a "national body" in the media spectacle of AIDS derives from this very order of things established in the exhibitionary complex of the nineteenth century. *Zero Patience* thus understands the museum, like its descendent, contemporary mass media, as a visual apparatus in which the subject comes to recognize his or her national identity and sexual citizenship through the spectacle of the other.

When the activists break into the museum at midnight ("zero hour"), it is the pathological figures of the dioramas that they first target, reframing their mise-en-scène to highlight nineteenth-century progressive activism and science. As they sing defiantly of their "zero patience" for the politics of blame and scientific arrogance, they replace the exhibit's pathological archive with a progressive one, swiftly transforming Typhoid Mary into the feminist health activist Fanny Wright and the Tuskegee sharecropper into George Washington Carver, the African American scientist and teacher.[45] The exuberant dynamic of the song number replaces the sobriety of the museum space with a transgressive energy that even causes the bound-up security guards to break free, strip off their uniforms, and dance like go-go boys. The activists make no attempt, however, to destroy or alter the Patient Zero display, the ultimate target of their protest, leaving Burton and Zero the opportunity to complete the transformation of the space as the number switches from a group number to a duet.

Zero stands in front of a huge electronic image of himself on the video screen. The frozen, pathologized image of Zero's Kaposi sarcoma–marked face is shattered as his ghost ruptures the boundary separating the historical world from the realm of visual representation. Zero's ghost fuses with the image, allowing him to exit the historical world and return to the space of representation, transforming it from a still image into a moving one. The sexual vitality of his buff, naked torso replaces the passive, objectified, and diseased face of the still image. Once reinscribed in the world of the electronic image, Zero looks directly at the camera, content and seductive. Shot-reverse-shot reveals the object of his gaze to be his lover, Burton, who stands in front of the video screen looking back at him. Thus Zero's direct address to the camera positions our gaze within the queer desire of Burton's gaze at Zero. Taking out a cigarette, Zero asks a candle-holding Burton for a light, a classic cinematic trope for seduction, but also a reference to Zero's earlier superstitious warning to Burton that with each cigarette lit by a candle, a sailor dies at sea. Zero blows the smoke from his cigarette in the direction

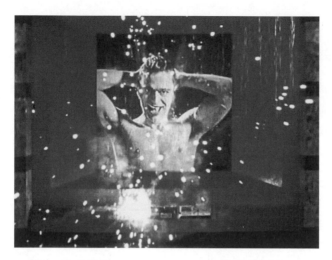

45. Frame capture from *Zero Patience* (John Greyson, 1993).

of the sprinkler system above, which eventually releases its water, showering Zero and short-circuiting the video display as water breaks through the surface of the image and into the historical world (figure 45). Sparks fly, the screen goes blank, and Zero disappears. This conclusion blatantly overturns the Hollywood musical's conventional closure of romantic union, opting instead to affirm the integrity of queer sexual culture and identity. Zero's final pose draws heavily from the iconography of gay porn: hands behind his head, Zero seductively displays his glistening naked torso under the stream of water.[46] The final image reframes the duality of sex and death produced by the spectacle of AIDS, in that it visualizes the sexual body that must be affirmed if it is to be properly mourned (Zero as the ordinary gay man) rather than the sexual body that begets death (Zero as the dying homosexual).

I discovered the continuing charge of that sexual body when I taught *Zero Patience* in my undergraduate course on the media of witnessing in April 2005. My millennial-generation students vehemently protested that the film was simply "too gay" to be taken seriously. Our subsequent discussion revealed several roots to this complaint. The contemporary invisibility of queer AIDS, the ongoing exigency of the global pandemic, and the students' liberal anxiety about equating AIDS and homosexuality encouraged them to want to "de-gay" AIDS and thus repudiate the film, even on the level of its historical significance of a different moment in the AIDS pandemic. Yet the sexual impudence of many of its song numbers also clearly succeeded in unsettling the ideological assumptions of this group of young people raised on the anodyne domesticity of *Will and Grace* and *Queer Eye for the Straight Guy*.

Refusing the Sanctity of the AIDS Hero

When Greyson returned to HIV/AIDS as a principal theme in his work in 2003, a decade after *Zero Patience*, the politics and structures of feeling around the epidemic had changed considerably. While the development of effective antiretroviral therapy against HIV prompted the notion of post-AIDS identities among gay men in the global North, the economic inaccessibility of such drugs to the exploding populations of the infected in the global South necessitated an emphasis on the global inequities of the pandemic and the assertion of health as a human right. Greyson became increasingly familiar with treatment activism in South Africa, and with Achmat personally, during the making of *Proteus* (2003), a queer historical feature set in eighteenth-century South Africa that he codirected with Jack Lewis (who lives with Achmat). As Achmat's pledge gained increasing national and international attention, Greyson and Lewis teased him with the suggestion that he would soon be known as Saint Zackie and that someone would write an opera about him. At some point the jest for Greyson morphed into a creative idea to stage an interrogation of the ethical and political dynamics of Achmat's pledge and its transnational mediation.

As a seasoned gay and antiapartheid activist well versed in the legacies of AIDS activism elsewhere, Achmat understood that his act of embodied witnessing would serve different functions nationally and globally. In South Africa, his pledge garnered him enormous respect among those infected with HIV and concretized his mandate to lead their movement in the public struggle against both the Mbeki government and the multinational drug companies over treatment access. The organization he led, TAC, fought simultaneously on two domestic fronts: to force the companies to lower the exorbitantly high prices of their AIDS drugs and to challenge the government's embrace of dissident AIDS scientists who continued to question the connection between HIV and AIDS.[47] An African nationalist reaction to the neocolonial discourse of "African AIDS" manifested itself in Mbeki's resistance to established AIDS science. He favored a cofactorial theory of AIDS that emphasizes the conditions of poverty as the underlying cause of the disease syndrome. Mbeki's denialism blocked the development of effective national strategies for both HIV treatment and prevention and has continued to hamper the rollout of antiretroviral treatment programs since political and legal pressure forced the ANC government to adopt them.

Outside South Africa, the audacity of Achmat's pledge undoubtedly caught the attention of international journalists, but the narrative hooks used to frame Achmat in the international press mythologized the story in ways well beyond Achmat's control. The first pitted him in a David-and-Goliath battle against Big Pharma, which elided the major role played by the mobilization of mass protest on a scale not seen since the days of apartheid. The second posited him as the "real" successor to Mandela in terms of his political integrity and symbolic power to embody a struggle. This frame not only invoked comparisons between Achmat's pledge and Mandela's famous 1964 speech after being sentenced to life imprisonment, in which he asserted his willingness to die for the struggle against apartheid, but it also positioned Achmat in absolute contrast to Mbeki, whose international media representation increasingly painted him according to the neocolonial trope of an irrational, paranoid, and authoritarian African leader. When Mandela publicly sided with TAC by visiting Achmat in his Cape Town home in 2002 after Achmat had missed the Fourteenth International AIDS Conference in Barcelona due to sickness, Samantha Powers reported it in her widely read *New Yorker* profile of Achmat as "a kind of coronation."[48] Achmat's quip that it was the meeting of the "sinner" and the "saint" revealed how sharply he understood the dynamics of his public profile in South Africa.

Achmat had long been very open about his sexuality, writing a frank essay about his sexual development in the Cape Town colored community for one of the first books about gay and lesbian life in South Africa.[49] Yet it was not specifically Achmat's queerness that generated controversy, since the new South African constitution reframed the public discourse on sexuality as a site of rights and political freedom and thus as one no longer beholden to the apartheid state's ideological moralism rooted in the imperatives of Afrikaner nationalism.[50] But as the South African sociologist Deborah Posel argues, this general acceptance of gay men and lesbians in postapartheid public culture has often been in tension with a broader cultural anxiety about sexuality in the era of the AIDS pandemic: "The imagery of sex as freedom, as the symbol of a virile new lease on life, jostles with that of sex as menace, sex as death."[51] Mbeki's denialism has been understood by critics like Posel as precisely a refusal to address the issue of sex in the AIDS pandemic for fear of conceding to the colonial imaginary and its sexualization of race. Thus Achmat's consistent openness about his own queer sexual history has been less concerned with contesting the stigmatization of homosexuality on its own and more with challenging the larger disavowal of sexuality per se in the South African government's approach to the AIDS pandemic. Moreover, TAC has necessarily focused a substantial amount of activism on destigmatizing the public discussion of sex in South Africa.

The fundamental challenge for Achmat in discussing his pledge with the media has been negotiating the journalistic pressure to privatize it in the name of individual heroism or of the pathos of martyrdom. Following Mandela's model of speaking of himself always in relation to the ANC, Achmat has chosen repeatedly to speak about his pledge and other aspects of his activism in terms of his ethical responsibility to others: to his fellow TAC activists, to HIV-positive South Africans. Nevertheless, news reports and articles have demonstrated a recurrent preference for framing Achmat in categorical tropes of the exceptional individual: "The AIDS warrior"; "the AIDS rebel"; "a good man in Africa"; and "a hero measured by the advance of a deadly disease."[52] An episode in Brian Tilley's documentary about Achmat, It's My Life (2001), perfectly encapsulates the tension in play between Achmat's commitment to collectivism and the individuating drive of the media. Just as Achmat is about to explain the ethics of his pledge to journalists from the Washington Post and the South African magazine Fair Lady during an interview at his home, Lewis interrupts with news that the magazine's photographer is waiting to do his photo shoot with Achmat. The icon trumps the ideas. Shot over a period of five months, Tilley's largely observational documentary follows the constant stream of interviews, meetings, and press conferences that fill Achmat's daily routine.[53] At the end of the documentary, Lewis openly argues that Achmat's pledge would be ineffective if it did not seek to exploit the widest possible publicity, "because to die in silence or to get extremely sick to the point of death while maintaining this purely moral position would seem to me to be really throwing your life away." Although it focuses primarily on Achmat's own negotiation of his personal and public life as the leader of TAC, the documentary repeatedly pulls back to reveal the technological media apparatus framing Achmat's presence in the public sphere. These scenes of photo editor meetings and television news editing suites self-reflexively emphasize how the institutional mechanisms of the national and international media do not merely facilitate the public awareness of TAC and Achmat's pledge but also function to frame them according to their own ideological prerogatives. As the magazine editor from Fair Lady notes as she looks over the photographs of Achmat, "I want to see the symbolism of the David and Goliath metaphor, which is very clichéd, but in fact this is very much what we're seeing here."

In stark contrast to the observational realism of It's My Life, Fig Trees turns to the vocabulary of opera and video installation for the aesthetic means to interrogate Achmat's pledge and its relationship to the social movement from which it emerged. Yet Fig Trees could in no way be mistaken for a conventional work of either opera or video. Greyson's collaboration with the queer avant-garde composer David Wall aimed to produce what Wall calls "video-ized opera" in which "each scene of our piece would employ a different compositional 'game': a technological aspect embedded in the actual composition which would render it both more interesting within a video context and inherently unperformable in the traditional sense."[54] Fig Trees was installed in eight different rooms at the Oakville Galleries in Oakville, Ontario, between November 2003 and January 2004, allowing visitors to choose their own path through the opera's episodic structure. Only the eight major scenes of the opera were installed at Oakville, lending further autonomy for each scene from the organizing narrative of the libretto. Inspired by the book Prepare for Saints, Steven Watson's historical account of Four Saints in Three Acts as a unique moment in queer modernist collaboration, Wall and Greyson were both fascinated by Stein and Thomson's dedication to playing with linguistic and musical form to the point of nonsense. Hence Fig Trees is filled with appropriated texts, alphabets, inversions, repetitions, and palindromes that radically reframe the episodic narrative of Achmat's pledge. Although Greyson's signature intertextual density and anachronistic encounters run throughout the work, they are subject to a rigorous separation of the elements and are thus less narratively integrated than in Zero Patience. The visitor to the installation would encounter an abundance of sound, image, and text in each room, but these elements retain relative autonomy and interact in dialectical rather than integrative ways. Much of the opera's narrative framework remained in the libretto, which was made available to gallery visitors as they moved through the installation. Typical for Greyson's densely constructed work, Fig Trees is not easily summarized on narrative, thematic, or aesthetic levels. Since the unique complexity of each scene precludes a detailed analysis of all eight room installations in the scope of this chapter, I have chosen to closely discuss four scenes that best characterize what Fig Trees achieves in the context of witnessing AIDS.

Borrowing the title of Kostenbaum's treatise on the queer love of opera, "The Queen's Throat," the opening scene of Fig Trees was installed in a small makeshift screening room, thus initially presenting visitors with a rather conventional mode of video exhibition — rowed seating before a large screen with individual headphones for each visitor.[55] The scene also invokes an archetypal Romantic trope of nineteenth-century opera — the "deathbed" aria of consumptive heroines like Antonia (Les contes de Hoffman), Violetta (La traviata), and Mimi (La bohème), whose lungs fight their crippling disease for one final glorious song before death.[56] Yet as the scene proceeds, these orthodoxies begin to unravel. On the screen the curtain rises to reveal Zackie (Van

Abrahams) sitting in a hospital bed holding papers as he begins a speech. As the libretto explains, Zackie is to give the closing keynote speech to the Fourteenth International AIDS Conference in Barcelona via satellite link because he is too ill to leave Cape Town. Footage of Achmat's actual speech can be seen and heard in the upper right-hand corner of the frame, but the satellite feed cuts out intermittently, causing ruptures in the sound and image (the full text of Achmat's original speech is printed in poster form and hung on the walls of the screening room).[57] The audible snippets form a new text that constitutes the initial words sung by Zackie on his bed: "I am not able to have medicine with dignity / nor speak to you / I hope to break the system." These words become the basis for translations in French, German, Italian, and Spanish, which other voices sing in counterpoint. These singers are shown in horizontal split-screen shots with ticker tape subtitles providing English translations of their words, which increasingly make less syntactic sense. As the image cuts to a largely white audience watching Zackie on-screen and listening through headphones, the ticker tape subtitles note that the translations are brought courtesy of "Google Simu-Lang Auto-Trans.™" The on-screen audience begin to forget their confusion as Zackie's performance intensifies emotionally. He gets out of bed, walks to the front of the stage, and sings "I appeal to the world: we want drugs, and I need hope itself." Through repeated translation in counterpoint, the line eventually becomes, "I form the world for the resemblance: we wish that drugs and need for I the interior of hope if have." Zackie then switches to his own Cape dialect of Afrikaans to sing his final line of the scene: "Ek is krities en sing liedjies: St. Zackie" (But I won't let them call me: Saint Zackie). However, the contrapuntal voices reply in unison with only the phrase "Saint Zackie," just as Zackie clutches his throat and collapses on the stage. Struck by the catharsis of the moment, the on-screen audience bursts into emotional applause. Flowers are thrown at Zackie's lifeless body on the stage.

Setting the tone for the whole work, the opening scene is structured as a palimpsest of polyphony and multiple layers of staging. In its rejection of opera's Romantic model of the singular hero, the contrapuntal fracturing of Zackie's voice into a polyglot multiplicity of voices points to an understanding of Achmat and TAC that embraces the collective rather than the individual impetus and agency of political change. "Musical polyphony in our context," notes Wall, "represents the ultimate democratization of history's rich and layered narrative."[58] Yet in repeatedly feeding its own words through automatic translation software, Greyson's libretto also implies the multiple ways in which testimony can be reframed through the process of mediation to the point of meaningless entropy. This critical skepticism about what happens to Achmat's testimony in its global transmission becomes similarly apparent in the scene's multiple layers of staging. Throughout the scene, the relationship between Zackie and his audience subtly slips back and forth between a staging that positions him, on the one hand, as a live performer on a stage in front of them (as in an opera house) and, on the other, as a mediated talking head on a large screen (as in a satellite transmission to an international conference) (figures 46 and 47). This slippage insinuates that the principal challenge for AIDS activists bearing witness to a global pandemic still remains the ability to sustain an ethical address while avoiding the pathos of privatizing historical trauma (here epitomized by opera's narrative conventions). Thus to bear witness required Achmat to move back and forth between an affirmation of the principled position from which he spoke and a resistance to his media canonization, which merely individualized the struggle. Both are acts of refusal, and such acts are never merely a matter of negation. The individual refusal of a treatment that should be available to all affirms the social right to it, while the refusal to recognize individual heroism or sanctity affirms the collective agency and achievement of the social movement.

The fourth scene of act 1, "Cut Throat," develops the theme of refusal further as Stein and Thomson initiate their search for suitable contemporary saints as subjects for a new opera. The libretto informs us that they approach four South Africans in an Oakville record store, yet the staging of the scene in the gallery presented an abstracted, denarrativized space in which Stein and Thomson are neither seen nor heard. The visitor enters a cellophane-covered square room in which a video monitor is placed in the middle of each wall. The monitors each display a singer portraying a well-known South African AIDS activist: Gugu Dlamini, who was stoned to death after she came out as HIV-positive on South African television; Christopher Moraka, a key TAC leader who gave highly persuasive testimony before Parliament in the campaign for treatment access; Nkosi Johnson, the twelve-year-old boy who fought the Johannesburg school that refused to admit him because of his seropositive status; and Simon Nkoli, the legendary gay activist who became the first South African to publicly reveal his seropositive status in 1995. Each screen presents three horizontally divided sections: the singer's head, the turntable of a record player, and a close-up of the tattooed musical notes of the song that "cut" all around the singer's throat.[59] Subtitles containing contextual information about the activists scroll along the bottom of the screen. All the elements in the frame revolve at different speeds in an endless loop,

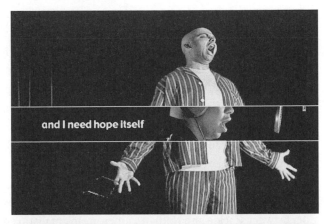

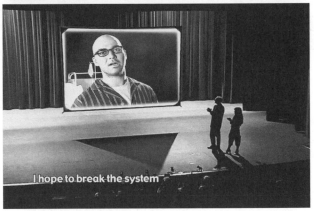

46–47. Stills from the video installation *Fig Trees* (John Greyson and David Wall, 2003). Courtesy of the artists.

mirroring the staggered-entry vocal polyphony of the scene's music, in which the activists each sing against the suggestion of their possible canonization. Although they surround the visitor from all four directions, their looping bodies and voices enact an address that refuses, that keeps turning away from the visitor, visually, textually, and acoustically. The polyphonic structure of the scene also retains the activists' firm but patient refusals as acts that are simultaneously individual and collective.

Visitors were caught in a different kind of tension as they entered the palindromic space of "Pils Slip," the sixth scene of act 1. Just as "Cut Throat" builds every formal element around a loop structure, so "Pils Slip" exploits the aesthetic symmetry of the palindrome in its music, text, and visuals for a duet between Zackie and Nathan Cameron, an amalgam character combining Nathan Geffen, the national coordinator of TAC, with Edwin Cameron, the gay AIDS activist and South African Appeals Court judge. The scene uses Geffen's and Achmat's illegal importation of the generic antifungal drug Biozole from Thailand as an opportunity for Zackie and Nathan to articulate private doubts about the medications they are taking, or refusing to take. Although Achmat flew back from Thailand in 2000, Greyson's libretto portrays Zackie's return on a train (which allows the partial staging of the duet in a tunnel) and changes the date of the event, so that the scene occurs at "the last perfect palindromic moment of the Roman calendar": 20 February 2002 at 8.02 p.m.[60] The installation of the scene was structured around two large video screens at each end of the room, one presenting Zackie, the other Nathan. Standing before a mirror and clad in pajamas of similar design but contrasting colors (Nathan in white, Zackie in black), the two men each hold a handful of pills that they accidentally drop at the same instant, then bend to pick up. After several shots of pills on a conveyor belt and of toy trains laden with pills, Zackie and Nathan appear at either end of a tunnel, slowly moving toward each other and singing a perfect palindrome together:

> Pils slip, pils on no lips
> Lips name no devil
> Pils did I live, never odd or even
> No devil is as selfless as I lived on
> *In girum imus nocte*
> Are we not drawn onward, we few?
> Drawn onward to new era?
> *Et consumimur igni*
> No devil is as selfless as I lived on

Never odd or even, evil I did slip
Lived one man spil
Spil on no slip, pils slip[61]

Seeming to pass through each other, they end up back at opposite ends of the tunnel (figure 48). Reversed footage returns the spilled pills to their hands, but when they look back at the mirror, Zackie now wears the white pajamas and Nathan the black. Nathan quickly swallows his pills, while Zackie holds them tight in his clenched fist—a gesture caught between dire need and determined refusal.

By holding similitude and difference in continual tension, palindromic form permits "Pils Slip" a rich density of meaning. Its forward-and-reverse dynamic subtly resonates not only with the political and medical pressures bearing down on Achmat but also with private equivocation, doubt, and anxiety about the effects and effectiveness of antiretrovirals. Its symmetrical structure, on the other hand, underlines the demand for equity of treatment access. The switch in costume at the end of the scene may even suggest a certain queer reciprocity between Nathan and Zackie, but their racial difference complicates any automatic homo-solidarity in this male-male duet. In the new South Africa, newly won political equality, across both race and sexuality, nevertheless belies persistent social and economic inequality, which remains the key factor in the country's AIDS crisis.

Solidarity emerges as the principal theme of "T-Shirts," the second scene of act 2, which Waugh also considers the opera's "most programmatic AIDS number."[62] After Dlamini was brutally murdered for coming out as HIV-positive, TAC began wearing and distributing white T-shirts with a simple purple logo—"HIV Positive"—as an act of solidarity that transcends the wearer's actual serostatus. "T-Shirts" draws on two important events in the history of TAC: its occupation of a Durban police station in March 2003 (as part of TAC's civil disobedience campaign against the ANC government's AIDS denialism), when TAC activists, led by Achmat, demanded the arrest of the minister of health, Manto Tshabalala-Msimang, and of the minister for trade and industry, Alec Erwin, for culpable homicide (figure 49); and Mandela's heavily publicized solidarity visit to Achmat's home in July 2002, during which the former president famously donned an "HIV Positive" T-shirt alongside Achmat.

As does the opening scene of the opera, "T-Shirts" presents a duality of documentary and operatic audiovisual tracks. To construct the scene, Greyson first edited a short documentary about the two events, which Wall then

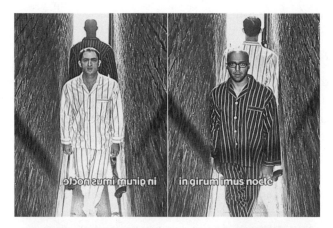

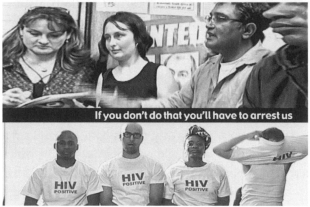

48–49. Stills from the video installation *Fig Trees* (John Greyson and David Wall, 2003). Courtesy of the artists.

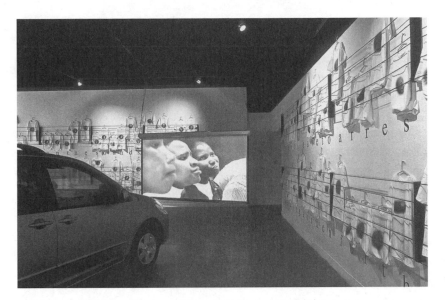

50. Gallery installation of *Fig Trees* at Oakville Galleries, Oakville, Ontario, 2003. Photo by Peter MacCallum. Courtesy of Oakville Galleries.

proceeded to "opera-cise" for a quartet of characters (Christopher, Gugu, Zackie, and Nathan) to sing on a separate audiovisual track.[63] The installation of the scene invoked a drive-in movie theater, with visitors getting into a parked minivan to watch the documentary track on a large video screen through the windshield and the operatic track on a small digital monitor on the minivan's dashboard (figure 50). As Greyson suggests, "The inescapable feeling of safari was ever present"; "you were forced to be 'safe' in the van with the music—but outside was the real life, the real experience, the words of the street, of the plague, of the world."[64] Separating the documentary and operatic tracks spatially in the mise-en-scène of the installation begs the visitor to consider what it means in ethical terms to "opera-cise" activism—to appropriate a historically contingent political act of witnessing and transform it into a Western musical form steeped in transcendental aesthetics. Such a question is amplified by Greyson's inclusion in the documentary track of clips showing the Generics, TAC's musical group, perform a tribute song to Achmat, which Wall's operatic track similarly opera-cises. How should we read such polyphony between a deeply local song performed in a popular musical idiom and its high-art transformation into modernist opera? As an act of Western mythification, or as one of global solidarity? One of the great achievements of *Fig Trees* is that it keeps open the question of its own ethical position in relation to its subject—Achmat and TAC. To answer the question if opera can bear witness to the magnitude of the AIDS crisis in South Africa and the activist response to it, Greyson and Wall raid the operatic tradition for some of its most affectively charged techniques, but they ultimately render an "impossible" opera in the conventional sense—a video installation of song spaces charged with as much self-reflexive difficulty as affective impact.

Greyson has acknowledged that the complexity and difficulty of Fig Trees came from a deliberate decision to avoid what he believed to be the mistakes he made in Zero Patience, "which have to do with trying to occupy a popular genre wholesale—though it's meant to be a meta-musical, in fact it became merely a musical, and therefore could be judged on those terms (quality of music/dance/production value, but most of all, narrative simplification . . .)."[65] Shorn of its representational self-reflexivity and historical intertextuality, Zero Patience loses its ability to genuinely bear witness to the life and death of Dugas, "an ordinary gay everyman in the age of AIDS," and becomes a merely cheeky, postmodern backstage musical.[66] On the other hand, the very form of Fig Trees—a self-reflexive series of audiovisual song spaces in an art gallery installation—renders it impossible to experience it as anything but a refusal of opera's transcendental aesthetics. But Greyson ultimately paid a price for sharpening the political, intellectual, and aesthetic rigor of his work in Fig Trees. Despite numerous negotiations with contemporary art institutions in Canada, such as the Musée d'Art Contemporain de Montréal, Greyson and Wall have been unable to fully remount Fig Trees since its premiere in Oakville.[67] They subsequently decided to write new material and to rerecord the existing scenes to rework Fig Trees as a single-channel digital feature film, so that it may reach a wider audience than those able to visit suburban Oakville during its mere two-month installation there. The additional scenes of the expanded version allow Fig Trees to address TAC's continuing battle with the ANC government over the rollout of antiretrovirals, Achmat's Nobel Prize nomination, Canada's role in legalizing generic antiretroviral drugs for the global South, and the ongoing battle with AIDS denialists in the ANC government, people who prescribe lemon and garlic as treatment for AIDS, and with powerful quacks like the German doctor Matthias Rath, whose vitamin supplements are a lucrative business in South Africa.[68] The feature film version, which premiered at the Berlin International Film Festival in February 2009, also focuses on the Canadian AIDS activist Tim McGaskell, who has been at the forefront of AIDS activism in Canada and internationally for over twenty years.[69]

Although Fig Trees self-reflexively problematizes opera far more than does Zero Patience, both works rely heavily on queer anachronism to sustain the witnessing dynamics in their use of vocal genres. Greyson's queer anachronism involves not only the incorporation of anachronistic queers (Burton, Stein, and Thomson) but also, and more important, the use of anachronism and its camp incongruity as a means to queer the space in which witnessing HIV/AIDS may occur. Paradoxically, the historical impossibility of the anachronistic encounters in Zero Patience and Fig Trees interrupts any transcendental or universalizing dynamic and pushes the very historicity of the witness into view, while still retaining song's claim to affective authenticity. The song numbers built around Burton's anachronistic presence allow us to discern the discursive genealogy that facilitated Dugas's disappearance during the first decade of the epidemic behind the spectral figure of Patient Zero. Zackie's refusal to be Stein and Thomson's operatic subject provides both an allegory of Achmat's relationship to the international media at the turn of the millennium and a meditation on the relationship between aesthetics and activism in the global pandemic. In their construction of deeply historical and self-reflexive spaces of song, Zero Patience and Fig Trees repudiate the kind of abstracted testimonial space of song proffered by Philadelphia, a space cut only to hold the universalizing message of love carried by the "Mamma Morta" aria.

□

CHAPTER FIVE

Gay Cinephilia and

the Cherished Body of

Experimental Film

In *Positiv* (1997), the opening short film in Mike Hoolboom's six-part compilation film *Panic Bodies* (1998), the viewer is faced with a veritable excess
of the visual. The screen is divided into four equal parts, suggesting a wall
of video monitors, but also Andy Warhol's famed simultaneous projections.
Hoolboom appears in the top right-hand frame as a talking head, tightly
framed and speaking directly to the camera. At once poignant and wry, his
monologue explores the corporeal experience of living with AIDS: "The yeast
in my mouth is so bad it turns all my favorite foods, even chocolate–chocolate chip ice cream, into a dull metallic taste like licking a crowbar. I know
then that my body, my real body, is somewhere else: bungee jumping into
mine shafts stuffed with chocolate wafers and whipped cream and blueberry
pie and just having a good time. You know?" Each of the other three frames
is filled with a montage of images from contemporary Hollywood films,
B-movies, vintage porn, home movies, ephemeral films, as well as Hoolboom's own experimental films.

These multiple frames feed the viewer with a plethora of visual sensations. They include disintegrating and morphing bodies (from *The Hunger*
[Tony Scott, 1983]; *Terminator 2* [James Cameron, 1991]; and *Altered States* [Ken
Russell, 1980]); the terrified, diminished body of *The Incredible Shrinking Man*
(Jack Arnold, 1957), teeming microscopic cells and viruses (from old instructional films), mundane shots of the repetitive medical tests taken by Hoolboom, scratched and bleached-out footage of a family Christmas, and melodramatic reaction shots of horror and pathos (from classic silent films).[1] The

imbrication of private and public spheres becomes clear in the film through the way in which the shifting array of images visualizes and renders into metaphor the personal testimony of the film's talking head. Bodily crisis pervades both the sound- and image tracks. Pop culture's diverse iconography of bodily fragmentation accompanies Hoolboom's testimony to the alienation from his own body that he endures due to the physiological effects of HIV infection. The corporeal fragmentation in these images, the sense of a body in parts, is amplified by the film's formal design: the frame is dissected into smaller frames, and the short film itself constitutes one of six separate parts of the compilation film. Yet these images do more than merely illustrate a testimonial performance, for *Positiv* powerfully illustrates how we come to use popular culture, and popular cinema in particular, to articulate our sense of self. This engagement with the image is not a simple identification with the visual signifier as a transparent reflection of lived experience, but a complex process of identification, appropriation, and negotiation. Hoolboom's film registers how identity and personal memory are continually inflected by the vocabularies of popular culture.

Despite their systematic marginalization by media institutions and their representational practices, gay cultural producers have consistently turned to the material archive of popular culture in search of an affective and aesthetic vocabulary for articulating and sharing lived experience.[2] Their attitude is, however, often inscribed by ambivalence about the possible toxicity of the culture they appropriate. Gay skepticism toward popular culture increased during the first decade of the AIDS epidemic when the dominant media, particularly network television and the popular press, consistently pathologized and demonized gay men. But alongside works explicitly contesting the dominant representation of AIDS, many of which I analyze in other chapters, one may also find a significant number of experimental films and videos that approach the material archive of popular culture as a rich source of affectively charged images.[3]

This chapter analyzes and contextualizes a number of these films, including Michael Wallin's *Decodings* (1988), Matthias Müller's *Aus der Ferne* (*The Memo Book*) (1989) and *Pensão Globo* (*World Hotel*) (1997), and Jim Hubbard's *Memento Mori* (1995). Whereas films and videos like *Zero Patience*, *Voices from the Front*, and *No Regret* engage with the pathologizing and phobic practices of dominant media representation, these experimental films demonstrate a critical fascination with the kind of images and iconography from postwar U.S. mass culture that are more associated with the positive, exemplary affirmation of the mainstream, the popular, and the normal. This can be seen, for instance, in their appropriation of 1940s instructional films, 1950s Technicolor melodrama, and the spectacular technology of widescreen cinema.

In bearing witness to experiences of loss and alienation caused by AIDS, these films differ from many of the other works I discuss in that bearing witness is not performed through the visual inscription of the witness generating a testimonial narrative, argument, or performance. Like the images they offer, the voice-over testimonies of these experimental films are fragmentary and elliptical, poetic and elegiac. This formal emphasis on the fragment and the gap between voice and bodily image reflects the corporeal crisis of the traumatized gay subject. These films supply the habeas corpus of testimony, but it is one riven by psychic and physical trauma. They bear witness to AIDS through the aesthetic articulation of specific gay structures of feeling around loss and alienation.

In using Raymond Williams's term *structures of feeling*, I am drawing from the conceptualization he offers in *Marxism and Literature*, where he describes them as "specifically affective elements of consciousness" and "meanings and values as they are actively lived and felt."[4] Williams understands them as historical and contingent, elements of "a social experience which is still *in process*, often indeed not yet recognized as social but taken to be private, idiosyncratic, and even isolatory" (132; emphasis original).[5] Although it is clear that the social and psychological upheaval experienced by gay men during the first two decades of the epidemic transformed their structures of feeling, it is important to recognize the simultaneous scope and diversity of the effects that AIDS has had on such structures. Thus when the clinical psychologist Walt Odets argued in 1995 that all gay men are living with HIV and AIDS, that "being gay means being profoundly affected by the epidemic," he was actually doing so in the service of articulating the specific needs of HIV-negative gay men.[6]

Seropositive and seronegative gay men must both deal with feelings of loss, anxiety, guilt, and isolation, yet in often strikingly different and socially polarizing frameworks. Some of these experiential differences derive from generational distinctions, with many older gay men suffering multiple loss with the deaths of many friends and lovers, as well as the loss of a sexual culture they helped create in the post–gay liberation years before AIDS. These polarized dynamics have been poignantly and succinctly articulated in Nguyen Tan Hoang's experimental video, *K.I.P.* (2001), in which the young gay videomaker records his faint reflection on a television screen that is showing a condom-free sex scene from classic gay porn starring Kip Noll (the iconic gay porn star of the late 1970s).[7] *K.I.P.* recalls Warhol's *Blow Job*

(1963) in that we only see Nguyen's head and shoulders as he responds eroti-cally to the images before him. Like those of Warhol's actor, Nguyen's facial expressions remain deeply ambiguous, suggesting at times ecstasy, pain, and sorrow. As the on-screen sex moves toward climax, Nguyen opens his mouth wide. The ghostly reflected image of his open mouth waiting to catch Noll's cum in the money shot crystallizes the sense of loss experienced by gay men of Nguyen's generation, who have never tasted another man's cum or enjoyed condom-free sex without the specter of HIV.[8] Nguyen presents a fantasy of intergenerational sexual communion, but one that, as the title's mournful connotation suggests, tragically exists only in the superimposition of images on a screen.

Yet even in their differences, determined by age and serostatus, these specific experiences of both physical and cultural loss resonate further with the prior experience of loss endured in the process of gay socialization or of coming out, which almost all gay men share in a heteronormative society. As Odets points out, loss is first experienced early in the proto-gay child's life as the "unattainability of a real self," since this self is connected to forbidden homosexual feelings.[9] This "anticipatory" loss of an authentic and meaning-ful life inscribes gay male subjectivity with indelible traces of loss and nos-talgia. The repeated and varied reinscription of such traces by the experience of the AIDS epidemic has profoundly shaped gay structures of feeling over the past twenty-five years. Even during those two and a half decades, gay structures of feeling have transformed as the epidemic among gay men has evolved from the dire crisis of the early 1980s through the years of activist empowerment to the current muted optimism emerging from the arrival of effective antiretroviral drug combinations.

To now look at the films of Hoolboom, Müller, Wallin, and Hubbard is to be reminded that below the emergent structures of feeling around the cur-rent notion of AIDS in the global North as a "chronic manageable disease" are deeper, residual structures of loss. As works of experimental cinema, the films invest stylistic form with greater significance than narrative, relying on the expressivity of their distinctive cinematic devices to engage their audi-ence, rather than on the conventional identificatory functions of narrative and character. This is a cinema of intense moments, or to borrow Derek Jar-man's term, "a cinema of small gestures," in which cinematic form momen-tarily suspends ephemeral gestures or movements captured by the camera.[10] Fashioned out of the archive of industrially produced cinema, these moments carry the unmistakable traces of loss and nostalgia that have come to be in-scribed in classical Hollywood cinema, and postwar U.S. mass culture more generally. It is this affective relationship to the cinematic archive that renders these films works of cinephilia. Cinephilia becomes the dynamic through which AIDS-related structures of feeling around loss and alienation come to be articulated. It is, however, manifested in different textual forms. Decodings and Aus der Ferne incorporate found footage from ephemeral and popular cinema, whereas Pensão Globo and Memento Mori appropriate widescreen cinema and Technicolor, two specific film technologies indelibly associated with classical Hollywood.

While each of the films analyzed in this chapter performs its own distinctive engagement with industrially produced cinema, the films do share a common artisanal mode of production and similar circumstances of distribution and exhibition. The contexts producing these films involve a number of different discursive frameworks. Aesthetic ones include American underground film, found-footage filmmaking, autobiographical film, and contemporary queer cinema, while cultural ones include forms of AIDS mourning, gay spectatorship, and the cultural space of lesbian and gay film festivals. This chapter examines the relationships between these various contexts since the textual address of the films needs to be read through the optic of the cultural practices that condition both their production and reception. Central to these practices is what I am calling gay cinephilia—the set of gay cultural practices that revolve around a collectively shared passion for cinema and its history.[11] While this chapter concentrates on cultural practices performed by gay men (predominantly forms of spectatorship and filmmaking) and acknowledges the specificities attendant to such a focus, it will also draw, when necessary, from ideas and theories relevant to other lesbian and gay cultural practices.[12] The specific advantage in deploying the concept of gay cinephilia in the analysis of these films lies in its ability to account for their cinematic meaning and affect in terms of a set of cultural practices shared by both filmmakers and audiences. Moreover, cinephilia is a dynamic that, I would argue, structures the reading practices of gay viewers and the formal techniques taken up by queer filmmakers.

The Context for Gay Cinephilia

Over the past two decades, lesbian and gay film scholarship has focused as much attention on the social and psychological relationship lesbians and gay men have to cinema as it has on the representation of homosexuality and queerness in film texts.[13] Judith Mayne argues that film spectatorship has become "a component of the various narratives that constitute the very notion of a gay/lesbian identity, from coming out stories to shared pleasures in camp to speculations about the real lives of performers."[14] Gay spectatorship embodies an array of performative manifestations incorporating social, cultural, and psychological components. First and foremost among them is the issue of gay men's and lesbians' psychic engagement with cinema. Brett Farmer and Patricia White have both emphasized the complexity of these engagements, which include the dynamics of identification, desire, and fantasy. As White notes, same-sex star-crush narratives shared by lesbian or gay subjects involve a complex negotiation between identification and desire and between idealization and recognition. Not merely psychological but also social, they facilitate the constitution of lesbian or gay identity through an identification with others who share one's own preferences. As Farmer elaborates, Hollywood and its products became a "veritable lingua franca" in urban gay male subcultures in the postwar era, providing a "capacious reference system" for gay subcultural appropriation and recoding.[15] Farmer's comments here indicate the very historicity of gay spectatorship: classical Hollywood cinema facilitated a specific form of spectatorship performed by gay men during this period.

Daniel Harris contrasts this historically marked spectatorship of classical cinema to gay men's current engagement with popular culture: "In the absence of the gay-positive propaganda in which contemporary gay culture is saturated, film became a form of 'found' propaganda that the homosexual ransacked for inspiring messages, reconstituting the refuse of popular culture into an energizing force."[16] Interestingly, Harris frames his discussion of gay spectatorship in terms similar to those used in describing the practice of found-footage filmmaking, which has become a major formal tendency in contemporary experimental filmmaking.[17] These similarities include the treatment of popular culture as "found" material; the fascination with material deemed ephemeral, with refuse, or with trash; and the process of reconstitution or the reworking of such material. His comments suggest the kind of confluence of reading strategies and aesthetic practice that I will investigate more extensively later in this chapter.

The processes of fragmentation and reconstitution are stressed by Al La Valley in his characterization of gay men's textual reading practices of classical Hollywood. La Valley was one of the first critics to emphasize gay men's willingness as viewers to ignore narrative linearity and closure: "They treasured film not so much for its narrative fulfillments as for its great moments, those interstices that were often, ironically, the source of a film's real power."[18] The moment with all its constituent sensory pleasures—gesture, spectacle, and excess—offered gay men a means to resist the typically normative trajectory and closure of the heterosexual romance fundamental to Hollywood narratives. Whereas Harris argues that this form of spectatorship has largely died away as gay men's engagement with popular culture increasingly shifted to television and popular music, Farmer insists that the "older traditions of gay cinematic capital" remain alive in repertory screenings, television broadcasts, gay video stores, and the abundant discourse on classical cinema in gay publications.

Farmer mentions lesbian and gay film festivals as spaces that have enlivened gay cinematic capital with a "wealth of new texts and pleasures."[19] Yet these film festivals have also been a major factor in sustaining the older tradition of which he speaks. In fact, many of the new pleasures to which Farmer alludes are derived from forms established in that older tradition of gay spectatorship. Not only have lesbian and gay film festivals continued to program classical Hollywood films, much as gay-oriented repertory theaters have, but they have also pioneered and developed a newer form of gay film spectatorship: the clip show. Presented by a film critic or academic, the clip show offers its audience a collection of cinematic moments organized around a particular theme and accompanied by a live and often witty commentary. Many of these shows combine the presenter's personal narratives and memories with political and subcultural textual readings. Clip shows constitute perhaps the most transparent instance of cinephilia at the festival. They are events in which gay reading practices are transformed into an autonomous text in that they rework a form of spectatorship into a new form of attraction or spectacle.

This preoccupation with classical cinema in such counterpublic spaces is not restricted to the recontextualization of its exhibition. Many of the films and videos that have come to be associated with New Queer Cinema appropriate and cite historical forms of popular cinema, especially Hollywood, both explicitly and implicitly. While many of these works, such as Todd Haynes's *Poison* (1991), usurp the stylistic and generic conventions of popular film, others, such as Cheryl Dunye's *The Watermelon Woman* (1997), take up specific historical contexts of filmmaking and moviegoing as their subject matter. The explicit quotation of popular cinema frequently takes the form of the found-footage film that consists predominantly or entirely of existing filmed material. Kaucyila Brooke and Jane Cottis's *Dry Kisses Only* (1990), Cecilia Barriga's *Meeting of Two Queens* (1991), Mark Rappaport's *Rock Hudson's Home Movies* (1992), and Barbara Hammer's *History Lessons* (2000) are only some such works to have screened in the film festival circuit. In detaching popular film images from their original context and remodeling them, these works play with the dynamics of gay spectatorship to constitute their aesthetic form.

In their support and development of these types of experimental films and videos as a major part of their programming, lesbian and gay film festivals have nurtured a space in which the dynamics of gay spectatorship—including fantasy, appropriation, fragmentation, and reconstitution—continue in a variety of different forms. The lesbian and gay film festival constitutes an important space of confluence for lesbian and gay reading strategies and lesbian and gay aesthetic practice in that many film- and videomakers demonstrate in their work an engagement with cinema that their festival audiences share and sustain. The name of such an engagement, I would argue, is *cinephilia*.

Celebrating the Moment

Although classical film theory is filled with concepts and arguments derived from the pervasive cinephilia of its writers, only recently have film studies begun to develop a sustained critical discourse on and around the concept of cinephilia itself.[20] This discourse shares striking similarities to the theoretical frameworks used to describe gay spectatorship. Both entail a rejection or neglect of narrative linearity and trajectory; a fetishistic preoccupation with the moment, the detail, and the fragment; and a performativity that contributes to identity formation. However, what appears particularly useful about the discourse on cinephilia for an examination of the experimental work circulating in the lesbian and gay film festival circuit is its applicability across various forms of cultural practice converging in such a space: spectatorship, criticism, and filmmaking.

Paul Willemen points out that "cinephilia itself describes simultaneously a particular relationship to cinema and a particular *historical period relating to cinema*."[21] The concept of cinephilia thus remains crucial to the historical understanding of postwar cinema, especially in the two and a half decades between the end of the war and the late 1960s. The postwar film cultures of Western Europe, which would help produce an international art cinema and a host of new wave cinemas, were grounded in an obsessive attachment to moviegoing. The career trajectories of many important directors such as Jean-Luc Godard and François Truffaut—from fan to critic to filmmaker— attest to the creative energies unleashed by cinephilia. It is no coincidence, then, that the waning of a theatrical market for such international cinema has prompted a return to the consideration of cinephilia by many film critics, most famously by Susan Sontag. In a much debated article published in 1996 during the centenary of cinema, she lamented the demise not of the medium itself but of movie audiences' intense loving relationship to it, which she claimed had faded away over the previous two decades. For her, what has been lost is the notion that "films are unique, unrepeatable, magic experiences."[22] While one may dispute Sontag's prognosis for the future of either cinema or cinephilia, her lament does suggest the degree to which contemporary discourses of cinephilia are structured by loss and nostalgia.

Cinephilia has been characterized as a cultish practice, imbued with a religiosity that shapes the kinds of ritual viewing habits followed by its devotees. Roger Cardinal distinguishes the cinephile's panoramic gaze from the single-minded gaze of what he calls the "literary mode," which is directed toward the obvious gestalt or narrative focus of the film, grounded as it is in a conformity to the continuity system. Cardinal summarizes the cinephile's panoramic gaze in sensuous and spatial terms: "The [panoramic] mode roams over the frame, sensitive to its textures and surfaces—to its ground. This mode may be associated with 'non-literacy' and with habits of looking which are akin to habits of touching."[23] Willemen's approach to cinephilia is rather more temporal, focusing on the way it privileges the capture of "fleeting, evanescent moments" in cinema. Cinephiles fetishize a particular moment in a film, isolating "a cystallizingly expressive detail," be that a facial expression, a bodily gesture, or some other detail. Significantly, most details are grounded in some form of movement. For example, Willemen singles out the moment at which the mechanical toy falls off the table in Douglas Sirk's *There's Always Tomorrow* (1956) as one of his own cherished cinephiliac moments. These are not the conventional memorable moments of cinema that one sees in compilations dedicated to the magic of movies. Rather, as Willemen argues, "What is being looked for is a moment or given that a moment is too unitary, a dimension of a moment which triggers for the viewer either the realisation or the illusion of a realisation that *what is being seen is in excess of what is being shown*. Consequently you see something that is *revelatory*. It is produced *en plus*, in excess or in addition, almost involuntarily."[24] In considering the cinephiliac moment as a revelatory supplement or excess to the image, Willemen turns to what one might regard as the first historical flourishing of cinephilia, in French impressionist film theory. He acknowledges his intellectual debt to Jean Epstein and his understanding of *photogénie*—the essence of cinema lies in its fleeting intensities of time, space, and movement that defy rational explanation.[25] By invoking *photogénie*, Willemen is interested less in Epstein's attempt to define the specificity of cinema than in its usefulness in describing a potential relationship between viewer and image, what he calls "that momentary flash of recognition, or a moment when the look at something suddenly flares up with a particularly affective, emotional intensity."[26]

It is precisely this drive for such revelatory moments in cinema that motors much found-footage filmmaking. While plenty has been written and theorized about the ideological unhinging and resignifying of images in found-footage work, little attention has been paid by the scholars of this work to its sensuous and affective dimensions.[27] Found-footage filmmaking bears many of the marks of cinephiliac behavior. Its practitioners tend to act as collectors, scavenging extant film material in search of those "fleeting, evanescent moments." As a form of montage, most found-footage work is, like the cinephile's ethos, fragmentary and nonlinear, resisting, and at times, actively working to subvert the narrative structures of documentary and fiction film. Many works also demonstrate an obsessive return to a particular shot or sequence that holds the artist in its grasp. Found-footage films and videos frequently display a paradoxical tension between the attempt to deconstruct or decode the found image and the desire to draw on its photogenic force. Such a tension can certainly be traced in Wallin's *Decodings*, which meticulously and lovingly edits found images from postwar ephemeral film together with a poetic, first-person voice-over to articulate gay male structures of feeling in the first decade of the AIDS epidemic.

Lost and Found

The use of found footage in *Decodings* constitutes a highly personal and melancholic appropriation of industrially produced film from the 1940s and 1950s. The variety of subjects included in the film's shots proves to be as broad as in Bruce Conner's classic of found-footage filmmaking, *A Movie* (1958). *Decodings* incorporates images as divergent as daredevil feats, children's play, classroom experiments, extreme weather, religious gurus, and stop-motion shots of seed germination. Yet Wallin's appropriation of these found images from discarded industrial and instructional films does not share Conner's playful postmodern irony toward its mass-mediated material. Through the film's editing strategies and sound-image relations, these abandoned remnants of mass culture come to bear witness simultaneously to the psychosexual alienation of growing up gay in the postwar period and to the experience of loss in the midst of the AIDS epidemic.

In speaking about the process of making a film entirely with found images,

Wallin revealed a distinctly cinephiliac disposition: "I'm very powerfully drawn to the statement a very simple, unadulterated image can make . . . just in terms of the composition in the frame, what occurs in a few seconds in that image, how it can join other images."[28] For Wallin, these found images appear to embody an ambivalent attraction—offering a certain pleasure of uncanny recognition, but one that also ignites an affective charge of loss. In another interview, Wallin commented that these industrially produced images had appeared terribly evocative of his own past, filled with "all the resonances and subtexts of things we were forbidden to talk and think about when I was growing up."[29]

One could argue that *Decodings* is simultaneously a film about AIDS and one *not* about AIDS. It makes no explicit references to the disease, only inferential and allegorical ones in its voice-over text and images. This presence/absence of the epidemic does not function as the form of blanket disavowal that has become increasingly commonplace in gay culture; rather, it serves as an articulation of the continuing and pervasive haunting of contemporary gay male desire by loss and alienation. Through its cinephiliac appropriation of powerfully simple found images, *Decodings* is able to construct an affective address to its audience that does not depend on an empathetic identification with particular bodies represented on the screen. However, while the film's referential elusiveness and fragmentary structure forestall the sentimentalization of its affective address, they in turn limit the recognition of AIDS as a subject of the film to those who can feel the resonance of such images, namely, those directly affected by the epidemic.

The heterogeneous montage of visual fragments, moments, and details on the film's image track is mirrored by its complex soundtrack that combines elegiac music by Dmitri Shostakovich with a poignant voice-over commentary. Although spoken by a single voice using the first-person register, the voice-over consistently avoids the linear narrativization and audiovisual suture found in conventional voice-over. Rather, the voice-over shifts between various stories, myths, memories, and observations, constructing associations on micro and macro levels of the text, but never resorting to a linear narrativization of either the speaking subject or the profilmic events. The montage of fragments in the voice-over contains its own logic that is neither wholly subservient to the visual montage of the image track nor determinative of it. Rather than frame or pin down a particular meaning in the other, these autonomous tracks seem to brush up against each other, suggesting metaphoric and metonymic connections and hinting at the disclosure of se-

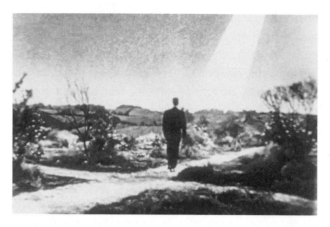

51. Still from *Decodings* (Michael Wallin, 1988).
Courtesy of the artist.

crets and other personal meanings, but always resisting that of a finite meaning. The fluidity of the sound- and image tracks implies the very structure of
desire itself with all its slippages, displacements, and transformations.

The film opens and ends with the image of a man following a ray of light
from the sky, with a quote from Confucius running underneath the image:
"The way out is via the door: Why is it that no one will use this method?"
(figure 51) This framing image/text addresses questions of ease and of difficulty that the following images and the voice-over subsequently take up
in relation to the codes of social behavior. The often tortuous assimilation
of normative masculinity emerges as a central concern of the film, through
the juxtaposition of images of boyhood camaraderie and homosocial discipline with spoken accounts of the wanderings of Joshua's "impure" tribe and
narratives of autistic withdrawal. While certain archival images in *Decodings*
suggest a preoccupation with sexual awakening and bodily contact (boys'
homoerotic horseplay on a beach, stop-motion footage of a seed germinat-
ing, and hands folding up a rope and knotting it), other images visualize the
social conditioning of the body (a group of blindfolded boys boxing, a mass
of people moving in unison on several escalators, and children skipping rope
in formation). The vulnerability of the body is also emphasized in images of
risk (a skydiver, a daredevil pilot crashing into a house, and open heart sur-
gery) and in images of isolation (a man alone in bed, an autistic child eating
a bowl of cereal, and a snow covered bench).

Although most of the imagery in the film is generically familiar as the
visual detritus of postwar U.S. mass culture, Wallin's editing in *Decodings* pro-

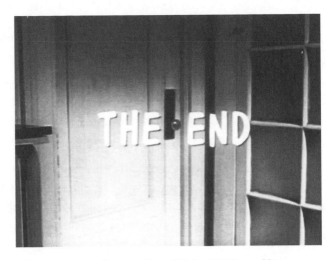

52. Frame capture from *Decodings* (Michael Wallin, 1988).

duces an uncanny sensation in viewing them. He captures a movement or gesture and, in tearing it from its original context, creates the kind of fetishistic and excessive moment celebrated by cinephiles. In one particular shot, for instance, a middle-aged man enters a bedroom from a hallway, where the camera is positioned. As he walks farther into the room and wearily lies down on the bed, the camera tracks in as though it will follow him, but stops short of the door, and soon the door itself shuts. The camera movement in this shot may well foster our desire for contact, but then thwarts it in its arrest. Without the original narrative context, the shot produces a powerful affective charge of alienation and isolation. Soon after the door has shut, the words "The End" appear over the image (figure 52). Since the shot has been torn from its original location at the close of a film, this familiar titling convention appears jarring, especially since *Decodings* continues for several minutes more. The title thus suggests not the end of *Decodings* but another end, the end of the middle-aged man's life. Shots of this man have appeared earlier in *Decodings*, at the beginning of the film. The man lies impassively in the same bed, followed by a shot of someone taking a rigorous pill regime, then succeeded by another shot of the man leaving a medical building. For an audience and a community familiar with pervasive illness and mortality, these images distinctly resonate with the experience of the AIDS epidemic, as does the simultaneous voice-over with its allusion to dementia: "If the brain becomes disorganized, a person may forget how to eat, he may walk in circles, or become rooted in a single spot."

Although the voice-over commentary in *Decodings* is read by a single, ruminative voice, it is markedly polyvocal on a discursive level as it casually moves between an ironic imitation of the pseudoscientific discourse of instructional films and the narration of mythical and fantastic tales:

> Pseudocutaneous linkage is believed to be involuntary, occurring when the strength of excitatory stimuli overcomes neuronal inhibition. . . . Investigators feel that the linkage reflex represents a primitive attempt on the part of the male organism at attachment and bonding.

> Unaccountably, the tribe is now all men. And each century they have grown younger, so that the men are now no older than boys. They have been blinded by the desert sun, deafened by the wind, but they have wandered together for so long that they know each other by touch. Most have now lost the capacity to speak or perhaps they simply lost the will, it doesn't really matter.

Through such strange mythical narratives the film allegorizes and connects two forms of alienation experienced by gay men—the self-estrangement caused in childhood by their failure to assimilate the codes of gender and sexual conformity and also the alienation rooted in illness, loss, survivor guilt, and emotional burnout related to AIDS. These tales of dementia and decimated tribes surviving great loss can be read in a number of ways—there is a veritable openness to them. In an interview, Wallin has commented that he felt his original voice-over commentary was "too confessional, too obvious," so he turned it over to an old friend, the science fiction writer Michael Blumlein, to refashion it so that it would no longer close down the images, but rather open them up (27).

In his review of the film, the gay filmmaker Tom Kalin contended that it offered "a reminder of how we become alienated from our skin even as we live in it."[30] The film's montage of sound and image insinuates a particular doubling of such alienation. The frequently traumatic experience for gay men around sexual discovery and identity formation in a heteronormative society has revisited many of them with the psychic and bodily crisis brought about by AIDS.[31] The simultaneous melancholy and nostalgic tone of *Decodings* resonates with an ambivalence felt by many gay men toward the difficult and painful childhood they endured. Moreover, AIDS came to transform gay structures of feeling with a new configuration of sadness and nostalgia around the loss of not only friends, lovers, and family but also of the sexual culture enjoyed in the postliberation era before the epidemic.

This particular resonance carried by the film was highlighted when *De-*

codings first screened in New York at the Lesbian and Gay Experimental Film Festival in 1988. The film was programmed with an earlier film by Wallin, *The Place between Our Bodies* (1975), a tender and sexually explicit autobiographical depiction of Wallin's experience in San Francisco at the height of the gay liberation era. Despite the frustration and alienation of what he calls "the endless hunt," Wallin unexpectedly finds a boyfriend, and the latter part of the film follows an extended sex scene between the two lovers. As reviewers of the festival, both Kalin and his fellow filmmaker Haynes noted the chilling sadness felt by the audience while viewing the ecstatic expressions of two men fucking without a condom.[32] The historical dissonance experienced by the audience in seeing *The Place between Our Bodies* would illuminate the somber historical pertinence of *Decodings*, the film that followed in that night's program.

The Cherished Body of Film

There is a sequence in Müller's AIDS elegy *Aus der Ferne* that appropriates that most conventional of shots from classical narrative cinema—the final inscription of "The End"—in a manner strikingly similar to Wallin's *Decodings*. On a television screen, Fred Astaire and Gene Kelly are seen dancing together (in *Ziegfeld Follies*). Cut to an end title announcing the finality of "The End." An eye blinks in close-up. A montage of different end titles follows. Although they differ in the size and style of their typeface, their language, and the markings of their studio origin, they all appear deeply familiar as the marks of closure for classical narrative cinema. The montage expands to include shots of a young man standing under a glimmering crystal chandelier, another young man (Müller) looking off-screen at a glaring light, a phonographic record revolving on a platter, and further shots of Astaire and Kelly. The footage of the young man under the chandelier bears the distinct traces of a home movie. The grain of the image is course; the subject looks directly at the camera with affectionate familiarity; and the roughly framed camerawork appears hand-held. As Michael Renov has argued in a different context, the "attenuated indexicality" of such an image may constitute a powerful inducement to desire.[33] A male voice intones on the soundtrack: "This was a false creation, an imitation of life." An anonymous hand then delicately fondles a handful of loose crystals.

This sequence of the film performs a mesmerizing imbrication of images drawn both from the personal and from the public archive. The memory of a deceased lover (seen in the home movie footage) is refracted through texts and images borrowed from classical Hollywood cinema. The repeated shots of end titles interrupt the queer pleasure of the Astaire-Kelly coupling (one of those Hollywood moments particularly treasured by gay popular memory) with the implication of finality, closure, and death. The words spoken on the soundtrack invoke lines from the theme song to Sirk's classic melodrama *Imitation of Life* (1959): "Skies above in flaming color / Without love, they're so much duller / A false creation, an imitation of life." In the original film, Earl Grant sings the song over its opening credit shots, in which cut-glass crystals fall from the top of the screen and gradually amass at the bottom. The quoted song phrase thus connects the personal cherished images of a lost lover to the lush iconography and emotional vocabulary of Sirkian melodrama, a group of films renowned for their popularity among gay men. But the film's appropriation of the song phrase also recasts its meaning, suggesting the bittersweet pleasure of memory in the face of irrecoverable loss. The light of the crystals may have the power to induce a cherished memory, but their tangibility serves as a reminder of the lover's absence—a hand is left merely fondling a few crystals in the final shot of the sequence.

As one of Germany's leading experimental filmmakers, Müller has developed a sophisticated and wide-ranging engagement with found material over the past two decades. A self-confessed cinephile, Müller maintains a formal interest in a wide array of found-footage film, including home movies, classical Hollywood, and ephemeral films. As a gay man, he also demonstrates a particular fascination with Hollywood melodramas. His most well-known film is *Home Stories* (1990), a six-minute film entirely constructed of footage from postwar Hollywood melodramas. Dubbed "experimental melodrama" by its maker, *Home Stories* contains a rigorously organized montage of heroines from 1950s and 1960s domestic melodramas who are involved in small but expressive gestures and movements—looking out of the window, switching on a light, or simply turning their head. Accompanied by a tense, complex soundtrack of found sounds and musical snippets from those same postwar melodramas, the image track gradually builds up a claustrophobic sensation of paranoid anxiety in these women's actions. The film incorporates clips already pregnant with quiet hysteria, but their decontextualization and carefully edited repetition intensify their excess as moments of cinema. *Home Stories* rises to a climax of collective hysteria as the women hurry down hallways and anxiously shut doors behind them. Ominously, the source of their apparent terror remains nowhere to be seen. While *Home Stories* undoubtedly elaborates a shrewd ideological critique of gender construction and the home, it also draws much poetic and affective power from the cinematic excess embedded in these narratively insignificant moments from popular cinema. In an interview, Müller has argued that Home Stories is in fact a deeply personal film motored by a strong sense of identification and fantasy: "I myself have an affinity to hysteria. I have always envied those leading ladies for having the privilege of expressing their emotions through grand gestures."[34]

Like Home Stories, Aus der Ferne summons the affective and visual vocabulary of classical Hollywood cinema to create a piece of first-person cinema that meticulously builds a personal narrative from footage shot on Super-8 and snatched moments from home movies and popular cinema. The film opens up as a work of recollection and mourning. A voice-over announces that "death had come to a young man." Hands gather up and tie together a stack of letters and photographs that appear to be a mixture of personal photographs and what we later come to realize are stills of later shots in the film, including several images from popular film. Typical of Müller's disposition toward metaphor, the imbrication of the personal and the popular is made concrete in this simple profilmic gesture. Müller himself appears as the film's young male protagonist, its witness-survivor, literally descending into memory on the stairs of an abandoned building and entering a basement room aglow with the crystalline memories of his former lover marveling at the chandelier. Presumably frightened by the realization of his own mortality, the young man absconds to a hospital to undergo tests and medical procedures, only to once again flee from the scene on seeing his own blood. Holed up in his apartment, he drifts into sleep, entering the dream realm of Jardim Botanico, Lisbon's botanical garden.

Intercut with the young man's entrance into the garden is a shot from Fritz Lang's Siegfrieds Tod (Siegfried's Death) (1923), in which Siegfried rides into the dark forest of Odenwald where the dragon is guarding his treasure.[35] In the mythic narrative, Siegfried discovers the magical powers of the dragon's blood after he has slain it. While he bathes himself in the magic blood, a single leaf falls from a linden tree onto his shoulder covering a small area of skin, which does not subsequently become invulnerable through contact with the dragon's blood. Aus der Ferne is less interested in the specific national and historical signification of the footage than in the mythology of vulnerability that Siegfried invokes, since the following shots show the young man rather than Siegfried with the linden leaf on his naked shoulder. Siegfried's mark of unknowing and fated vulnerability becomes a fitting motif for the contingency of survival felt by gay men in the midst of the epidemic, particularly as many had become infected long before knowledge of HIV existed. Close-up, solarized images of male genitalia superimposed on shots of the garden vegetation, which follow the inserted shot of Siegfried, emphasize this allegorical dimension. The young man bathes in a stream of blood that flows over his body and onto the surrounding vegetation. His pursuit of invulnerability is broken by the discovery of an open wound on his stomach, as the mythic dream turns to nightmare. After moving into more urban spaces, the young man finally awakens and reenters the social world.

The final sequence of the film returns to the concern for memory and mourning that had opened the film. The young man gazes at a spinning zoetrope, with its movement casting flickering shadows on his face.[36] Superimposed on the shot of the zoetrope are home-movie images of children playing and of the deceased lover carrying heavy luggage. A hand suddenly stops the zoetrope. Sheets fly off a stack of paper on a table. Papers blow about on a windy street (figure 53). A close-up shows a still photograph of the lover carrying the luggage. Wind blows open the pages of a notebook, revealing the words on its cover: "Memo Book." A hand writes text in the memo book. The film ends on a train with the young man looking out of the window, his face illuminated by the bright sun. Flickering shadows cast on his face by passing obstacles invoke the spinning zoetrope and perhaps its descendent, the film projector's shutter.

This complex sequence epitomizes Müller's visual patterning, which is based on relations of displacement and metaphor. As a nineteenth-century optical toy and precursor to cinema, the zoetrope invokes the animation of discreet images into an illusion. Its inclusion in Aus der Ferne suggests the animation of memory from an image.[37] The hand that stops it suddenly underscores the ephemeral nature of such illusion. Arrested movement materializes into still images imprinted on sheets of paper, which are then open to the fate of the wind. Images, especially moving images, promise the pleasure of the deceased's presence, but ultimately they can only provide a material reminder of his permanent absence. Müller's affective allusion to the zoetrope and its historical relation to cinema points to the multifaceted cinephilia that informs Aus der Ferne.

In addition to its incorporation of found footage and its historical references to a cinematic precursor, Aus der Ferne is saturated with the cinephilia of Müller's artisanal filmmaking techniques. By working with Super-8, Müller was able to hand-process the entirety of his own footage. The refilming of all the footage, whether appropriated or his own, allowed the film stock to be altered in a number of different ways: through tinting, bleaching, scratching, solarizing, or slowing the motion of the image (figure 54). It is not the destructive urge of the iconoclast that drives Müller's manipulation of the

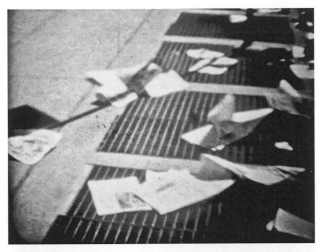

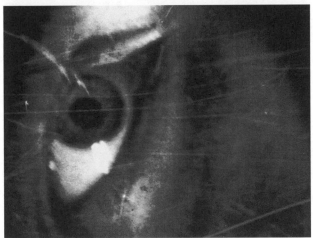

53–54. Stills from *Aus der Ferne (The Memo Book)* (Matthias Müller, 1989). Courtesy of the artist.

film image, but rather the transformative ethos of the alchemist. Furthermore, Müller weaves numerous alchemical references into the sound- and image tracks of *Aus der Ferne*, most notably with the sounds and images of the four elements.[38] Alice Kuzniar adeptly reads this treatment and transformation of the celluloid image as a means of rendering the processes of memory and mourning by mimicking "the movement of the unconscious, or as Freud describes it, the displacements and condensations of the dreamwork."[39] But it is also important to acknowledge how these treatments emphasize the very materiality of the film itself. However much the gorgeous red- and sepia-tinted footage suggests "a faded, melancholic world brought only momentarily back to life," it nevertheless also testifies to its own material existence as a carefully manipulated piece of celluloid (209). In the various hand-processed treatments undertaken on its image, *Aus der Ferne* displays an emphatic tension between the aesthetic expression of ephemeral states, like dreamwork and memory, and the stark reminder of the film's materiality.

By emphasizing the materiality of the film, Müller sets up one of its most striking metaphors—the film as body. The metaphor is enacted through both the celluloid filmstrip and the camera. Müller's reshooting and hand-processing techniques demonstrate a fetishistic attitude to the medium. The film materializes as an object to be cherished, but one that can be touched and felt, subsequently undergoing a variety of transformations at the hands of its filmmaker. There is indeed a distinct eroticism to Müller's treatment of the film footage, particularly in the way his transformations of the film appear as imprints on a sensuous surface. Müller has commented, "In my 'bodily films' I have wanted to give the shot a corporeal quality. The 'epidermal' effect of the shot influences one's sensory perception. Besides, you encounter a different relationship to the shot when you process it with your own hands rather than have it developed commercially."[40]

Furthermore, the film's corporeality is also manifested in its hand-held camerawork, which induces a sense of embodied vision in the shots in which its particular mobility replicates the movement of the human body. As a staple technique in the avant-garde film tradition that P. Adams Sitney dubbed the "trance film," this effect is enhanced in shots incorporating hands or feet that appear attached to the body/machine that sees or films them.[41] Shots of the protagonist's body that do not involve embodied vision nevertheless retain senses of proximity and fragmentation since the camera consistently remains close to the protagonist's body, often shooting in extreme close-up, capturing only a fragment of his body in the frame. By alternating between the embodied vision of its point-of-view shots and the fragmented, claustro-

phobic shots of the protagonist's body, Aus der Ferne fosters a complex identification between the film and the body it represents, subtly shifting between
internal and external witnessing positions. The inscription of Müller's own
body (as the protagonist) thus comes to bear witness to the psychic dynamics
of alienation and anxiety engendered by the loss of one's gay lover to AIDS.

The Color of Gay Cultural Memory

In Pensão Globo (1997) Müller returned to the city of Lisbon and to the subject
of AIDS. The perspective has shifted from a gay man's experience of mourning a lost lover, and the paranoid fears of infection it incites, to the struggle
with illness and the contemplation of mortality by a gay man with AIDS. Pensão Globo retains a similar combination of a dreamlike visual structure and a
voice-over interior monologue read by Müller's friend and fellow filmmaker,
Hoolboom. Although the fifteen-minute film makes less use of found footage
than Aus der Ferne, it nevertheless shares the earlier film's engagement with
cinephilia.[42] Pensão Globo constitutes its cinephiliac address through two distinct means. First, the film's editing undercuts the linearity of its rudimentary
narrative through the haunting repetition of gesture and action, placing emphasis on the cinematic moment and its emotional texture. Second, the film's
lavish use of color recites the nostalgic pleasures of Technicolor cinema in
general, and the chromatic stylization of Sirkian melodrama in particular.

The film's narrative structure follows a simple design. A young man with
AIDS travels to Lisbon for perhaps his last journey, staying at the Pensão
Globo. He spends time in his hotel room contemplating his own mortality
as he recalls painful medical treatment and reflects on his precarious future.
His sojourn is filled with the banalities of waiting: looking out of the window,
watching television, tossing and turning on a bed (figure 55). On venturing
out into the city, he encounters a seductive stranger who entices him into
the secluded domain of the botanical garden. Recalling a similar sequence in
Aus der Ferne, close-ups of the prickly vegetation jostle with roaming close-up
shots of his naked body. The film ends elusively with his return to the hotel
room. The young man repeatedly covers his naked torso with a red robe. The
chambermaid removes the bed linen in the empty hotel room and closes the
shutters. These final small gestures offer succinct metaphors for the closure
of his life, his final departure.

Extending the formal exploitation of repetition developed in his previous
films, Müller refilmed two sets of images projected onto a screen of frosted
glass to produce the effect of a fragmented and unstable double exposure.

In each scene, two slightly different shots of the same action or gesture are thus nonsynchronously superimposed. This staggered effect splits the young man's body into two, creating a doppelgänger.[43] Since no one image layer is prioritized, the two bodies maintain the same visual density. The body's unity collapses as the film's fragmented layers hover over one another. The slight temporal gap between the two layers of the scene generates a sense of spatial and temporal dislocation, which is exacerbated by the way in which the image layers appear unhinged, floating about in the frame (figure 56).

Kuzniar reads this technique of "pulsating beauty and sadness" as the visual concretization of the young man's mental and physical dissociation brought on by his illness and its treatment.[44] This spectral doubling of the image visualizes the sporadic, dislocated phrases of the voice-over: "Sometimes it's like I'm already gone, become a ghost of myself." Furthermore, the voice-over replicates the visual doubling in its overlapping repetition of phrases, generating an echoing, hollowed-out voice, doubly disconnected from the body on the screen. Kuzniar stresses the temporal aspect of this dislocation, observing that his lonely present has been emptied of significance by the inescapable psychic oscillation between the past and the future. The voice-over bemoans, "Then the attacks would start. You'd go a few weeks without thinking about it, and then it starts again, and you think it will never end, because you don't know. Waiting. Wondering when it's going to happen, and hoping it will, so it will be over." Temporality compresses as his disposition shifts from sensing that he is becoming a child again to suddenly feeling old. In his acutely perceived mortality, he is haunted by prior fatalities: "I can't go to bed alone. I bring them all with me, the ones who came before."

Peter Tscherkassky posits that this manipulation of linear temporality constitutes a foundational element in Müller's filmmaking: "The flow of time is replaced by simultaneity of happenings that gives depth to the images, from which springs forth the desired ambience" (173). Although his films construct basic narratives, Müller's cinematic practice aims for "the paradigmatic representation of elements" associated with poetic form, rather than for the syntagmatic chain of events constructed in prose form. He condenses and rarefies narrative elements that are connected in his films "like loosely threaded beads." Tscherkassky construes this disposition toward the paradigmatic forms of poetry as Müller's embrace of the cinematic moment and all its affective potential: "His scripts focus on moments designed to capture the synthetic expression of a specific feeling. These moments generally acquire depth, to become *impressions* like those expressed in poetry; they are condensed feelings, glimpses of a state of mind" (173).

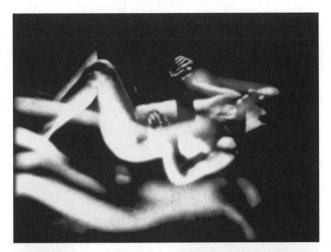

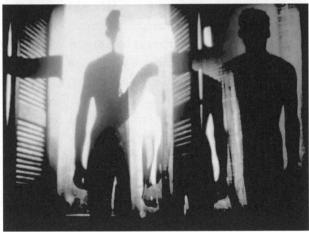

55–56. Stills from *Pensão Globo* (Matthias Müller, 1997).
Courtesy of the artist.

Tscherkassky's comments illuminate the relevance of poetic form for an understanding of cinephilia. Müller's poetic cinema is indeed steeped in the cinephiles's ethos of capturing "fleeting, evanescent moments." Whereas Wallin demonstrates this ethos through his montage of unhinged fragments of mass culture in Decodings, Müller articulates it in the layering, blending, and superimposition of his paradigmatic style in Aus der Ferne and Pensão Globo. In the visual excess of their haunting repetition, the young man's gestures and movements in Pensão Globo can generate an intensified emotional effect that potentially resonates with the multiplicity of loss experienced by those in the midst of the epidemic. The film's rich metaphorical vein, generated by its narrative condensation and paradigmatic style, provides significant resistance to a descent into the kind of pathetic sentimentality that many mainstream AIDS films have produced through their recourse to an affective address. Unlike Philadelphia, which attempts to reintegrate its melodramatic excess into the structures of sentimental identification it has set up, Pensão Globo employs melodramatic excess to articulate the magnitude of trauma, which defies the kind of narrative containment offered by Jonathan Demme's film.

Visual excess in Pensão Globo is not limited to its palimpsestic editing; elements of mise-en-scène, namely, the use of props and color, also render the kind of aesthetic supplement that pushes attention onto the cinematic moment rather than the narrative trajectory of the film. Both the sound- and image tracks accentuate the presence of particular objects in the hotel room: the net curtains by the window, the red lamp and the fan on the table, and the brightly patterned mattress. Shot in close-up, the succulent but prickly cactus leaves in the botanical garden also overwhelm the frame. Many of these objects provide metaphors and metonyms for the film's thematic structure. The net curtains and the cactus leaves, for instance, engender differing epidermal metaphors. While the gentle movement of the translucent curtains swaying in the wind echoes the hovering instability of the young man's bifurcated skin as he stands before them, the intercutting between the spiky cactus leaves and the surface of his skin insinuates the epidermal sensitivity and pain commonly experienced by people with AIDS. Yet these objects retain a certain excess beyond their specific metaphorical functions, which lies in their sensual components of sound, texture, and color.

Müller employs a rich color design in Pensão Globo that calls to mind the nostalgic pleasures of Technicolor cinema. Although deep red predominates in the color design (the bed, the man's shirt, the wallpaper, the lamp), other rich, luminous colors abound as well, including the lush green vegetation of the garden and the glowing blue reflection from the television screen. What connotes the postwar film technology in particular is the film's distinct chromatic quality, the result of Müller's hand-processing of the film stock; the plastic, postwar color palette appears minimally faded and slightly washed out, as though it had aged gracefully and lost only marginal pigmentation and density.[45] The lack of any contemporary references, save a bottle of Retrovir (an AIDS drug), furthers the allusion to postwar classical Hollywood. In its costuming, set design, and found footage, *Pensão Globo* exudes the look and feel of the 1950s without ever offering any specific verifying detail.

These historical accents in the film's visual design hint at the more specific cinematic references to be found in the film's use of color. In its lush, expressive use of contrastive colors, particularly the abrasive clash of red and green elements, and in its brooding low-key lighting, *Pensão Globo* cites the distinctive chromatic stylization of Sirk's Technicolor melodramas from the 1950s, such as *All That Heaven Allows* (1955) and *Written on the Wind* (1956). Sirk's use of color has attracted critical attention throughout the historical reception of his films. Truffaut highlighted Sirk's employment of "industrial colors that remind us that we live in the age of plastics."[46] Emphasizing the expressionist aspect of the director's color design, J. Hoberman described *Written on the Wind* as "the original Technicolor noir."[47] But it is Thomas Elsaesser who comes closest to articulating the exact qualities of Sirk's chromatic stylization that Müller appropriates in *Pensão Globo*: "Sirk has a peculiarly vivid eye for the contrasting emotional qualities of textures and materials, and he combines them or makes them clash to very striking effect, especially when they occur in a non-dramatic sequence."[48] In discussing a minor scene in *Written on the Wind*, Elsaesser describes how the interaction of color with texture in Sirk's films can produce a powerfully dissonant emotional effect. In *Pensão Globo*, Dirk Schaefer's haunting soundtrack supplements the visual expression of texture with its repetitive use of precise sound effects. For instance, at the beginning of the film, creaking floorboards overlay the sounds of the crisp white bed linen as the chambermaid stretches it across the elaborately patterned red mattress. The especially intense conjunction of color, texture, and sound throughout the film further emphasizes the sensual excess of its scenes above their narrative content.[49]

Müller's earlier piece of "experimental melodrama," *Home Stories*, made his preoccupation with the genre evident, and his judicious sampling from Sirk's features in that film hinted at a deeper affection for the director's work. In fact, Müller submits that *Imitation of Life* is indeed his favorite film.[50] When asked about his relationship to popular cinema as an experimental filmmaker, he enthusiastically declared himself a passionate moviegoer, mentioning melodrama as his favorite genre. He added that "the films of Douglas Sirk are some of the most beautiful that I have ever seen."[51] Interestingly, Müller's words of admiration for Sirk echo the phrasing of his countryman and fellow gay filmmaker, Rainer Werner Fassbinder. In his well-known critical commentary on six films directed by Sirk, Fassbinder concludes with the following line: "I've seen six films by Douglas Sirk. Among them were the most beautiful in the world."[52] Whether he was deliberately alluding to Fassbinder or not, Müller certainly shares in a similar appreciation of Sirk—Fassbinder treated Sirk's oeuvre as a model for making a politically and socially critical cinema that nevertheless retained an emotional address to its audiences.[53]

The significance of these specific influences and affinities is less about establishing the foundation of Müller's status as an auteur and more concerned with situating his filmmaking practice within the historical context of gay cinephilia and its engagement with Hollywood melodrama. It has become a critical commonplace in lesbian and gay film studies to cite melodrama's privileged relationship to gay audiences.[54] Farmer adroitly summarizes the foundations of this association: "With its scenarios of sexual and social transgression and its highly stylized mise-en-scène, the melodrama opens a space for queer and otherwise aberrant formations of meaning and desire that 'most Hollywood forms have studiously closed off.'"[55] Müller's quotation of Sirkian melodrama creates a cinephiliac address that produces a distinct resonance among gay audiences. The nostalgia invoked in *Pensão Globo* by its allusions to Sirkian melodrama is not the playful postmodern variety, but a bittersweet one in which the recognition of loss cuts across the sensual pleasures of melodramatic form. The sensuality of its melodramatic aesthetics allows the film to eroticize a gay male body with AIDS while simultaneously underlining the magnitude of loss—not only numerous lives, but also the sexual culture developed in the post–gay liberation era. Since they are filtered through the prism of a collectively maintained gay cinephilia, the emotional effects of melodramatic form avoid being reduced in *Pensão Globo* to sentimentality and pathos.

The Intimate Spectacle

Like *Pensão Globo*, Hubbard's short experimental film *Memento Mori* also explores AIDS-related mortality through an engagement with a film technology closely associated with postwar Hollywood cinema. To shoot the footage for his personal and poetically structured meditation on death and mourning, Hubbard designed his own anamorphic lens attachment for a 16mm camera.

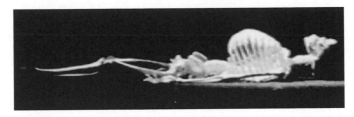

57. Still from *Memento Mori* (Jim Hubbard, 1995). Courtesy of the artist.

The resulting seventeen-minute film thus bears the expansive aspect ratio of widescreen cinema. Expressing the historically accrued double meaning of *memento mori*, the film serves both as a work dedicated to the memory of two deceased loved ones and as a contemplative reminder of mortality.[56] Images of mourning rituals, including the preparation of ashes and their scattering in a river, are combined with more metaphorically inflected shots: a skeleton (figure 57), a woman sweeping and tidying, painterly still-life arrangements, and seasonal landscape shots of a cemetery. As an artisanal filmmaker like Müller, Hubbard processed the film by hand, allowing him to draw out distinct color temperatures in the seasonal images that provide an overarching temporal structure for the film. The nonsynchronous soundtrack incorporates a montage of simple everyday sounds—a clock ticking, water dripping, a broom sweeping a stone floor—that simultaneously evoke the aural texture of the domestic space and amplify the metaphorical resonance of the images. A single voice (Hubbard's) recites the kaddish, the Jewish mourning prayer, sporadically across the soundtrack. At other points, the voices of different mourners repeat an untitled elegy by Emily Dickinson, each time with a different tempo and inflection:

> The Bustle in a House
> The Morning after Death
> Is solemnest of industries
> Enacted upon Earth—
> The Sweeping up of the Heart
> And putting Love away
> We shall not want to use again
> Until eternity.[57]

The decision to use a widescreen image in *Memento Mori* marks a definite departure from Hubbard's previous films. Like Müller, Hubbard established his cinematic practice in the context of narrow-gauge filmmaking. Since the

1960s, 8mm film formats have offered experimental filmmakers a variety of advantages over 16mm, as the larger gauge became increasingly professionalized with the proliferation of a commercially viable independent cinema. Established as amateur formats, 8mm, and later Super-8 film, granted experimental filmmakers an opportunity to work with an extremely cheap format that could be hand-processed and therefore manipulated to a greater degree. In addition, their amateur status and technical limitations provided greater scope than 16mm film for an aesthetic disidentification with the polished spectacle of popular narrative cinema. The flexibility gained from the hand-held mobility of the Super-8 camera, combined with the constraints of its narrow focal range, would provide the perfect medium for feminist and gay filmmakers to develop what Daryl Chin has called an "aesthetics of intimacy": the exploration of the political construction of the personal by seizing the "home movie" machine.[58] Moreover, Patricia R. Zimmermann adds, "This work envisions the potentialities of amateurism for exploration of the self and the private sphere. These amateur formats exorcise familialism from the discursive construct of amateurism; they insist on specificity, difference, and voice."[59] Hubbard's short film Elegy in the Streets (1989) is a perfect example of this tendency in gay experimental cinema. This silent film interweaves two strands of Super-8 footage: intimate, candid shots of a deceased friend, Roger Jacoby, and footage of the collective response to the AIDS crisis as it develops from the mourning ritual of the candlelight vigil to the militant direct action of ACT UP. Crosscutting between the two strands, the film coincidentally problematizes the ideologically maintained distinctions of public and private, individual and collective, and mourning and militancy.

We can thus read Hubbard's replication of the widescreen format in Memento Mori as a curious inversion of his earlier experimental appropriation of the "amateur gauge" of Super-8. In its artisanal reconstruction of the widescreen image, the film confiscates a technology of the spectacular, contrasting with the earlier films' reworking of a technology of intimacy. The postwar U.S. film industry promoted widescreen processes as an enhancement of cinema's spectacular capabilities. Equating the aesthetic expansionism of widescreen technology with the ideological fantasy of a panoramic "canvas of history," Hollywood promoted widescreen cinema through the genre of the historical epic. Blockbuster productions like The Robe (Henry Koster, 1963), Ben-Hur (William Wyler, 1959), Lawrence of Arabia (David Lean, 1962), and Spartacus (Stanley Kubrick, 1960) ensured that widescreen cinema would come to enter popular memory as a technology of mass spectacle, constructing history through its "sweeping panoramas" and its "cast of thousands."[60]

But *Memento Mori* deploys widescreen space for altogether more intimate subjects: the process of personal mourning and the contemplation of mortality. In reclaiming a spectacular form of cinema technology, the film counters the pathology performed by the "spectacle of AIDS" circulating in mass culture. Since Hollywood heavily exploited widescreen formats in its battle with the emerging competitor of television, it seems perhaps a fitting irony that, in working to construct an understanding of contemporary gay mortality beyond the sensationalist and pathologizing framework perpetuated by the small-screen medium of television, Hubbard would turn to the spectacular technology of widescreen cinema. *Memento Mori* harnesses the technology's affective potential (found in its excess), but places it not in the service of generating spectatorial awe, as it had been used in the historical epic, but rather uses it to provide viewers with a sensual articulation of magnitude in the form of grief's sublimity.

Subjectivity and the Material Archive of Popular Culture

Each of the experimental films analyzed in this chapter exhibits a distinctly cinephiliac engagement with the industrially produced image. *Decodings* and *Aus der Ferne* both focus that engagement on the incorporation of the found image. *Decodings* rescues the obsolete images of postwar ephemeral films for their complex resonance with gay structures of feeling in the first decade of the AIDS epidemic, while *Aus der Ferne* embeds found images from classical cinema into the psychic landscape of loss and alienation through which its witness-survivor journeys. Cinephilia takes a different form in *Pensão Globo* and *Memento Mori*. Rather than working with found images, these two films turn to specific postwar Hollywood technologies and their aesthetic legacies, namely Technicolor and widescreen cinema. While the invocation of these two historically bound film technologies summons the nostalgic aura of a long-deceased cinematic era, it brings with it, more important, the spectacular dynamics established by Hollywood's exploitation of these technologies. Since both color and widescreen processes were identified as much with spectacle as with realism in the postwar film industry, they offer contemporary experimental filmmakers like Müller and Hubbard a rich and popularly recognized aesthetics of excess from which to draw.[61] *Pensão Globo* uses the Technicolor style of Sirkian melodrama to forge emotionally intensified cinematic moments that articulate the corporeal and psychic crisis of AIDS-related illness through the hysterical excess of the film's mise-en-scène and cinematography. Although visually more subdued than *Pensão Globo*, *Memento*

Mori deals with spectacle and excess through the element of scale, fashioning the widescreen aspect ratio into a more intimate spectacle of mourning.

In their different manifestations of cinephilia, these experimental films about AIDS mediate the relationship between individual and collective experience through the appropriation of industrially produced cinema. This work is thus situated at the intersection of two distinct contexts in which the articulation of subjectivity finds its address through explicit recourse to the material archive of popular culture — gay cultural practices around AIDS and contemporary experimental cinema. The films examined in this chapter constitute an element of the diverse cultural practices developed by gay men in response to the psychic burden of AIDS and the losses it has caused. The archive of popular culture has played a significant role here. Pop songs played at gay funerals perform vital emotional and community-sustaining functions; movie and pop memorabilia have become part of the affective material literally incorporated into the AIDS Quilt; and many gay visual artists have turned to "the raw materials of pop culture" to construct an address that moves between individual experience and collective structures of feeling around AIDS.[62]

Despite the long-standing efforts of many filmmakers and academics to disavow experimental cinema's relationship to industrially produced film to maintain its status as an autonomous, modernist avant-garde, recent film histories have firmly established the necessity of recognizing the wide range of discursive and material relations between experimental and popular cinema. American underground cinema has long been the *locus classicus* for this historiographic debate. The only relation to experimental cinema that P. Adams Sitney's seminal history, *Visionary Film*, allows Hollywood is one of absolute otherness. Sitney historicizes American underground cinema as an avant-garde project defined by its artisanal autonomy and its aesthetic independence from industrially produced cinema, a personal cinema with a Romantic commitment to new forms of perception. In *Allegories of Cinema*, his revisionist history of alternative U.S. cinema in the 1960s, David James argues that although the desire to create an alternative to Hollywood constituted a foundational aspect to the American underground, it nevertheless retained a complex dialogue with popular cinema, plundering and reframing its forms and its actual images (often as found footage).[63] As James demonstrates, the films of Kenneth Anger, Jack Smith, Warhol, Bruce Conner, and the Kuchar brothers abound with such intertextual dialogues. The experimental AIDS cinema of Hoolboom, Wallin, and Müller, with its articulation of sexual identities through the idiom of popular culture, indicates a deliberate affinity with the earlier gay cinephilia of underground filmmakers such as Smith and Anger.[64]

In a survey of experimental film practice in the 1980s and 1990s, Paul Arthur summarized its prevailing ethos in a way that seems particularly apt for the films I have analyzed in this chapter: "The talisman through which the avant-garde has conducted its sweeping synthesis is the notion of recovering history, enmeshing the prerogatives of personal experience — memory, autobiography, direct observation of everyday life — with the constraints of a socially-shared past, recasting radical subjectivity as the interpenetration of public and private spaces."[65] The gay cinephilia of these films is precisely a recovery of history, a means to articulate historically specific gay structures of feeling in the AIDS epidemic through the material archive that has played a significant role in the constitution and maintenance of postwar gay identities and subcultures.

Since the gay cinephilia from which these films draw is a shared cultural practice among filmmakers and spectators, their affective address constructed through the dynamics of such cinephilia would thus find its greatest resonance among gay audiences. This is a "cinema of small gestures" in an institutional as well as an aesthetic sense. In the lesbian and gay film festivals where these films were widely shown, they could bear witness to AIDS in community space, producing ephemeral opportunities for gay men to collectively recognize and engage their shared structures of feeling in the midst of the epidemic.

◻

CHAPTER SIX

Sound, Image, and the

Corporeal Implication

of Witnessing

The chapters of this book have elucidated the diverse means by which queer
AIDS media have visually reframed the bodies of its witnesses through
self-conscious performance, embodied immediacy, doubling effects, queer
anachronism, and corporeal metaphor. But what happens when the body is
not merely reframed but displaced from vision altogether? What new testimonial dynamics arise from the refusal to provide a visual figuration of the
body? How can sound function to produce a mediated space of witnessing
in the context of such visual abstraction? These questions are at the heart
of Derek Jarman's final film, Blue (1993), which will constitute the focus of
this final chapter. Whereas the experimental AIDS cinema of Matthias Müller, Jim Hubbard, and Michael Wallin displaced queer corporeality onto the
materiality of film itself, Jarman undertook an even more radical move in
Blue, creating what Patrizio Lombardo has called the "most bodyless film ever
produced."[1] We never see Jarman (and only hear his own physical voice once)
during the film, since Blue performs a radical visual ascesis by removing all
images from the frame. For the film's entire seventy-six-minute duration, the
screen is filled only with a luminous monochrome blue, while the soundtrack
incorporates a complex sound montage of poetic and testimonial spoken
text, music, song, and sound effects. Created during the final years of his life,
at a time when Jarman was struggling with the onset of AIDS-related blindness, the film both visualizes blindness on its monochrome screen and the-
matizes it in the spoken script. The image and the word thus come together
in Blue to explore the boundaries of visuality itself. As the film's spoken script

asks at one point: "If I lose half my sight, will my vision be halved?" Time and again in the film, Jarman prioritizes the visual imagination over the physical realm of perception as the ethical space in which the act of bearing witness to AIDS can most effectively take place. Blue thus rejects the conventional visual components of cinema that render its impression of reality: cinematography, editing, and mise-en-scène. The film image not only denies any sensuous or material figuration of the witness's body it also negates the profilmic itself (the time-space in front of the camera). In fact, Blue is one of those rare analog films made without a camera, for the monochrome blue was produced from an electronic color field created in the lab.[2]

The film's provocative visual form has prompted many critics to frame Blue as an integral part of avant-garde cinema's long-standing iconoclastic dedication to what William Wees has termed "a fuller and much more revealing visualization of sight."[3] Epitomized by the films of Stan Brakhage and Michael Snow, this tradition has pursued a modernist self-reflexivity around the cinematic apparatus, challenging the perspectivist tradition of the photographic camera in the service of liberating the spectator's vision, of forging new experiential relations between seeing and knowing the world. Noting Jarman's rejection of cinematic language, Paul Julian Smith contends that in Blue, we are "thrown back on the cinematic apparatus itself, on the projection of light onto a screen and our own physical presence before it."[4] The chromatic constancy of the blue screen also prompts us to notice the scratches and nicks on the celluloid, distinct reminders of its historical materiality. Chris Darke argues furthermore that the soundtrack, especially the film's spoken script, transfers the responsibility of visualization from the filmmaker to the spectator: "The soundtrack works to spark the spectator's own images off the silent blue canvas: this is a film that takes place as much in the spectator's head as it does onscreen — 'an infinite possibility becoming tangible,' as Jarman puts it in one of the monologues."[5] In this sense, Blue draws on the visual aspects of radio as a medium: it stimulates the mind's eye to imagine images rather than have the eye perceive them physically. The spoken word carries the witness and his world into the mind of the spectator. Indeed, the ascetic denial of sensually perceptible images provides the very stimulus for the rich visual imagination of Blue. But Blue is more than a "radio film" such as Walter Ruttmann's Weekend (1930), because the spectator's experience of his or her own visual perception during the projection of Blue is crucial to the stimulation of the mind's eye.[6] By attending to the significance of the film spectator's embodied perception and cognition, Smith and Darke demonstrate how Blue is not in fact the "most bodyless film" that Lombardo claims it to be. Although the film's spectators are denied any explicit visual figuration of the witness's body on the screen, they do become distinctly aware of their own body in the theater during the screening of the film. The body of the witness that has disappeared from the screen returns through the corporeal experience of the spectator. In the following sections of the chapter I examine how *Blue* uses the relations between visual and aural perception to implicate the body of its spectator in the act of bearing witness to AIDS. This process of what I call "corporeal implication" allows the film's spectator to become a witness to AIDS through a simultaneously visceral and imaginative encounter with Jarman's subjectivity.

"The Attrition between the Private and Public World"

To fully understand the power of the film's visual ascesis at the time of its original exhibition in the United Kingdom, we must also consider Jarman's career-long aesthetic preference for image over narrative and his related political investment in visibility, which would appear, at first sight, to contradict the iconoclastic, antispectacular drive of the film. The visual *poesis* of Jarman's films, exemplified in *The Angelic Conversation* (1985), *The Last of England* (1987), and *The Garden* (1990), is built around the nonlinearity of their crystalline montage, tableau staging, and sensuous spectacle, thus placing them within British cinema's antirealist countertradition, at the center of which stand the films of Michael Powell and Emeric Pressburger.[7] Indeed, Jarman is now recognized as a major figure of English Romanticism's twentieth-century legacy, as much for his influence on the new Romantic movement of the 1980s, with its foppish sensibilities of the aesthete, as for the direct influence of Romantic visionaries like William Blake on his own work.[8] Jarman's films are imbued with the kind of oneiric subjectivism that also characterizes much of the queer avant-garde canon (Jean Cocteau, Jean Genet, Gregory Markopoulos, and Kenneth Anger).[9] They refract autobiographical material through the iconographic archive of history, myth, literature, and art. In his 1987 book *The Last of England*, Jarman characterized his work as a form of archaeology that moves between the private and the public through the dynamics of retrieval, projection, and ignition:

> My world is in fragments, smashed in pieces so fine I doubt I will ever reassemble them. So I scrabble in the rubbish, an archaeologist who stumbles across a buried film. An archaeologist who projects his private world along a beam of light into the arena, till all goes dark at the end of

the performance, and we go home. . . . Now you project your private world into the public arena and produce the flashpoint; the attrition between the private and public world is the tradition you discover. All you can do is point the direction that everyone in the audience who wishes to "travel" has to take.[10]

This "attrition between the private and public world" would constitute a central pivot in the critical evaluation of Jarman's oeuvre. For some, his endowment of the "most intimate and subtle nuances of individual experience" with aesthetic form exemplified the moral and political function of art, while for others, particularly for conservative art critics in the Tory press, Jarman's works never achieved the transcendental status of art, because they were "all ornaments to his own life, arrangements of his own milieu, which is why they will ultimately vanish with him."[11] Whether celebrated or dismissed, Jarman was widely understood to be a key British cultural figure during the Thatcherite era of the 1980s and early 1990s, a flashpoint for the intersection of the personal, the political, and the aesthetic.

Moreover, when Jarman died on 19 February 1994, he was the most publicly prominent person with AIDS in the United Kingdom. Both the *Guardian* and the *Independent* carried the story on their front page, with the latter's headline connecting Jarman's death to the imminent vote in the House of Commons to lower the age of consent for gay men from twenty-one to sixteen: "Gay Champion Dies on Eve of New Age; A Vigil outside the Commons Tonight Is Likely to Turn into a Wake for Derek Jarman."[12] Jarman had campaigned hard for this legal reform in the final year of his life, but he died two days before he could witness the Tory government's last-minute compromise of lowering the age to eighteen. In his obituary for Jarman published in *Artforum*, Simon Watney described Jarman's demise as "a self-consciously political death."[13]

A year after being diagnosed as HIV-positive in 1986, Jarman decided that he could no longer keep his serostatus a secret. Shortly before the publication of *The Last of England*, in which he explicitly reflected on his diagnosis, Jarman gave an interview for the *Guardian* in October 1987 with his close friend Nicolas de Jongh and arranged for the issue of his serostatus to be mentioned, almost in passing.[14] Jarman's decision to voluntarily disclose his HIV status while he was still asymptomatic distinguished him from other public personalities, such as Rock Hudson and Arthur Ashe, who had been pulled out of the HIV closet by the increasingly visible onset of AIDS. Furthermore, in contrast to public personalities like Magic Johnson or Elizabeth Taylor, Jarman consistently refused to institutionalize his public discussion of HIV/AIDS through an affiliation with an established organization or public agency. He preferred to remain a peculiarly English dissident and queer outsider, persistently provoking the establishment.[15] As his longtime collaborator and close friend Tilda Swinton has noted, he was not, however, an obscure or marginalized figure from the worlds of British art and film, but "a proper tabloid figure in the '80s, involved in constant argy bargy with moral arbiters like Mary Whitehouse and Ian McKellen."[16] Jarman would address his contentious relationship with the tabloid press and its representation of AIDS and gay sexuality in the iconoclastic painting Blood (1992), in which he painted over collaged photocopies of a ludicrous tabloid headline from the Sun ("AIDS Blood in M&S Pies") with monochromic red and then repeatedly and angrily etched the word blood across the whole painting.[17]

Like his fellow artist David Wojnarowicz, he embraced the opportunity to play the role of the queer outlaw, yet what made Jarman's public intervention in the AIDS epidemic so distinctive was his ability to address multiple publics in his writing, his artwork, his filmmaking, his political activism, and his diverse engagements with the British press. His avowed Romantic conservatism tapped into a broad-based high Tory anxiety about the Thatcherite modernization of Britain: "Politically I am not a Tory. Culturally I am. My art has always been Tory art."[18] Appearing regularly in the tabloid and broadsheet press, Jarman wrote letters to the editor and op-ed articles on a wide range of subjects related to AIDS and gay rights, including the threatened closure of St. Bartholomew's Hospital in London, Ian McKellen's knighthood, the politics of HIV disclosure by public figures, and the popular representation of AIDS. Many of his interviews barely touched on his creative work, instead concentrating on how he dealt with his diagnosis, the experience of medical treatment for his opportunistic infections, his religious outlook in the face of terminal illness, and even the spiritual value of gardening at his cottage in Dungeness on the bleak Kent coast.[19] When the journalist Lynn Barber argued in an interview that he should be spending more energy on his "real work" (that is to say, his art) than on public "squabbles" with figures like McKellen, Jarman countered, "It is my real work. I have to say. It would be wonderful if it was unnecessary but it's not yet even possible to imagine a situation where I didn't have to do it. For me to talk into your tape recorder is as important as making a film because these things have to be communicated and they are actually, believe it or not, a matter of life and death."[20] Even among those who knew little about or thought little of his artistic practices, Jarman was widely admired for his courageous honesty and disarming wit in serving as the most public person with AIDS in Britain during the Thatcherite era. Although the visual ascesis of Blue contrasts sharply with the persistent cultural visibility of Jarman in the early 1990s—whether depicted smiling impishly in his customary blue work overalls or as "Saint Derek of Dungeness" canonized by the Sisters of Perpetual Indulgence—the film script's repeated engagement with contemporary political commentary and its sustained description of the physical and psychological experience of living with AIDS reveal a profound continuity with Jarman's public image in the early 1990s.[21]

Hybrid Origins

The idiosyncratic characteristics of Jarman's final film owe much to its long genesis. Dedicated to an imagistic rather than a narrative mode of filmmaking with little commercial appeal, Jarman struggled throughout his filmmaking career to secure funding for his projects. The first trace of the work's conception is to be found in one of Jarman's notebooks from 1974 in the tantalizing but enigmatic phrase, "the blue film for Yves Klein."[22] Jarman had long been fascinated with Klein and his work. Like many of the other artists, filmmakers, and writers, such as Caravaggio, Pier Paolo Pasolini, and Genet, from whom Jarman drew inspiration, Klein provided not only an influential body of work but also, and perhaps more important, an artistic and public life with which Jarman could identify. It was the kind of public life from which he would borrow for the performance of his own public life as an artist. Thus the subsequent shift in the project from a biography of Klein to a personal and frequently autobiographical exploration of AIDS appears less a displacement or rupture and more an intelligible conceptual development, a more complete identification with Klein.

In the late 1950s Klein began to produce a series of monochrome paintings. Derived from specially developed luminous pigment, Klein's paint was applied uniformly with a roller. By rejecting the paintbrush, Klein gestured to a radical evacuation of artistic expression in the material trace of the paint. By 1958, Klein narrowed his monochrome interest to one color: blue. In a masterful gesture of artistic self-promotion, Klein adopted a particular hue of ultramarine blue and branded it with his name: I.K.B. (International Klein Blue). Appropriating the notion of "a blue period" à la Pablo Picasso and evacuating the color of its expressive function, Klein celebrated blue for what he believed to be its status beyond the signifying dimensions of other colors. Gaston Bachelard's claim that blue offers poetic knowledge that precedes rational knowledge was profoundly influential on Klein, who often quoted a line from the French critic as a testimonial for his own art: "First there is nothing, then there is a deep nothing, then there is a blue depth."[23] Klein himself stressed that even in its most material and concrete associations, namely, the sea and the sky, blue signified "the most *abstract* aspects of tangible and visible nature" (78; emphasis added).[24] Through his monochrome blue canvases, Klein strove to deobjectify the work of art, a goal that has become an important aspect of conceptualism.[25] As the art historian Sidra Stich notes about Klein's use of blue, "This is then a realm in which imagination thrives without images; it is a realm of solitude, transparency and dematerialization that prospers within and by means of effacement. It is therefore a realm of nothingness that is, however, alive with possibility."[26] Throughout the spoken script of *Blue*, Jarman invokes notions of blue that draw heavily from Klein's conception of the color: "Blue transcends the solemn geography of human limits." Elsewhere, the script invokes "the fathomless blue of bliss" as "an infinite possibility becoming tangible."

Jarman's idea for "the blue film for Yves Klein" only materialized into a concrete project in 1987. Following the success of his film *Caravaggio* (1986), Jarman began to build a funding proposal for an experimental biography of Klein, tentatively titled "International Blue." Jarman described the project as "a film without compunction or narrative existing only for an idea."[27] Funding discussions with the Sony Corporation dried up after the company realized that Jarman remained committed to a radically antinarrative film. The project resurfaced in 1991, but not as a film. Titled *Symphonie Monotone*, after Klein's famous single-note symphony, the event functioned as a prescreening performance before a special AIDS benefit premiere of *The Garden*.[28] A film loop of one of Klein's blue monochromes owned by the Tate Gallery was projected onto the cinema screen, while Jarman and the actress Swinton, dressed in blue, sat at a table on the stage running their moistened fingers around the rims of wine glasses and reading Jarman's personal and poetic reflections on the color blue. Musicians sat at the front of the theater playing an ethereal score by the contemporary British composer and longtime Jarman collaborator Simon Fisher Turner. From time to time, a young boy would run out into the audience and hand out blue and gold painted stones.[29] Jarman was simultaneously researching and writing a book of reflections on color that he would subsequently publish as *Chroma* (1994). Typical of Jarman's writing style, the book draws together a montage of philosophical reflections, historical anecdotes, edited journal entries, and personal memories all centered around the colors of the spectrum. Although most of the chapters included recent memories and journal entries dealing with Jarman's illness, it was the chapter on blue that most fully explored such experience. This chapter subsequently became the foundation for the film script of *Blue*.[30]

The filmed loop of Klein's painting was replaced by a 35mm filmstrip of electronically generated luminous blue once Jarman's producer, James Mackay, finally secured the majority of funding for the film in 1992 from Channel Four, the Arts Council of Great Britain, Brian Eno, and the Japanese producer Takashi Asai. The blue image was no longer a photographic image of an object in the spatiotemporality of the historical world, albeit an abstract image. It now existed only as a nonrepresentational color field generated through the alchemy of modern filmmaking technology.[31] Mackay secured completion funds for the production from BBC Radio Three, which facilitated the simultaneous broadcast of *Blue* on British public radio and national television. The *Radio Times*, the BBC's listings magazine, invited listeners to send in for a blue postcard if they decided not to watch *Blue* simultaneously on television.[32] Coinciding with the theatrical release of *Blue* in the United Kingdom, the film script was published as a book and the soundtrack released on compact disc. Mackay also planned a special interactive CD-ROM version of *Blue*, but lack of funding prevented it from being completed. The CD-ROM was to include the film along with Jarman's previously unreleased Super-8 films, materials from the live performances, video interviews with principal participants, the complete script, HIV prevention information, and a segment entitled "The Void," which would invite participants into an interactive exploration of *Blue* in which they could potentially manipulate sound and image.[33]

Clearly this history of the work's genesis challenges any attempt to privilege the origin and status of the work as quintessentially cinematic. This hardly seems surprising when we consider that throughout his career Jarman self-identified as a painter and an artist far more than as a filmmaker, despite the critical and popular perception of him as first and foremost a filmmaker. *Blue* not only emerged from but was also disseminated in multiple media forms, including live performance, film, television, radio, a book, a book chapter, a sound recording, a gallery installation, a public art event and, at least conceptually, a CD-ROM. Each of these media offers a different opportunity to mediate the act of bearing witness. Each produces a varying dynamic of reception and can render the impression of the witness's presence through often starkly differing means. Live performance and cinema, for instance, rely heavily on the visual presentation of bodies in front of their audiences, even though cinema functions through a paradoxical presence/ absence of such bodies.[34] Radio privileges the auditory qualities of the voice and its presentation in both private and public acoustic spaces, whereas books articulate presence through a linguistic understanding of voice that is tied to structures of address and discursive register. However, none of the manifestations of Blue signified uniquely through a single medium. They each implied a relationship to one another. For example, the performers in the live performance Symphonie Monotone acted as both a corporeal supplement or excess to the abstract monochrome film and as a bridge closing the gap between the spectator and the screen. While the film screen lacked the impression of corporeal presence, the performative aspects of the event "filled in" that absence of represented bodies with live ones in the auditorium. Blue is certainly a work of cinema, but it is also far more than that. This multiplicity frames the ways it produces meaning, thus suggesting that it need not necessarily be understood as either quintessentially cinematic or as a self-reflexive critique of the cinematic apparatus. The film's hybrid origins indicate how its visual iconoclasm cannot be understood outside of a consideration of the complex dynamics between sound, word, and image, especially those borrowed and adapted from other media.

Corporeal Implication

The spoken script of Blue acknowledges at several points its own iconoclastic impulse in the face of the visuality of AIDS: "For accustomed to believing in image, an absolute idea of value, his world had forgotten the command of essence: Thou Shall Not Create Unto Thyself Any Graven Image, although you know the task is to fill the page. From the bottom of your heart, pray to be released from image." As Peter Schwenger notes, the injunction against the image in this passage is paired with an implicit command to write.[35] It is not the screen, nor the canvas, that is filled, but the page. Language in Blue not only facilitates the means by which to bear witness, to construct a testimonial address to an other, it also serves as the form through which the witnessing body may be imagined. In combining an abstract monochrome image track with a rich and multilayered soundtrack structured around verbal performance, Jarman inverts the hegemony of image over sound that has shaped the history of both popular narrative and experimental cinema.[36] The film sound theorist Michel Chion argues that the very notion of the "soundtrack" misleadingly implies an autonomy to the perception of sound during film spectatorship: "A film's aural elements are not received as an autonomous unit. They are immediately analyzed and distributed in the spectator's perceptual apparatus according to the relation each bears to what the spectator sees at the time."[37] In what Chion calls "an instantaneous perceptual triage," many aspects of film sound are merely "swallowed up" in the image's false depth, often in the service of enhancing a conventional narrative film's realistic impression of spatiotemporality (3).[38] *Blue* shatters this conventional triage by denying the image track figuration and rendering its impression of spatial depth as either infinite or zero. The blue screen presents itself as either pure surface or a depthless void, neither of which provide suitable perceptual anchors for sound, and in particular, for the voice. This ambiguous perceptual status of the blue screen problematizes the term *voice-over* as a means to describe the spoken script in *Blue*. A voice-over implies a phenomenological separation from the spatiotemporality figured on the screen, *over* which it may speak. Such conventional relations between sound and image remain deliberately absent from *Blue*.

The unanchored, seemingly disembodied quality of the voice in *Blue* functions as a particular and idiosyncratic example of what Chion calls the "acousmêtre," the speaker who cannot be seen.[39] While certain modern media, like radio, the phonograph, and the telephone, rely completely on "acousmatic listening," cinema has been able, since the arrival of sound film, to explore the tension between seeing and not seeing the source of a voice or other sound. A film spectator may frequently oscillate between such visualized and acousmatic listening during the course of a film. Chion points out that the placement of the loudspeaker behind the cinema screen produces a specific perplexity in the spectator's perception of an acousmêtre during the film: "For the spectator, then, the filmic acousmêtre is offscreen, outside the image, and at the same time *in* the image. . . . It's as if the voice were wandering along the surface, at once inside and outside, seeking a place to settle" (23; emphasis original). *Blue* complicates these dynamics by denying any figuration or perspectival depth and breadth to the image. There is therefore simply no place on the screen where the voice can be located.

Citing the voice of God and the maternal voice as its precedents, Chion finds significant power in the film acousmêtre: "The acousmêtre has only to show itself—for the person speaking to inscribe his or her body inside the frame, in the visual field—for it to lose its power, omniscience and (obviously) ubiquity" (27). During the first ten to fifteen minutes of *Blue*, film spectators may strongly anticipate the imminent appearance of the witness's body in the film frame—and with it, a reassuring phenomenological relation to the witness—but eventually they submit either to their own boredom or to the obstinacy of the film's visual abstraction. But the anticipation of figuration, or at the very least of change, in the monochrome screen is never extinguished. As

John Paul Ricco argues about the film, "one is never free from the sense that a visual accompaniment to the audio has gone missing."⁴⁰ The monochrome blue field may also prompt the association of being on the wrong channel, failing to locate a signal or awaiting its input, given the standard use of a blue screen in video equipment to indicate the absence of a video signal.⁴¹ The image track of the film could present the body, but it resolutely does not. This refusal is at the heart of what Ricco calls "a disappeared aesthetics" in Blue, which "visualizes nothing but a potentiality or a preference to not-visualize, and thereby points to the ethical-political dimensions of visuality itself" (42). To understand why the film refuses to visualize the body of the witness on the screen, we need to examine more closely how the film script's language and its spoken performance allow that same body to be imagined.

The spoken script of Blue engenders an elaborate collage of different themes, discourses, and modes of address. While it frequently journeys into poetic and philosophical ruminations on the color blue, often through a mythical boy character called Blue, the film's script consistently returns to the subject of the body and the ravage inflicted on it by AIDS: "I have a sinking feeling in my stomach. I feel defeated. My mind bright as a button but my body falling apart—a naked light bulb in a dark and ruined room." Blue records in great detail the painful and arduous treatment that Jarman undergoes to fight the cytomegalovirus (CMV) gradually blinding him: "The shattering bright light of the eye specialist's camera leaves that empty sky blue afterimage. . . . The process is a torture, but the result, stable eyesight, worth the price and the twelve pills I have to take a day." The address of the spoken script shifts at times from such first-person testimony to citing the impersonal pharmaceutical small print of the drugs Jarman is taking, or to his doctor's diagnosis: "The white flashes you are experiencing in your eyes are common when the retina is damaged." After reading out the over forty possible side effects of the CMV treatment drug DHPG, which include its proven capability as a carcinogen, the spoken voice sarcastically parrots the advice at the end of the small print on the packaging: "If you are concerned about any of the above side effects, or if you would like any further information, please ask your doctor."

The script spoken across the film is read by four different voices: Nigel Terry and John Quentin, occasionally Swinton, and for one brief, compelling passage, by Jarman himself, as he describes what his partner H. B. sees for him in the waiting room of the hospital eye department (another moment of proxy for Jarman's subjectivity). Rather than suggest a polyphonic or heteroglossic structure, these voices imply a subtle diffusion of the author's voice. We hear no overlapping or dialectic engagement between these distinct voices; they each enunciate as part of an ongoing monologue that is passed from one voice to the next. Moreover, these shifts in voice follow no apparent pattern or logic, whether thematic, discursive, or affective. The often sudden shifts in the spoken script between different emotional states—despair, anger, sadness, black humor, and acceptance—bear out the experience of discontinuity and radical unpredictability that people living with AIDS have time and again articulated: "The worst of this illness is the uncertainty. I've played this scenario back and forth each hour of the day for the last six years." This often vertiginous alternation in the film's tone is supported by a complex and shifting soundtrack that mixes recorded sounds of natural landscapes, medical machines, street life, and the low hum of fluorescent lighting with a diverse range of music including Coil's disco-inflected industrial electronica, the haunting ambience of Brian Eno, Erik Satie's *Les gnossiennes*, and Fisher Turner's ethereal scoring. As listeners of *Blue*, we thus come to feel a distinct tension between this relative coherence to the testimonial subjectivity of the script—its literary voice—and the multiple layers of differentiation that begin with the four voices who perform it. A brief sung section of the script wittily acknowledges this dispersed subjectivity through a queer embrace of polymorphous perversity:

I am a cock-sucking
Straight-acting
Lesbian man
With ball-crushing bad manners
Laddish nymphomaniac politics
Spunky sexist desires
Of incestuous inversion and
Incorrect terminology
I am a Not Gay

Those familiar with Jarman's other films and his books will recognize several aspects of *Blue* as continuities in his oeuvre. First, all three of the actors who Jarman used in the film—Terry, Quentin, and Swinton—had become closely associated with his film oeuvre as members of his informal ensemble by 1993. Since Jarman's films had consistently been framed (by both himself and his critics) as personal visions, the use of his ensemble actors in his last film ensured that the performance of the testimonial script through several voices could disperse, but not completely dissipate the subjectivity articulated in *Blue*. Second, the complex collage-like script of *Blue* follows the free-flowing and digressive, nonlinear structure of his books *Dancing Ledge* (1984), *The Last of England*, *Modern Nature* (1991), and *At Your Own Risk: A Saint's Testament* (1992), all of which drew heavily from the content and form of his personal journals, with their penchant for imagistic fragments, quotidian observations, and aphorisms.

The specific techniques of sound recording in *Blue* also play an important role in determining how the film's testimonial voice is articulated, and how it is subsequently perceived by the audience. All the different voices are closely miked (the mouth positioned close to the microphone), creating a sense of intimacy between the speaking voice and the listening spectator similar to the auditory dynamics of listening to radio commentary. In *Blue*, we thus sense virtually no distance between the voice and our ears. At certain points, the voice even whispers the script. Close-miking also reduces reverberation, the sonic quality that situates a voice in physical space. This recording technique gives a strong impression of aural presence to the voice, hinders the perception of distance, and thus closes up any identifiable space that would facilitate the clear delineation between speaker and listener. Chion argues that this technique, what he calls "the I-voice," structures the spectator's identification in a particular manner: "All you have to do is add reverb in the mix to manipulate an I-voice; the *embracing* and *complicit* quality of the I-voice becomes *embraced* and *distanced*. It is no longer a subject with which the spectator identifies, but rather an object-voice, perceived as a body anchored in space."[42] To hear the difference in aural quality between these two modes, one need only compare the soundtrack of the film *Blue* to the live recording of the Rome performance of *Blue* in July 1993. In the Rome recording, the reverberation of the live performers' voices presents their bodies as anchored in a specific place.[43]

By liberating the speaking voice from its body through both visual and aural disembodiment, *Blue* produces the effect of corporeal implication in the spectator: "The voice makes us feel in our body the vibration of the body of the other."[44] This visceral, mimetic component to the spectatorial experience of *Blue* generates a potential transformation in the dynamics of bearing witness to AIDS. The film's visual and aural techniques negate the space in which a stable phenomenological relationship between the viewer/listener and the witness with AIDS may be constructed. In foreclosing my ability to imagine the body of the person with AIDS "out there," I come to witness the witness through my very own body. The body of the other, the witness's body, is implicated in my own. I want to distinguish this process from conventional forms of cinematic identification in which the difference of the other is written over by an identification of the viewing subject *as* the viewed other. As much as *Blue* permits me access to the subjective space of the witness, the acoustic and optical qualities produced by the film's screening in physical space prevent me from either pinning down the other with my eyes and my ears or forgetting my own embodiment. Such witnessing dynamics reveal a resonance between Jarman's film and Felix Gonzalez-Torres's AIDS-themed installation art, which foregrounds corporeality just as it displaces the visual figuration of the body onto metaphor and trace.[45] For instance, Gonzalez-Torres's candy-pile portrait of his lover, *Untitled (Portrait of Ross in LA)* (1991), invites gallery visitors to partake in their literal consumption, an act of both dismemberment and communion that blurs the distinction between the body of the artwork and its beholder.

"An Infinite Possibility Becoming Tangible"

The profound significance of such corporeal implication cannot be underestimated during a pandemic in which people living with HIV and AIDS have consistently been subject to the spatial techniques of abjection, including pathology, stigmatization, social isolation, quarantine, and even incarceration. Cultural hysteria about the presumed contagion of the retrovirus has demanded that HIV-infected bodies be contained at a "safe distance." *Blue* reverses the visual attention of the spectacle of AIDS from the body with AIDS out *there* back onto the spectator's own body right *here* before the blue screen.

I felt this transformative moment during the first time I saw the film at Film Forum in New York City in 1994. Sitting in the movie theater gazing at the monochrome blue screen, I gradually began to pay attention, like Smith, to my own presence in the cinematic apparatus, to my phenomenological encounter with a screen of reflected blue light.[46] And the object of my gaze continually spilled over beyond the edges of the screen. Blue light seeped out of the rectangular frame and into the space of the theater, bathing the normally darkened space of the theater's seats in diffuse illumination. In the blue light in which Jarman's body, the witness's body, remained unfigured, the spectator's body, my own body, now became visible as the reflected light of the film touched it. In the blue aura around me I had begun to notice my own seated body (as well as the bodies of other viewers nearby). Such diffusion of light threatened to absorb the distance between spectator and screen, preventing my very ability to grasp precisely the object of my visual perception. Was I looking at a screen or merely, and incredibly, at light? On the one hand, the rectangle of light on the screen resisted definitive perceptual identification as either a frame (delimiting two-dimensional space) or an aperture (opening up to infinite space).[47] This ambiguity snagged my visual perception in that impossible gap between surface and depth. If, on the other hand, I was looking at light, then I was already looking at both nothing and everything. It was thus my own body that emerged as the surest presence to be sensed by my own visual perception. I could see myself engaged in the act of seeing at the same time that I felt myself losing control of it.

This embodied spectatorship engendered by Blue operates through the combination of seeing and hearing. The spectator's vision is denied an external body on the screen to either misrecognize in the phantasmatic process of identification or to repudiate through a disidentification with it as an abject other. The monochrome screen reflects back merely light, bathing the spectator's body in an illumination that arouses the perception of his or her own embodiment. Vision in this instance relies less on the spectator's perceived distance from the world and its otherness than on his or her felt incorporation within it. Hearing similarly frames the spectator's relation to otherness in terms of proximity and corporeal implication. The film's employment of the aural I-voice produces a perception of such closeness to the ear that the boundary between inside and outside the spectator's body seems to dissolve as he or she listens and watches. Light and sound envelop him or her in a space-diminishing embrace.

We may comprehend these particular spectatorial dynamics in terms of what Laura U. Marks has called "haptic visuality."[48] Drawing from the work of the nineteenth-century art historian Aloïs Riegl, Marks distinguishes two modes of visuality: optical and haptic. On the one hand, optical visuality relies on a separation between the viewing subject and the world, thus allowing the former to distinguish the latter as distinct objective forms in deep space. This is how we conventionally think of seeing in an everyday capacity. However, we must be aware that it is also the foundation of instrumental and disciplinary modes of seeing. Haptic visuality, on the other hand, posits a relationship of proximity and contact (rather than distance) between the viewing subject and the world; it allows our eyes to function like organs of touch. Haptic visuality presupposes a different mode of seeing, one that tends to move over the surface of the world and its objects, rather than focus on specific objects or bodies situated in deep space. Marks draws such distinctions to explain how works of diasporic and exilic filmmaking, such as Rea Tajiri's History and Memory (1991) and Mona Hatoum's Measures of Distance (1988), come to represent experience and memory. The haptic visuality engendered by such "intercultural cinema" facilitates the representation of cultural difference through embodied knowledge rather than through the rational, disciplinary epistemologies of Western modernity.[49]

Although not a work of intercultural cinema in the sense proposed by Marks, Blue certainly does invoke the dynamics of haptic visuality when it bears witness to the filmmaker's experience of AIDS by rejecting the disciplinary gaze of the spectacle of AIDS. In fact, the ways in which Marks describes the spectatorial dynamics of haptic visuality in intercultural cinema could equally be applied to Blue: "The works I propose to call haptic invite a look that moves on the surface plane of the screen for some time before the viewer realizes what she or he is beholding. Such images resolve into figuration only gradually, if at all" (162–63). In its process of displacing the body of the witness from the screen to the auditorium, Blue takes this ambivalent relationship to figuration to an extreme. Spectators are suspended in the simultaneous contemplation of the material surface of the projected image and the infinite depth of the representational image. As our eyes graze across the screen, we come to detect in the monochrome frame the minor scratches and marks that accrue on the film print as it is repeatedly projected. Marks understands such attention to the film's materiality to be a major distinction between optical and haptic visuality: "While optical perception privileges the representational power of the image, haptic perception privileges the material presence of the image" (163). In Blue, that material presence is dual: both the monochrome rectangle of reflected blue light on the screen and the diffuse blue light that bathes the auditorium. When our eyes attempt to sustain an optical perception of the monochrome image in Blue—to focus on it as representation—we gradually succumb to the perceptual effects of continuously gazing at a homogenous visual field, the phenomenon known as the Ganzfeld effect: "It is as if the mind cannot endure pure ground, but must always play figures against it, if only those of its own erratic physical vision. So, irregular movements of the eye produce a sense of irregularities in the perceived field, which are then interpreted by the mind's eye as images."[50] Degrees of visual figuration in the image thus arise in Blue from the physical qualities of both the film itself and the spectator's own act of seeing.

Of course, these dynamics do not function in isolation from the film's use of sound. The film's spoken words and nonverbal sounds generate a complex array of synesthetic effects that allow Blue to figure the lived experience of AIDS in ways that resist optical visuality. This resistance to the optical is at the core of Jarman's radical call to the spectator as witness because with it are rejected the risks of pathologization and abjection.[51] Such synesthesia abets the process of corporeal implication that allows the viewer to become a witness to the witness with HIV/AIDS. Jarman's film script for Blue abounds not only in rich sets of literary imagery but also in poetic language that continually fuses the senses of seeing and hearing. The script invokes an "archaeology of sound" that is witnessed by the character Blue: "A word or phrase materialized in scintillating sparks, a poetry of fire which casts everything into darkness with the brightness of its reflection." This synesthetic imbrication of light and sound runs throughout the film, often used powerfully in the scenes when grinding electronic sound effects convey the visually painful effects of the eye treatments described by the testimonial voice. An early passage of the script (read by Quentin) explicitly spatializes this synesthesia as Jarman posits his own subjectivity through the metaphorical figuration of an empty, sunlit room filled with the echo of voices:

> I fill this room with the echo of many voices
> Who passed time here
> Voices unlocked from the blue of the long dried paint
> The sun comes and floods this empty room
> I call it my room
> My room has welcomed many summers
> Embraced laughter and tears
> Can it fill itself with your laughter
> Each word a sunbeam
> Glancing in the light
> This is the song of My Room
> (in whispers) David. Howard. Graham. David. Paul. Terry . . .
> (repeated refrain) Blue stretches, yawns and is awake.
> (simultaneously in whispers) David. Terry. Paul. Howard. Graham . . .
> Blue.[52]

This passage figures Jarman's remembrance of individual friends and lovers who have died of AIDS as, at once, rays of light and echoed voices, unlocked from the "long dried paint" of death. Each metaphor is imbricated in the other: "Each word a sunbeam / Glancing in the light." The synesthetic effect is here enhanced by the musical score, which introduces sharp, high-note percussive rings that evoke such glinting rays of sunlight. This accompanying music and the sound effects of summertime (birdsong, buzzing insects, and a trickling stream) do not provide an aural anchor so that the audience may situate Quentin's voice in an objective spatiotemporality. Like the closely miked I-voice, these accompanying sounds are presented as interior, as the subjective sensations of memory.

In imagining Jarman's subjectivity through the image of the empty room, the film not only implies the psychological and physiological toll of an impending death brought about by AIDS but also suggests how subjectivity is filled with the traces of other subjectivities who have "passed time" in it. Jarman cannot bear witness to his own experience of AIDS without also remembering those close friends who have died before him. This is not merely an ethical commitment to speak on behalf of those who have already been silenced by death. The knowledge of their painful fate haunts Jarman's experience of illness and mortality with the anticipation of his own as he follows their path.[53] Jarman's particular spatial figuration of subjectivity here enables an intricately complex relationality that shatters the binaristic dynamics of dis/identification in the name of the witness's radical alterity. Yet this passage of the film script resuscitates hope by awakening the mythical boy Blue, the film's embodiment of infinite possibility in the face of death.

By simultaneously figuring subjectivity *as a space* filled by the presence and effect of other subjectivities and as something existing *in a space* that renders its differentiation from other subjectivities, *Blue* suggests new possibilities for shaping the intersubjective encounter at the heart of the act of bearing witness. The film clearly refuses conventional means for mediating acts of bearing witness in cinema, such as the talking head or the observational mode of documentary. Jarman rejected the optical visuality that allows such conventions to generate a strong visual impression of the witness's presence in the deep space of the image. He preferred the haptic visuality that implicates the viewer's own body in the dynamics of bearing witness through an audiovisual medium like cinema. The power of the film lies in the embodied spectatorship it generates, "in the infinite possibility becoming tangible." The interaction of the film's visual asceticism with its acousmatic qualities enables the viewer to experience the subjectivity of the witness "passing time" in his or her own embodied subjectivity. The intersubjective encounter in which the viewer/listener becomes a witness to the witness thus comes to occur within bodies as well as between them. It is in this aspect of the film that *Blue* most fully articulates the tension between the internal and external dynamics of bearing witness that characterize queer AIDS media. This inside/outside dynamic also seemed to have shaped the reception of *Blue* for radio listeners during its initial broadcast in 1993, albeit through different means. Commenting on hearing *Blue* on BBC Radio Three while looking at the blue postcard provided by the *Radio Times*, the filmmaker Clive Myer notes, "The experience was intense and enabling as we were surrounded by the sound not the image and visual and mental concentration was self regulatory rather than potentially imposed by the size of a large screen. . . . The viewer/listener was not subjected *to* the piece but rather became the subject *of* the piece."[54]

Afterlife in the Art World

The trope of "passing time" came to shape the conditions of exhibition for *Blue* in the years following Jarman's death as it was increasingly shown in gallery spaces as an installation.[55] After its limited theatrical run in the United States, the Walker Art Center in Minneapolis presented *Blue* from June 1994 until October 1996 as a free-standing black-box installation in one of the galleries devoted to the museum's permanent collection.[56] By installing *Blue* next to works by Andy Warhol, Sigmar Polke, Mark Rothko, and Carl Andre in a gallery dedicated to the themes of light and transcendence, the Walker affirmed both the work's intermediality and its resonance with various postwar art movements, particularly minimalism and conceptualism. The gallery visitor would pull back a black curtain to enter the 13×14ft space of the installation (figure 58). It was not just the relatively small size of the installation (compared to a movie theater) that rendered it a particularly intimate and immersive experience. The stereophonic soundtrack was also channeled through speakers embedded in the left, right, and rear walls, overturning the classical movie theater's placement of the sound source behind the screen image as noted by Chion. Hence Jonathan Kahana recalls the sound of the installation being "more prominent and proximal than it might have been in a theater."[57]

The installation's continuous looping of the film and its two year life span made it highly impractical to use the Walker's own 35mm print of *Blue*, which, even outside of technical impossibilities, would have become unprojectable in a relatively short period due to all the scratches and tears it would sustain from continual use. Thus Bruce Jenkins, the Walker's film and video curator at the time, asked the technician Peter Murphy to create a "simulated film presentation" using a color-gelled stage light, a metal gobo, and a flicker generating device.[58] *Blue* had literally become pure light. Its visual aspect was freed from the temporal bounds of the filmstrip, but it also now lacked the material foundation of a filmic body that registers its history through the marks left on its "skin." Unsynched from the image track, the CD soundtrack became the temporal foundation of the work, permitting its continual

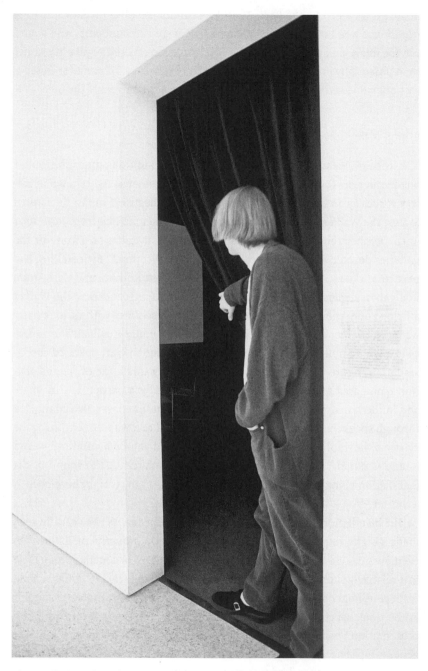

58. Installation of Derek Jarman's *Blue* (1993), Walker Art Center, Minneapolis. Photo by Dan Dennehy for Walker Art Center, Minneapolis. Courtesy of the Walker Art Center.

looping through the simple programming of the player. The looping of Blue transformed its temporal experience for the viewer of the installation. Encountering a work with such a fragmentary structure in medias res opened it up to a more ephemeral mode of reception in which visitors could pass time briefly in Blue and then move on to other works in the gallery. Those visitors who remained for the entire duration of the loop would nevertheless miss two of the film's most intense moments: the cuts between black and blue screens at the beginning and the end of the film, moments that open and close our engagement with the figural void of Blue. In transforming the temporal and spatial qualities of the film, the Walker's installation of Blue subtly shifted its witnessing dynamics. The solidity and relative permanence of the installation allowed it to function as a memorial space for Jarman, who had died six months before its opening, but those same qualities also shifted the ephemeral aspect of the work from the film to the viewer. Cinema's ephemeral nature lies in the temporary occupation of the movie theater by not only the viewer but also the film itself. Cinema is a form of temporary cohabitation of the space by both parties. The looped installation in the gallery, on the other hand, is a physical space that the visitor encounters, chooses to enter, and, most important, decides how long to remain in. Given the searing testimony of Blue, that decision becomes an ethically charged one, framed by the question of how long the visitor is willing to stay and listen.[59]

Blue proved to be a popular choice as well among cultural institutions for programming during the annual Day with(out) Art, since the work's tension between denying image and giving voice aligned well with the event's objective to both mourn and to empower.[60] The installation of Blue on Day with(out) Art in 1999 at the University of Michigan's Museum of Art in Ann Arbor represents a typical example of such programming: Blue was screened on a medium-sized video monitor in the center of a gallery room where all the paintings and sculptures were draped in black cloth.[61] In such a context, the viewer/listener no longer enters the space of Blue, but rather encounters it as an aesthetic object in the space of the gallery, a temporary replacement for the shrouded art objects.

Scott Burnham's staging of Blue at the South Bank Centre in London the following year transformed the spatial dynamics of the work in a more radical fashion. The blue light of the film was projected onto one side of the National Theatre's concrete, cube-shaped Lyttelton Flytower, while the soundtrack was transmitted to wireless headphones available to visitors standing on the Thames embankment (figure 59). This open-air staging of Blue reversed the optics of its theatrical screening. Rather than reflect an intense blue aura

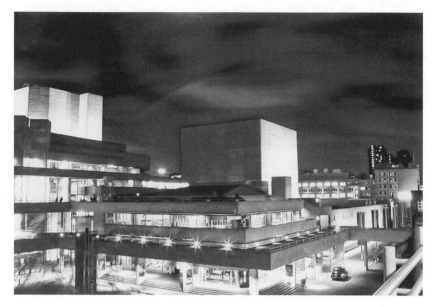

59. Public exhibition of Derek Jarman's *Blue* (1993), 1 December 2000, South Bank Centre, London. Photo by Clifton Steinberg. Courtesy of Scott Burnham.

that blurred the boundary between screen and space, the massive concrete screen appeared to absorb the light, creating an arresting blue-sided cube, a luminous sculptural object in the London cityscape orienting the attention of listener/viewers and passersby alike. Hearing the soundtrack on headphones in the open air provided a new articulation of the film's dynamic relationship between interiority and exteriority. To listen to the close-miked intimacy of Jarman's testimony amid the obliviousness of passing strangers and the wide-open space of the cold winter night provided an embodied sensation for the "incommensurability of experiences" in the AIDS epidemic that I discussed at the very beginning of this book.

In Derek Jarman: Brutal Beauty, the exhibition Isaac Julien curated for London's Serpentine Gallery in 2008, *Blue* returned indoors as part of a project to remember Jarman and to confirm his aesthetic legacy for contemporary British art. In his catalog essay, Julien notes, "It is significant how many of the developments in British art over the past three decades were prefigured in the work of Jarman, who prophetically refused to be tied to a single medium."[62] Julien argues that Jarman's work can function as "a fascinating archive that we can put to use to examine our present" (29). Drawing on the significance that Jarman placed on mise-en-scène in his work, Julien aimed to produce "an immersive environment" in which Jarman's works in

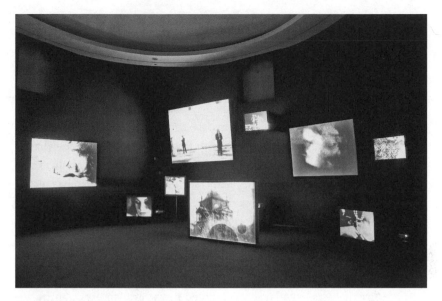

60. Gallery installation of Derek Jarman's Super-8 films in the exhibition Derek Jarman: Brutal Beauty, Serpentine Gallery, London, 2008. Photo by Sylvain Deleu. Courtesy of the Serpentine Gallery.

different media could be experienced in close relation to one another. The exhibition included three film installations. Blue was installed in the first room, while the adjacent room contained randomly placed screens of different size silently displaying Jarman's early Super-8 films (figure 60). The third room contained a projection of Julien's recently completed documentary portrait of Jarman, Derek (2008), which is structured around an extensive talking head interview that Jarman gave with Colin McCabe at Prospect Cottage in 1991 and a public letter Swinton wrote to Jarman in 2002 mourning both his personal loss and his mode of filmmaking practice, which she argues was buried by the wholesale commercialization of British cinema in the 1990s.[63] Rather than pose a problem for the exhibition, the bleeding of sound across the three installations contributed to the immersive effect sought by its curator. Moreover, on a visual level, Derek and the Super-8 films functioned to bring back into sight both the corporeal image of Jarman himself and the rich imagery of his film corpus.

The British DVD release of Blue in 2007 by the art-house distributor Artificial Eye also performed a similar restoration of Jarman's image and his images by packaging Blue together with Glitterbug (1994), a posthumous compilation of Jarman's visually ecstatic Super-8 fragments shot between 1970 and 1986. This archive of avant-garde home movies offers a celebration of his bohemian life and gay world before AIDS, often inscribing Jarman in the image as he captures himself filming in a mirror. But the DVD's digital transfer of *Blue* also functions as an archive of sorts in that it was struck from a used theatrical print and hence registers its own material history in the dirt and scratches preserved in the digital image. Reviewing the DVD release in *Sight and Sound*, Michael Brooke approvingly notes, "A DVD could easily generate a perfect image, but the occasional flashes of dust and dirt that speckle this film-sourced transfer chime well with Jarman's characteristically hand-tooled, defiantly analogue aesthetic."[64] The digital copy will not produce new layers of scratches and dirt on the "skin" of the image. Any scratches or dirt on the disk will produce an altogether different disturbance, a skipping in the playback that will register more noticeably in a fracturing of the sound-track rather than of the image track—a fitting material trope for the gaping historical disjuncture that separates the complex queer structures of feeling toward AIDS in 1993 from the "normalization" of AIDS in the early twenty-first century that has been largely prompted by the availability of antiretro-viral therapies (access to which Jarman missed by a few years).

□

Afterword

Just as the AIDS pandemic has transformed since the heyday of queer AIDS media in the late 1980s and early 1990s, so too has the media ecology in which social movements and moving-image media intersect. The rapid development of digital video technology in the late 1990s enabled greater access to media production. Higher-quality images could be shot on both consumer and semi-professional equipment, while nonlinear editing software gradually deskilled postproduction to the point of it now being a standard feature in software packages for personal computers. The distribution of digital video images has also been revolutionized by a range of online services and practices that include blogs, peer-to-peer file sharing (BitTorrent), video-uploading sites (YouTube), social networks (Facebook), and collaboratively authored sites (wikis). The processes of convergence involved in this new media ecology are not merely technical but also cultural, facilitating the emergence of what Henry Jenkins has dubbed a new "participatory culture" that has the potential to employ the "collective intelligence" of its users for "serious" purposes and not merely leisure activities.[1] Moreover, the hugely expanded capacity of non-professionals to "archive, annotate, appropriate, and recirculate media content" has permitted remix practices to extend well beyond the avant-garde, activist, and subcultural contexts in which they originated.[2] The media piracy now rampant throughout this new media ecology ranges from the radical appropriation of corporate intellectual property to the banality of endless Internet movie parodies and mashups.[3]

So what relationship do queer AIDS media hold to this new media ecology? First, we must acknowledge the variety of ways in which queer AIDS media pioneered practices that have become central to the convergence culture posited by Jenkins. As I discussed in chapter 2, AIDS video activists involved in ACT UP were among the first to exploit the consumer technology of the VHS camcorder for political purposes. Their lo-fi remix aesthetics spliced their own footage with sounds and images appropriated from broadcast news and music videos, a practice now endemic in the genre of the video mashup. In addition to their pervasive appropriation of mainstream media, AIDS video activists demonstrated a strong commitment to sharing resources and footage that could be reused and refunctioned in different tapes. This nonproprietary relationship to moving images has continued in Web-based grass-roots media networks like Indymedia. The circulation of queer AIDS media in different spaces of exhibition, including political meetings, courtrooms, cable-access television, film festivals, classrooms and art galleries, also anticipates the increasing drive toward the multichannel conception and the dissemination of witnessing projects in the new media ecology. For instance, in his discussion of the strategies developed by the human rights organization WITNESS, Sam Gregory cites the multiple media contexts through which NAKAMATA, a Filipino indigenous land rights organization, disseminated video images of human rights abuses against its members.[4] The footage was screened in the indigenous community, presented as direct evidence of the abuses to police authorities, sold to a prominent national news program, edited into a short video documentary uploaded to the WITNESS Web site for a global audience, and featured in Katerina Cizek and Peter Wintonick's Canadian public television documentary, *Seeing Is Believing: Handicams, Human Rights, and the News* (2002).

It is the archival function of the new media ecology that has proven most valuable to queer AIDS media themselves. Video-streamed virtual archives permit continued access to works without official distribution. For example, James Wentzy has maintained a small online archive of Quicktime files on the DIVA TV Web page, which includes Vito Russo's "Why We Fight" speech as well as other speeches, performances, and actions, while Bob Huff recently uploaded onto YouTube his AIDS activist shorts from the late 1980s and early 1990s, works long out of circulation.[5] But the archival practices enabled by the new media ecology are not limited to the construction of online open repositories of existing work. I want to conclude the present study by briefly considering two ongoing witnessing projects in this new media ecology that deploy specific archival practices not only to preserve the legacy of earlier AIDS activism but also to stimulate new forms of activism. The ACT UP Oral History Project and the SILENT|LISTEN project by the sound collective Ultra Red illuminate how radically different archival practices can bear witness to the present moment in the AIDS pandemic and its historically specific exigencies.

In this book, I have traced how queer AIDS media developed a versatile array of formal techniques to reframe the discursive space of testimony in the service of securing effective acts of bearing witness. Their wide-ranging experimentation with the fundamental formal elements of moving-image media—cinematography/videography, editing, mise-en-scène, and sound—demonstrate the absence of a singular formal model for the queer moving image to bear witness to the AIDS crisis. Furthermore, the act of bearing witness to AIDS retains a multiplicity of social, political, psychological, and cultural functions that cannot be reduced to a universal significance, even though they are all grounded in the ethical encounter of intersubjectivity. Queer AIDS media have remained complex acts of bearing witness even as the historically changing imperatives of the AIDS pandemic have transformed their original meaning and value. There is an oft-cited moment in *Fast Trip, Long Drop*, when Jean Carlomusto comments on how activist footage she shot during the heyday of ACT UP has now also become a record of loss.[6] What was once energizing and empowering has become difficult for her to watch, almost a burden. Time itself has reframed militancy as mourning. Thus one of the principal challenges for queer media makers in the third decade of the pandemic has become how to reframe the archive of AIDS cultural activism in ways that generate new acts of bearing witness to the present moment of AIDS and the ongoing historical trauma and crisis it constitutes. The two projects that I have chosen to discuss in this afterword engage that archive and reframe the act of bearing witness through two of the fundamental dynamics of the new media ecology: the logics of the database and the remix.

The ACT UP Oral History Project was initiated by Sarah Schulman and Jim Hubbard, two longtime collaborators who in 1987 founded MIX: The New York Experimental Lesbian and Gay Festival. On the twentieth anniversary of the AIDS pandemic in 2001, Schulman heard a radio story in Los Angeles that framed the history of AIDS in the United States along the lines of "At first, America had trouble with people with AIDS, but then they came around."[7] For Schulman, this story exemplified the country's prevalent cultural narrative about AIDS, which, she argues, has been sustained by highly influential cultural texts, such as Jonathan Demme's film *Philadelphia* (1993), Jonathan Larson's Broadway musical *Rent* (1993), and Tony Kushner's two-part theatrical opus *Angels in America: A Gay Fantasia on National Themes* (1991–92). This narrative of moral education, which allows straight America to overcome its fear of people with AIDS, completely disavows the collective mobilization against AIDS by lesbians and gay men.[8] To prevent such forgetting in the cultural memory of AIDS, Schulman worked with Hubbard to create an oral history of ACT UP, with the ultimate aim of interviewing every surviving member of the original New York chapter, the "mother church" as Schulman calls it.[9] The project's homepage emphasizes its present- and future-oriented acts of witnessing: "We hope that this information will de-mystify the process of making social change, remind us that change can be made, and help us understand how to do it."[10] An e-mail to Dudley Saunders, one of the interviewees, from Bethany Winkler, a quadriplegic activist in the group Unite 2 Fight Paralysis, indicates the practical value of the archive for building other social movements. She reports telling a fellow activist, "These people did it before us and they left an instructional manual!"[11]

Initial funding from the Ford Foundation enabled the ACT UP Oral History Project to interview over sixty members in the first two years, but since then lack of major grant funding has slowed down the project, leaving over one hundred members on the waiting list to be interviewed by 2005.[12] Lasting anywhere from two to four hours, the interviews are recorded on DVCAM, then transferred for preservation to digital Beta tapes, which are likely to last longer than the thinner tape stock of DVCAM. The preservation tapes and VHS viewing copies are then deposited in the New York Public Library. Working with James Wentzy, Hubbard then selects from each interview a short two-to-three-minute clip with a self-contained narrative or anecdote for uploading on the Web site. The clips they have chosen to stream both illuminate diverse aspects of the group and encourage users to order a VHS copy of the interview or to download a free transcript of the whole interview, the hyperlink to which appears next to each clip. This strategy appears to have been successful, since over forty thousand copies of interview transcripts had been downloaded across the globe by 2008.[13] The Web site was designed to be "clean, direct and easy to use," with the numbered testimonies arranged simply in chronological order, displaying a thumbnail image along with the interviewee's name, the date of the interview, and a subject heading to identify the topic covered in the short clip (figure 61).[14]

What happens to the mediated act of bearing witness when it enters the database structure of an online archive like this? Lev Manovich contends that the database has become the symbolic form of the digital age, displacing the linear, narrative logic of analog media.[15] The consequences for testimony are significant. The functional capacities of the database have the power to rationalize testimony into an information mass, which is then subject to the systematic operations of digital asset management, including description, segmentation, categorization, and indexing. This whole process therefore threatens to override or conceal the ethical, affective, and political dimen-

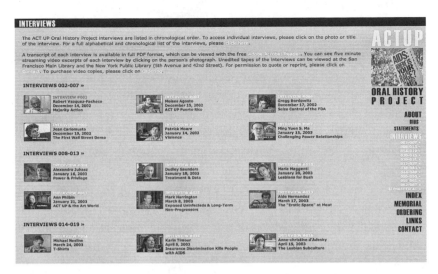

61. From the ACT UP Oral History Project Web site (www.actuporalhistory.org).

sions of testimony. Since these issues have been most extensively examined in relation to the video archive of the Shoah Foundation, it is worth briefly bringing this project into my discussion.[16] It also provides an impression of the kind of institutional production of testimonial databases that the ACT UP Oral History Project is attempting to counter.

Originally founded by Steven Spielberg after completing *Schindler's List* (1993), the archive of the Shoah Foundation now contains over fifty-two thousand testimonies in thirty-two languages. The scope of recording and cataloging this massive amount of testimonies led the foundation to systematize the structure of the interviews. First, the survivors were sent a forty-page preinterview questionnaire that was broken down into standardized narrative stages of Holocaust experience: prewar life, hiding, the ghetto, the camps, liberation, and postwar life. This linear narrative trajectory thus not only streamlined the attribution of catalog descriptors ultimately assigned to each interview but it also served as a de facto template for the interviews themselves. Supported by multimillion-dollar grants, the foundation researched the possibility of using automatic speech recognition technologies to catalog the archive, but ultimately concluded that it could not use them.[17] The foundation did, however, develop a cataloging system that segmented the testimonies at one-minute intervals. Attributing catalog descriptors to these automated sections proved to be a considerably faster process than cataloging by listening for the actual internal structure and integrity of the individual testimony.

These matters are more than mere technical issues of archivization, for they fundamentally shape the interface of the online archive, whether that be the small sample of clips available on the foundation's public Web site or the full archive on restricted access to specific educational institutions through Internet2. The "Online Testimony Viewer" on the public site offers twelve testimonial clips (two for each of the standardized narrative stages) and provides personal information about the witness in a standardized format on the right-hand side of the video window once a testimony has been selected. The very information and organization that makes such an interface supposedly user friendly also opens up the risk of compromising the intersubjective dynamics between witness and viewer, since the testimonial talking head is surrounded by standardized sets of contextualizing information and thumbnail menus of alternate testimonies, which can all foster a distracted mode of viewing.[18]

By contrast, the ACT UP Oral History Project provides a far more straightforward and uncluttered interface that encourages an unstructured browsing of the database far more than narrowly defined search functions. The site will eventually offer a full index of all the interviews, but it will constitute a supplementary means to navigate the archive rather than its primary one. Whereas earlier queer AIDS media used formal experimentation to reframe the discursive space of the speech act itself, particularly the talking head, the ACT UP Oral History Project's Web site reframes the conventional screen interface in which the user navigates access to those talking heads. With their medium–long shot, head-and-shoulders framing, the actual talking heads are not themselves formally radical. Rather, it is the organization of the archive's interface that embodies the radical ethos of ACT UP. Just like the group itself, this interface refuses to frame its participants in terms of hierarchy, role designation, or authorized expertise. Like the group's meetings, it brings together "a diverse, non-partisan group of individuals."

Admittedly, the very small size of ACT UP's testimonial archive in comparison to that of the Shoah Foundation partly explains why it can use a much simpler and less managed interface. But we must not forget that this issue of size is connected to the grass-roots ethos of Schulman's and Hubbard's project. Schulman acknowledges that, in researching video testimony archives during the planning stages of the ACT UP project, the Fortunoff Video Archive for Holocaust Testimonies at Yale proved more influential than the Shoah Foundation, which she characterizes as "a consensus response to Holocaust revisionism."[19] The Fortunoff archive was also established as a grass-roots initiative to counteract what many Holocaust survivors perceived as the distortion of their experience in NBC's landmark 1980 television mini-series *Holocaust*.

Both being long-term members of ACT UP, Hubbard and Schulman are clearly insiders to the testimonial community they are interviewing. The solicitation and collection of the interviews replicated ACT UP's own grass-roots organizing in existing social networks in that Hubbard and Schulman simply asked all the activists they knew and then asked those activists to suggest further names. The project therefore needed no public invitation to testify. Moreover, Schulman has been writing about ACT UP in a variety of literary genres for many years, while Hubbard has become the world's lead-ing authority on AIDS activist film and video, having collected, preserved, and cataloged the AIDS activist video collection now in the New York Public Library. In fact, both Hubbard and Schulman have planned documentary and literary projects based on the testimonial archive, confirming that effective acts of bearing witness beget further such acts. Hubbard is currently edit-ing a feature-length documentary entitled *United in Anger: A History of ACT UP*, which brings together archival footage with interviews from the project. Under a strict division of labor, Schulman carries out all the interviews for the project, while Hubbard oversees the preservation, cataloging, and dissemi-nation of the interviews. After every interview has been cataloged and tran-scribed, they meet to discuss the issues it has raised. In this way, Schulman explains, they are "constantly reconceptualizing the project." This process of ongoing feedback and assessment allows Schulman to incorporate new ques-tions into the subsequent interviews as she and Hubbard discover previously unacknowledged issues in the group's history.[20] Along with Schulman's al-ready extensive insider knowledge of the history and experience of ACT UP, this process ensures that the testimonial relation between Schulman and her interviewees is grounded in mutual respect, recognition, and a commitment to exploring the complexity of the group's political, social, and psychological dynamics.

Whereas Schulman and Hubbard practice a fluid, process-oriented inter-view technique to create a permanent testimonial archive of ACT UP's history and the experience of its members, Ultra Red has undertaken a set of rigor-ously constructed archival procedures to create SILENT|LISTEN as a project that paradoxically resists solidification into a permanent archival object. De-spite its systematic use of archival discourse — "testimony," "statements," "the record," and "the minutes" — the project remains thoroughly rooted in the durational process of conceptual art and the ephemeral quality of per-formance art. SILENT|LISTEN emerged from the attempt in 2004 to revive the Los Angeles chapter of ACT UP.[21] During a day-long organizing retreat, a screening of *Voices from the Front* elicited a melancholy response from the activists present: "For most of us, even the long-time survivors, the images of outrage seemed distant and remote."[22] The members of Ultra Red involved in this resuscitation of ACT UP concluded that the affective dynamics of the present moment had to be reflected on and analyzed before any direct action could be taken. Echoing Douglas Crimp in his critique of *Voices from the Front* a decade earlier, Ultra Red doubts that "restaging the art of outrage from the early '90s will succeed in an alchemical change in our disappointment" (90). The collective similarly remains suspicious of "cathartic performances of lament" for a lost radicalism in a post 9/11 culture where grief is quickly transmogrified into vengeance. Ultra Red thus pursues a spatial practice—what it calls an "affective architecture"—aimed at collectively constructing a critical discourse among PWAs, AIDS activists, case managers, and service providers through a collaborative process that resists resolution (92).

SILENT|LISTEN invokes the AIDS activist slogan "Silence=Death" but reframes it through Paulo Freire's pedagogic principle of the "discipline of silence," which avows silence as the condition for listening and listening as the condition for action, since it enables genuine reflection and analysis.[23] "Listening, if you engage in it actively," claims the Ultra Red member Robert Semper, "can reveal the structures of power that determine what actually exists in a space, what gets amplified in a space, what becomes the agenda for future action."[24] The project has thus involved a series of performances at art institutions across North America since April 2005, in which the collective creates procedures for activists, community organizers, care providers, and members of the public to bear witness to their experience of AIDS after twenty-five years of the pandemic.[25] With each iteration of the performance, its rigorous structuring procedure becomes modified to permit every new performance to engage with the testimonial record produced by the previous one.

To create the conditions for listening, the performances all start with John Cage's famous conceptual work of pure silence, *Four Minutes and Thirty-Three Seconds* (1952). The silence is then collectively evaluated as the facilitator asks four questions to individuals in the room: "What did you hear? When was the last time you were in this space or one like it? What is the relationship between this space and [the name of the city where the performance is held]? When was the last time you talked about AIDS in this space or one like it?" Such questions reveal how the silent, contemplative copresence of bodies in space can bear witness as powerfully as spoken words themselves. Four invited speakers from local AIDS organizations then individually come to the microphone table to "enter a statement into the record." After each statement has been completed, the facilitator plays back its recording through a variety of digital sound-processing filters that fragment, distort, and repeat the voice. Each time a statement is replayed electronically, it is mixed into the recording of the previous statement, so that by the end of the four statements, the recording has become a dense aural palimpsest, constituting the "minutes" of the performance. The performance concludes with an open invitation to the public to enter statements into the record, which are recorded but not played back during the performance. At each new performance the "minutes" (the remixed statements) of the previous performance are played back before new statements are entered into the record.

After the completion of seven performances of SILENT|LISTEN, Ultra Red reconfigured the performance for the Sixteenth International AIDS Conference in Toronto in August 2006 by inviting the speakers from the previous performances to join international conference participants assembled at seven separate tables. The "minutes" of the previous performance in Carbondale were played back simultaneously, but filtered and pitched differently at each table. Since the tables also had their microphones live during this "review of the minutes," the room filled with "a tremendous wall of feedback that circulated and phased between the audio-monitors placed on the tables."[26] The statements were then entered into the record simultaneously at each table, producing a cacophony of sound. Like Jarman's Blue, the participants' embodied experience of sound and the recognition of relationality and alterity it engendered were as important to the performances as hearing what each witness said. Remixing testimony in this manner permits the affective architecture of the project to be realized.

Moving the project beyond live performance to other platforms, Ultra Red released the minutes of the first seven performances of SILENT|LISTEN as a CD that could be freely downloaded from the group's online archive and produced a gallery installation in conjunction with the conference at the Art Gallery of Ontario in Toronto.[27] For the gallery installation, the collective listened to the raw recordings of every statement from the seven performances in search of "moments when the speaker enunciated some affect, a feeling, or registered affect within a metaphoric figure."[28] Seven of these moments were then ripped from their semantic and syntactic context, reduced to their most concise enunciation, and spliced into a repetitive loop. These excerpted statements included utterances such as "And this question frustrates me to no end [pause] [breath]"; "But every time I'm with a man I always worry [pause]"; and "I'm not pissed off or anything [short pause] it obviously still affects my life." In the installation, each looped utterance was played simultaneously on a single audio monitor placed on each of the seven tables in the gallery (figure 62).

Ultra Red subsequently used the transcriptions of six of these loops as the basis for a further gallery installation, Untitled (For Six Voices), in the Make Art/Stop AIDS exhibition at the Fowler Museum in Los Angeles in 2008. Introducing moving images into the project for the first time, the collective filmed six activist colleagues performing a continuous two-minute recitation of each loop, while the choreographer Taisha Paggett directed their visual gestures. Six flat-screen video monitors were hung in the exhibition space as though portraits on a gallery wall (figure 63). Facing the video monitors were six filing cabinets mounted on concrete plinths, each labeled with the name of a different "institution": politics, media, medicine, religion, scholarship, and business. Reframing a highly influential project from the archive of AIDS cultural activism, these labels are direct citations from Let the Record Show . . . , the AIDS activist installation mounted in 1987 in the window of New York City's New Museum of Contemporary Art. Whereas the six statements cited from each institution named in Let the Record Show . . . exposed the dominant ideological construction of AIDS in its first decade, the labeled cabinets in Untitled (For Six Voices) serve as a kind of anticipatory archive—a repository for conceiving new forms of AIDS activism in the third decade of the pandemic. Ultra Red has developed new collaborative performances using these six video testimonies that will collectively generate material to fill those filing cabinets.

The six talking heads of Untitled (For Six Voices) arguably constitute the most complex instance of reframing yet performed by queer AIDS media. Each utterance has resulted from a series of human and electronic processes of listening, recording, remixing, transcribing, condensing, and repeating. These utterances should not be seen as a sentimentalizing reduction to pure affect. Nor do they serve to produce catharsis, stipulate specific political demands, or correct the historical record. Rather, they demand that their audience listen to them and in listening to these dense audiovisual palimpsests of individual and collective affect generate the conditions for new acts of bearing witness that respond to the complex political, economic, medical, and cultural exigencies of the present moment in the AIDS pandemic. If Ann Cvetko-

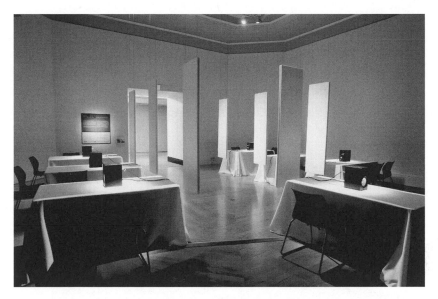

62. Ultra Red, SILENT|LISTEN: *The Record*, 2006, gallery installation, Art Gallery of Ontario, Toronto. Photo by Art Gallery of Ontario. Courtesy of Ultra Red.

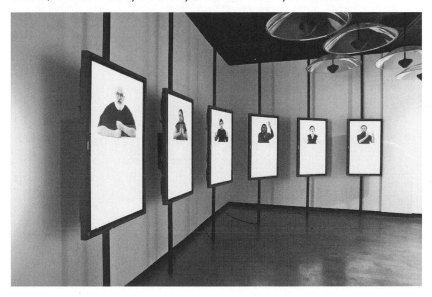

63. Ultra Red, *Untitled (For Six Voices)*, 2008, gallery installation, Fowler Museum at the University of California, Los Angeles, 2008. Photo by Reed Hutchinson. Courtesy of Ultra Red and the Fowler Museum.

vich is right in arguing that the affects associated with trauma may serve as the basis for new public cultures, such as the one that arose around AIDS activism in the late 1980s, then Ultra Red's SILENT|LISTEN project powerfully demonstrates how those public cultures must continue to acknowledge the historicity of those affects and to consider how they may be reframed if they are to become enabling rather than debilitating.

□

Notes

Introduction

1 Fever in the Archive: AIDS Activist Videotapes from the Royal S. Marks Collection was curated by Jim Hubbard and consisted of eight programs that ran between 1–9 December 2000 at the Guggenheim Museum in New York. The series was subsequently shown in Minneapolis, San Francisco, Milwaukee, and London.

2 Crimp noted in a 1991 interview how "the incommensurability of experiences" contributed to the traumatizing effect of the epidemic on queer people: "Certain people are experiencing the AIDS crisis while the society as a whole doesn't appear to be experiencing it at all. Richard Goldstein said that it's as if we were living through the Blitz, except that nobody else knows it's happening." Caruth and Keenan, "AIDS Crisis Is Not Over," 256.

3 The Estate Project for Artists with AIDS, a nonprofit organization dedicated to preserving the cultural legacy of the AIDS crisis, hired the filmmaker and archivist Jim Hubbard in the late 1990s to collect and oversee the preservation of AIDS activist video produced in the United States. Hubbard eventually collected over two thousand hours of completed works and video footage (mostly from makers in New York City), which were then deposited in the New York Public Library, the only institution willing to accommodate the collection in its entirety. One thousand hours of the collection were remastered in Beta SP for preservation and VHS dubs made available to the public for screening in the library. Full listings of the collection's holdings are available in the library's online finding aid (www.nypl .org/research/chss/spe/rbk/faids/aidsvideo.pdf).

4 Given that I move between analyses of films, videos, and moving-image installations, I am using the term *media* as the plural of *medium*, rather than in the totalizing (and vague) singularity often referred to as "the media."

5 For example, three of the major works of AIDS cultural analysis situate John Greyson's groundbreaking AIDS musical *Zero Patience* (1993) within specific battles over AIDS representation, but they offer only a brief critical analysis of the film itself. See Juhasz, AIDS TV, 129–30; Treichler, *How to Have Theory in an*

Epidemic, 312–14; and Crimp, Melancholia and Moralism, 125–28. On the other hand, most of the sustained analyses of Tom Joslin and Peter Friedman's Silverlake Life: The View from Here (1993) refrain from situating the film within queer AIDS media. See Phelan, Mourning Sex, 153–73; Egan, "Encounters in Camera"; and Lane, Autobiographical Documentary in America, 84–91.

6 Felman and Laub, Testimony, 80; emphasis original.

7 Caruth, Trauma, 8.

8 In the context of cultural memory, Marita Sturken makes a related argument about the distinctive temporality of AIDS as a historical trauma when she contends that "the politics of remembering AIDS can never be detached from the fact that the epidemic is still killing people. . . . Cultural memory in the context of AIDS is not about achieving closure but about keeping any sense of closure at bay." Sturken, Tangled Memories, 175–76. Like Ann Cvetkovich, I find Sturken's analysis of the cultural memory of AIDS within a national frame both useful and limiting to my project. Although it provides an important conceptual structure for understanding the dynamics of dominant AIDS representation, it also tends to marginalize or blur the distinctiveness of cultural production—such as queer AIDS media—that primarily circulates within counterpublics established in opposition to the "national public sphere." See Cvetkovich, Archive of Feelings, 162.

9 Cvetkovich, Archive of Feelings, 160.

10 When Frameline, the San Francisco–based nonprofit organization for lesbian, gay, bisexual, and transgender (LGBT) media arts, organized the "Persistence of Vision" conference in 2001 to assess the state of contemporary queer media, the single panel dedicated to AIDS media suffered the indignity of panelists outnumbering audience members. Furthermore, when the "Moving Image Review" editors of GLQ published a "Queer Film and Video Festival Forum" with ten international festival curators in 2005, not a single mention was made of HIV/AIDS. See Straayer and Waugh, "Queer Film and Video Festival Forum."

11 The topic was the subject of an online symposium, "The Unfashionability of AIDS," curated in 2000 by Robert Atkins for Artery: The AIDS—Arts Forum. See also Román, "Not-About-AIDS."

12 For a more detailed analysis of such advertisements, see Bordowitz, "Guest List for a Cocktail Party."

13 See Sullivan, "When Plagues End"; and Rofes, Dry Bones Breathe. Rofes's adoption of the term was inspired by the sociological research of Gary Dowsett and David McInnes, which observed how Australian gay men in the mid-1990s were no longer experiencing AIDS as "a communal crisis" and increasingly adopting "judicious risk-taking" as they adapted to "living with" the epidemic as a permanent aspect of gay identity. Dowsett and McInnes, "Gay Community."

14 Crimp offers an incisive critical response to these strategies in Melancholia and Moralism, 1–27.

15 See Dangerous Bedfellows, Policing Public Sex.

16 See Freeman, "In Search of Death"; Denizet-Lewis, "Double Lives on the Down Low"; and Specter, "Higher Risk."

17 See Tomso, "Bug Chasing." David Halperin has also boldly proposed the need to understand gay male subjectivity in the third decade of the AIDS epidemic outside the framework of psychology and psychoanalysis. In his recent book, *What Do Gay Men Want?*, he turns to Jean Genet's nonpsychoanalytic concept of queer abjection as a frame that potentially escapes the ever-present risk of repathologizing gay subjectivity.

18 For example, Anderson Cooper began a brief segment on CNN *News* about the documentary with the following sensationalist introduction: "Believe it or not, there are actually some people who want to get the AIDS virus. The name on the street for some of these people is bug chasers. And the virus itself, they call the gift. That's also the name of a new film that's getting a lot of attention. It's about a subject we are sure you may find uncomfortable, even shocking. But it's also a subject we should not ignore." CNN *News*, 6 June 2003.

19 Crimp, *AIDS Cultural Analysis*, 15.

20 See Green, "When Political Art Mattered"; Deitcher, "What Does Silence Equal Now?"; and Patten, "The Thrill Is Gone."

21 Some of these influences and continuities are discussed in Shepard and Hayduk, *From ACT UP to the WTO*.

22 In the introduction to their collection *Queer Looks* (1993), Martha Gever, John Greyson, and Pratibha Parmar declared, "When we started this book in 1989, three people from three cities, we knew we were living in three very queer places. Places of new possibilities and shocking repercussions. Places of unprecedented opportunities and unbridled repressions. In our particular cases: London, New York, Toronto. We knew from travel, from work, from networks of friends and colleagues, that there were lots of other queer places, north and south, east and west. Very queer places. Each particular, each idiosyncratic. Their experiences were nevertheless similar to ours" (xiii).

23 See Crimp, *Melancholia and Moralism*; Cvetkovich, "Video, AIDS, and Activism"; Danzig, "Acting Up"; Saalfield and Navarro, "Shocking Pink Praxis"; Greyson, "Strategic Compromises"; Bordowitz, *AIDS Crisis Is Ridiculous*; Fung, "Shortcomings"; Juhasz, *AIDS TV*; and Kalin, "Flesh Histories."

24 The establishment of Out in Africa, Cape Town's gay and lesbian film festival, in 1994 secured a South African presence in the transnational queer counterpublic.

25 Alexandra Juhasz uses the term *alternative AIDS media* to describe the "use of media to speak from within and to a politicized community" that formed in response to the AIDS crisis. Juhasz, *AIDS TV*, 6.

26 In an early analysis of the media representation of AIDS, Simon Watney argued that "Aids is not only a medical crisis on an unparalleled scale, it involves a crisis of representation itself, a crisis over the entire framing of knowledge about the human body and its capacities for sexual pleasure." Watney, *Policing Desire*, 9.

27 Greyson, "Strategic Compromises," 61. Whereas Greyson chose to use the term AIDS *tapes* to describe both videos and films as "a bit of revenge against decades of thoughtless critics who say 'film' when they mean both video and film" (73), I have chosen to use to the broader term *queer* AIDS *media*, since I not only move back and forth between film and video but I also examine several works, like Derek Jarman's *Blue* (1993), that moved across different media platforms.

28 Raw footage and audiovisual documentation accounts for a substantial portion of the AIDS Activist Videotape Collection at the New York Public Library. For Hubbard, finding an institution willing to accept this type of historically valuable but often institutionally neglected material became a major priority for the project. See Hubbard, "Report."

29 Juhasz, AIDS TV, 3.

30 Quoted in Gott, *Don't Leave Me This Way*, 28.

31 In her introduction to the show's catalog, Goldin indicated the dual drives to attest and to contest that were present in these acts of bearing witness: "I have also witnessed the community take care of its own, nurse its sick, bury its dead, mourn its losses, and continue to fight for each others' lives. We will not vanish." Goldin, *Witnesses*, 5. Goldin's show generated national controversy when John Frohnmayer, the chairman of the National Endowment of the Arts, attempted to pull funding from it, which he deemed "too political." See Meyer, *Outlaw Representation*, 244–47.

32 In legal and historical discourses, witnessing produces a form of evidentiary record; in various religious contexts, it performs faith through the believer testifying, at times to the point of martyrdom, to the truth of the sacred word or the existence of a divine being (for example, the life of Christ); and in certain psychoanalytic frameworks, it allows the witness to gain ownership and a level of psychic control over a traumatic past that has eluded narrativization and thus been denied prior psychic incorporation as an experience. For the major studies of testimony and bearing witness in these fields, see Felman and Laub, *Testimony*; Coady, *Testimony*; Loftus, *Eyewitness Testimony*; and Trites, *New Testament Concept of Witness*.

33 Video-mediated testimony has begun to be accepted in some courts, but only in special conditions, such as rape cases, when the bodily copresence of perpetrator and victim may cause psychological harm to the latter.

34 The Greek word for witness is *martis*, and it became closely associated in early Christian postcanonical literature with the persecution of believers, thus taking on the modern meaning of *martyr*. See Trites, *New Testament Concept of Witness*, 222–30.

35 McBride, *Impossible Witnesses*, 5.

36 My distinction here between bearing witness and confessing is indebted to Gregg Bordowitz's essay, "Dense Moments," in which he argues, "Through testimony one bears witness to one's own experiences to one's self. Through confession one relinquishes responsibility for bearing witness to and for one's self with the

hope that some force greater than one's self will bear away the responsibilities for one's actions. . . . The testimony is offered to an other, who listens. The confession is posed to an other, who has the power to punish or forgive. They are two distinctly different acts because the precondition for the testimony is a historical cause and the precondition for the confession is a subjective cause. . . . A testimony that leads to confession recapitulates repression. A testimony performed successfully can lead toward liberation. (An idealization.)" Bordowitz, The AIDS Crisis Is Ridiculous, 116–17.

37 Like Bordowitz's, my differentiation between testimony and confession is grounded in a Foucauldian conceptualization of the latter act that stresses its function as a regulatory and disciplinary apparatus of modernity. In his analysis of a number of "first person video confessions" that have been circulated in "nonhegemonic contexts," Michael Renov argues, on the other hand, for a critical reconsideration of confessional dynamics in independent video practices. He contends that "video confessions" in which the positions of self and other, confessor and confessant, remain fluid and reciprocal afford "a glimpse of a more utopian trajectory in which cultural production and consumption mingle and interact, and in which the media facilitate understanding across the gaps of human difference, rather than simply capitalize on those differences in a rush to spectacle." Renov, Subject of Documentary, 215.

38 Agamben, Remnants of Auschwitz, 17.

39 The debate in historiography about experience as evidence and the multitude of legal cases over "false memory syndrome" bespeak the contestation of the witness as superstes in the discursive fields of history and law. See Scott, "Evidence of Experience"; Haaken, "Recovery of Memory, Fantasy, and Desire"; and Walker, Trauma Cinema, 3–29.

40 In many religions, the believer's faith may compel him or her to bear witness to the event of a prophet's or a divine being's life as the means through which to share the truth of the Absolute, to pass it on to others. The religious concept of witness can be found in Christianity, Judaism, Buddhism, and Islam.

41 Dori Laub explains that "the emergence of the narrative which is being listened to—and heard—is, therefore, the process and the place wherein the cognizance, the 'knowing' of the event is given birth to. The listener, therefore, is a party to the creation of knowledge de novo." Felman and Laub, Testimony, 57.

42 For a more extensive discussion of the image as witness, see my coauthored introduction to Guerin, Image and the Witness, 1–20.

43 See Loftus, Eyewitness Testimony.

44 Bazin, What Is Cinema?, 1:13. As one recent photography textbook asserts, "Photography, as witness to history, gives testimony in the court of public opinion. Photojournalists are the bearers of that witness." Chapnick, Truth Needs No Ally, 13. See also Monk, Photographs That Changed the World.

45 It is for this reason that the historian Peter Burke calls images "mute witnesses." Burke, Eyewitnessing, 14.

46 Moreover, the discursive imbrication, particularly in television and photojournalism, of homosexuality and Africa as the moral etiology of the disease established a persistent conflation of AIDS with homosexuality and with Africa. In their analyses of AIDS discourses in the early years of the epidemic, Simon Watney and Cindy Patton have both examined the "metaphoric cross-inscription of bodies" around constructions of "black"/"heterosexual" AIDS in Africa and "white"/"homosexual" AIDS in the United States. White American homosexuals were posited as anally fixated, abject others who had transformed their bodies into the equivalent of a third world sewer overflowing with dirt and disease, while black African heterosexuals were queered through their allegedly greater practice of anal sex (sodomy being overdetermined by homosexuality). The cross-inscription of these cultural myths helped produce the long-standing psychic disavowal of white heterosexual AIDS in the United States. These highly specularized bodies were placed in the discursive service of making legible the healthy social body of the (white, heterosexual) "American nation." See Patton, *Inventing AIDS*, 77–97; and Watney, *Practices of Freedom*, 103–20.

47 Nichols, *Representing Reality*, 229–66.

48 Janet Walker makes a similar point in *Trauma Cinema*, 189–90.

49 See Watney, *Practices of Freedom*, 46–59.

50 Crimp, *Melancholia and Moralism*, 84–107; and Grover, "Visible Lesions," 39–42.

51 Quoted in Crimp, *Melancholia and Moralism*, 87.

52 Watney, "Representing AIDS," 185.

53 Juhasz, *AIDS TV*, 6.

54 Juhasz's critical redemption of such "reflexive realism" is grounded in the double movement she notes in its use by alternative AIDS media: "The mimetic representation of an alternative reality becomes a self-conscious or deconstructive act which challenges the 'naturalness' of the dominant reality. However in alternative documentaries the distance of realist style is as often self-consciously erased, just as it is in traditional documentary, so as to inspire identification with the reality being pictured." Juhasz, *AIDS TV*, 76.

55 Nichols quoted in Juhasz, *AIDS TV*, 78. Queer AIDS media are not unique in their reliance on a constitutive tension between contrary formal dynamics. In her analysis of how experimental documentaries about the Holocaust and incest necessarily articulate the irreconcilable contradiction between historiography and traumatic memory, Janet Walker argues that such "trauma cinema" ranges back and forth "across a continuum, with the most veridical forms of documentary to the right and fiction films in which there are invented characters and stories to the left." Walker, *Trauma Cinema*, 24.

56 See Sobchack, "Inscribing Ethical Space," and Nichols, *Representing Reality*, chap. 3. Sobchack writes, "What eventually gets on the screen and is judged by those of us who view it in the audience is the visible constitution and inscription of an 'ethical space' which subtends both filmmaker and spectator alike. It is a space which takes on the contours of the events which occur within it and the

actions which make it visible. It is both a space of immediate encounter and mediate action." "Inscribing Ethical Space," 298.

57 Levinas, "Ethics as First Philosophy."

58 Levin, *Philosopher's Gaze*, 251.

59 As Martin Jay puts it, "Levinas explicitly tied ethics to the Hebraic taboo on visual representation and contrasted it again and again to the Hellenic fetish of sight, intelligible form, and luminosity." Jay, *Downcast Eyes*, 555.

60 Levin, *Philosopher's Gaze*, 241.

61 Levinas elaborates this most fully in his late work, *Totality and Infinity*.

62 Levinas writes, "Knowledge as perception, concept, comprehension, refers back to an act of grasping." Levinas, "Ethics as First Philosophy," 76.

63 Michael Renov has suggested that documentary studies approach Levinas's notion of the encounter as a kind of "ethical asymptote, which as Webster's tells us is a straight line always approaching but never meeting a curve, a tangent at infinity." While he acknowledges that "no documentative practice can meet the ethical standards of the encounter, stimulating a mode of thought better than knowledge," Renov does contend that "it may be useful to measure particular instances against the metaphysical limit" of the encounter, given that there are "significant ethical distinctions to be made among media forms." Renov, *Subject of Documentary*, 156–57.

64 See Crimp, *Melancholia and Moralism*, 83–107. I also discuss the documentary representation of global AIDS and its discourse of faciality in my essay, "Face of AIDS."

65 Cvetkovich, *Archive of Feelings*, 195.

66 New social movement (NSM) theory prioritizes the significance of representational politics and identity formation over resource mobilization in the study of social movements. For an analysis of AIDS activism as a new social movement, see Gamson, "Silence, Death, and the Invisible Enemy."

67 To name this period as the "queer moment" in lesbian and gay history is not, however, to restrict practices that may be understood as queer only to this time period. Lesbian and gay studies have in fact dedicated much energy to tracing genealogies for queer social, cultural, and sexual practices.

68 Rich, "New Queer Cinema." Rich's initial conception of a New Queer Cinema has been both thoroughly contested and revised by queer makers, critics, and scholars: it prioritized narrative filmmaking (albeit inflected by experimentation); it emphasized the medium of film at the expense of video (a more financially accessible medium to more marginalized makers); it downplayed the significance of queer shorts (a form that seldom led to the kind of critical attention needed to recognize a "new cinema" movement); it marginalized works by women and people of color (by fetishizing white male film auteurs such as Tom Kalin and Todd Haynes); it underestimated the role played by lesbian and gay film festivals (by overstating the value of festival recognition at Sundance and Toronto); and it overplayed the newness of the work (by treating the abundant allusions to queer

and feminist antecedents like Jean Genet, Andy Warhol, Kenneth Anger, Chantal Akerman, and Yvonne Rainer as playful postmodern intertextuality rather than as aesthetic and thematic influences and continuities). The critique of Rich's article began with responses from British-based makers Derek Jarman, Prathibha Parmar, Isaac Julien, and Constantine Giannaris, which were printed in the same issue of *Sight and Sound* (Smyth, "Queer Questions," 34–35). For a wider range of critical perspectives on New Queer Cinema, see Aaron, *New Queer Cinema*.

69 Arroyo, "Death, Desire, and Identity."

70 See Reid, "UnSafe at Any Distance"; and Rhodes, "Allegory, Mise-en-Scène, AIDS."

71 I have also chosen not to discuss safer-sex videos in this book. With its complex relations between an ethical and a (dominant) pedagogic address, as well as its often fraught relations with public funders and the porn industry, the genre deserves its own separate study. For an important discussion of these issues, see Patton, "Safe Sex and the Pornographic Vernacular."

72 See Butler, "Critically Queer"; and Sedgwick, "Queer Performativity."

73 See Fuss, *Inside/Out*, 1–10.

74 Crimp, *Melancholia and Moralism*, 192; emphasis original.

75 See Cvetkovich, *Archive of Feelings*, chap. 5.

76 I am borrowing the term *structures of feeling* from Raymond Williams, who used it to name the affective aspects of social experience. I discuss this more fully at the beginning of chapter 5. See Williams, *Marxism and Literature*, 132–33.

77 Waugh, "Mike Hoolboom," 420.

78 Thomas Waugh remarks, "Hoolboom, the social subject may or may not be bisexual, but Hoolboom the filmmaker is here and queer." Waugh, "Mike Hoolboom," 426.

79 Although it borrows Russo's opening rhetorical gambit ("If I'm dying from anything . . ."), this part of the text was written by Hoolboom.

80 Viewers may not have recognized the precise words of Russo's 1988 speech, but they would nevertheless have recognized the rhetoric of combat and survival that marked that era of AIDS activism.

81 David Román argues that AIDS vigils and marches in the early 1980s should be seen as precursors to the radicality of ACT UP tactics rather than in contrast to them, as has often been claimed. See Román, *Acts of Intervention*, 1–43. For an analysis of the AIDS Quilt and its politics, see Sturken, *Tangled Memories*, 183–219; and Hawkins, "Naming Names."

82 For an analysis of this debate, see Crimp, *Melancholia and Moralism*, 196–202.

83 Grover, AIDS, 3.

84 Crimp, "Mourning and Militancy."

85 Laura U. Marks makes a similar point in her analysis of the film: "The identity of a person with AIDS [is] dispersed across many subjects with whom one might identify." Marks, *Touch*, 99. However, Marks fails to acknowledge how Hoolboom's own coming out as a PWA is refracted through his appropriation of Russo's speech.

86 Marks notes that "the look itself becomes dispersed in the way many of the images themselves break down or lose legibility. The battered sepia-toned film of a stumbling bride suggests an unrecoverable past time." Marks, *Touch*, 99.

87 Dovey, *Freakshow*.

1. Historical Trauma and Talking Heads

1 See Waugh, "Walking on Tippy Toes."

2 For a discussion of the significance of Austin's concept of the performative to poststructuralist theory and cultural studies, see the introduction to Parker and Segdwick, *Performativity and Performance*, 1–18.

3 Bruzzi, *New Documentary*, 153–54.

4 Nichols, *Blurred Boundaries*, 99.

5 It is arguably this faith in filmed testimony that Errol Morris submits to persistent skepticism in his films through their technological and rhetorical reorganization of the talking head interview. For a discussion of his films in the context of witnessing, see Orgeron and Orgeron, "Megatronic Memories."

6 Margaret Morse analyzes how direct address functions in the "discourse space" of television in her article, "Talk, Talk, Talk." For discursive analyses of the documentary interview, television news broadcasting, and the talk show, see Grindon, "Q & A"; Stam, "Television News and Its Spectator"; and Shattuc, *Talking Cure*.

7 Lesage, "Political Aesthetics of the Feminist Documentary Film."

8 Juhasz, AIDS TV, 233.

9 Paul Arthur has addressed the relationship between film and portraiture in his illuminating article, "No Longer Absolute," in which he argues that 1960s documentary and avant-garde cinema provided the specific contexts in which the portrait film could fully come into being as a distinct cinematic genre. While Arthur's analysis of films by Stan Brakhage, Andy Warhol, D. A. Pennebaker, and others elucidates the dynamics of performance inherent to modern portraiture, he says little about the equally important issue of the portrait as a function of modern disciplinary power.

10 Sekula, "Body and the Archive," 6.

11 See Tagg, *Burden of Representation*, 34–65.

12 Sekula discusses both scientists in depth in "Body and the Archive."

13 Although contemporary documentary constructions of otherness rarely take on explicitly repressive functions, as they did in nineteenth-century photographic pathology and ethnography, they do participate in the maintenance of the normative and nationalized social identity of the so-called general population, which subsumes the news anchor and his or her presumed audience, as well as the vox populi interviewees incorporated into news reports.

14 On the "victim tradition" in Griersonian documentaries, see Winston, *Claiming the Real*, 40–47.

15 John Tagg argues that the realist ideology of transparency in dominant modes of cultural representation depends on a continual process of citation and intertextuality: "Realism is a social practice of representation, an overall form of discursive production, a normality which allows a strictly delimited range of variations. It works by the controlled and limited recall of a reservoir of similar 'texts,' by a constant repetition, a constant cross-echoing. By such 'silent quotation,' a relation is established between the realist 'text' and other 'texts' from which it differs and to which it defers." Tagg, *Burden of Representation*, 99.

16 See Foucault, *Archaeology of Knowledge*. For an analysis of the concept of the archive that negotiates such empirical and abstract definitions, see Osborne, "Ordinariness of the Archive."

17 Foucault, *Archaeology of Knowledge*, 128–29.

18 Foucault, "Politics and the Study of Discourse," 63–64.

19 Foucault, *Archaeology of Knowledge*, 130.

20 The early years of Channel Four provided important opportunities for queer makers in light of the new channel's mandate to support independent producers and to address communities underrepresented on the three existing national channels in Britain. This included the first gay and lesbian series on British televison, *Out on Tuesday*, which broadcast new work by Pratibha Parmar, Stuart Marshall, and Isaac Julien. However, this commitment did not go unnoticed by Thatcherites and quickly became a significant political issue by the mid-1980s. For a discussion of these issues from the perspective of the filmmakers, see Chamberlain et al., "Filling the Lack."

21 Marshall, "Contemporary Political Use of Gay History," 65.

22 Martha Gever, "Pictures of Sickness: Stuart Marshall's *Bright Eyes*."

23 Marshall provides a more detailed account of this discursive genealogy in his essay "Picturing Deviancy."

24 White, "Stuart Marshall."

25 In addition, Marshall used much of the material from *Bright Eyes* in a multichannel video installation, *A Journal of the Plague Year* (1984), which was initially shown in the Video '84 exhibition in Montreal, and later in the Oxford Museum of Modern Art's 1990 survey exhibition Signs of the Times: A Decade of Video, Films, and Slide-Tape Installation in Britain, 1980–1990.

26 In 1989, *Bright Eyes* screened at two highly influential events on alternative AIDS media: Jan Zita Grover's exhibition AIDS: The Artist's Response at the Wexner Center in Columbus, Ohio; and "How Do I Look?," a conference and screening series organized by the Bad Object-Choices collective at Anthology Film Archives in New York.

27 The first memoir to recount the personal experience of the Nazi persecution of homosexuals, Heinz Heger's *Die Männer mit dem rosa Winkel* (*The Men with the Pink Triangle*), was published in 1972 and appeared in English translation in 1980.

28 For a historical account of such techniques of disguise in the early television representation of homosexuality in the United States, see Tropiano, *Prime Time Closet*,

1–12. Gever reads this scene's complexities in terms of the tropes of light and shadow in the historical representation of homosexuality and disease, a theme around which the video circles repeatedly in part 1 (Gever, "Pictures of Sickness," 122–23).

29 Marshall, "Contemporary Political Use of Gay History," 67.

30 Although the Vietnam War provided a powerful analogy for many AIDS activists to mobilize in the United States, both in terms of the appalling number of dead and the possibility of radicalization and mass protest against the state, I have found no works of queer AIDS media that substantially engage with this analogy. For an excellent analysis of the relationship between these two national traumas, see Sturken, *Tangled Memories*, especially 14–16.

31 Arlene Stein illuminates how activists have exploited the moral aspects of the Holocaust frame: "Gay activists have sought to revise the historical record to reflect the extent of gay victimhood during the Nazi period; they have also used the Holocaust as metaphor, comparing the plight of homosexuals today to the plight of victimized minorities during the German Reich. Through the use of the Holocaust frame, lesbians and gay men have positioned themselves as victims and situated their opponents—garden variety homophobes, negligent AIDS bureaucrats, and Christian right anti-gay campaigners—as perpetrators." Stein, "Whose Memories?," 523.

32 For an analysis of Kramer's use of the Holocaust analogy, see Long, *AIDS and American Apocalypticism*, 63–105.

33 See Crimp with Rolston, *AIDS Demo Graphics*, 14–16; Meyer, *Outlaw Representation*, 225–27; and Watney, "Art AIDS NYC," 59–60.

34 The photograph is also historically ambiguous since the lovers are both wearing plain white shirts that could indicate the 1980s just as much as the 1930s.

35 Gever, "Pictures of Sickness," 120.

36 Callen's speech was given at a time when the causation of AIDS was still a matter of scientific uncertainty and debate.

37 Landers, "Bodies and Anti-bodies," 23.

38 The Fear of Disclosure Project was produced by Jonathan Lee and ran from 1989 to 1994, producing five works: *Fear of Disclosure* (Phil Zwickler and David Wojnarowicz, 1989); *(In)visible Women* (Ellen Spiro and Marina Alvarez, 1991); *No Regret (Non, je ne regrette rien)* (Marlon T. Riggs, 1992); and *Out in Silence* and *Not a Simple Story* (Christine Choy, 1994). Zwickler's original grant proposal for the series stressed its primary address to HIV-positive people, their partners, and their communities: "Using real people, not actors, these culturally sensitive videos will explore real life situations involving the act of disclosure in various communities, and, as such can provoke discussion about the sexual and ethical responsibilities related to AIDS." Fear of Disclosure Grant Proposal, 1989, Phil Zwickler Papers, Human Sexuality Collection, Cornell University Library, box 18, folder 24.

39 Donald Woods, "Prescription," in Hemphill, *Brother to Brother*, 162.

40 W. E. B. Du Bois's essay "Of the Sorrow Songs" was one of the first attempts to politically redeem the spiritual tradition, which had long been considered only in a religious context. See Du Bois, *Souls of Black Folk*, 250–64.

41 See Spencer, *Protest and Praise*; and Sanger, *"When the Spirit Says Sing!"*

42 Quoted in Spencer, *Protest and Praise*, 104.

43 See Patton, "Refiguring Social Space."

44 As Maya Lin's Vietnam memorial and the Names Project demonstrate, naming is in fact an important mode of bearing witness in its own right. In the public exhibition of the latter, the names of those inscribed in each of the panels are read aloud in a memorial ceremony. For further discussion of these testimonial dynamics, see Sturken, *Tangled Memories*, 186–91; and Hawkins, "Naming Names."

45 See Corner, *Art of Record*, 128–32.

46 Riggs has himself used a textile metaphor to describe the poetic structure of his work: "In *Tongues Untied* I was dealing with the weaving, in terms of our lives, where truth, fiction, fantasy, fact, history, mythology really interweave to inform our character, psyche, values and beliefs." Quoted in Kleinhans and Lesage, "Listening to the Heartbeat," 122.

47 *Voices from the Front* (Testing the Limits, 1991) documents this convention in its sequence summarizing the history of mainstream AIDS representation.

48 The technique of the desynchronization of sound and image in *No Regret* demonstrates affinities with Trinh T. Minh-ha's *Surname Viet, Given Name Nam* (1989): "Direct address, which is predicated on the synchronization of image and voice, in Trinh's work points not to a singular cohesive female subject, but to a more complicated conception of subjectivity as multiple, shifting, and communal, indicating not only the psychological but the social heterogeneity of a talking head." Lawrence, "Staring the Camera Down," 177.

49 In an analysis of homophobia and race that demonstrates the need for interventions like Riggs's work, Phillip Brian Harper argues that "if, even today, response to AIDS in black communities is characterized by a profound silence regarding actual sexual practices, either homosexual or heterosexual, this is largely because of the suppression of talk about sexuality generally and about male homosexuality in particular that is enacted in black communities through the discourses that constitute them." Harper, "Eloquence and Epitaph," 256.

50 See Cohen, *Boundaries of Blackness*.

51 For a discussion of Fung's pragmatism, see Waugh, *Romance of Transgression*, 305–15.

52 Performance monologues such as Ron Vawter's *Roy Cohn/Jack Smith* and David Drake's *The Night Larry Kramer Kissed Me* were both transformed into films, while other artists and performers working on AIDS-related issues have been profiled in film and video works, such as Catherine Saalfield's *Hallelujah! Ron Athey—A Story of Deliverance* (1998), her documentary portrait of the controversial ritualist performer.

53 See Kotz, "Aesthetics of 'Intimacy'"; and Solomon-Godeau, "Inside/Out."

54 Kotz, "Aesthetics of 'Intimacy,'" 207–8.

55 Feneley, "William Yang."

56 Yang notes, "When I first started off taking photographs, I think there was an idea I had that the photographer should be objective and that was the only way to get any sort of truth or unbiased reportage, all those ideas. But in fact now, later on in my career, when I look back, I find that I write on photographs and as a performer too I'm putting myself in the picture more and I'm revealing my relationship with the subjects, be it an event or a person." Feneley, "William Yang."

57 In his seminal 1988 essay, "Portraits of People with AIDS," which first brought critical attention to Kybartas's video, Douglas Crimp argued that *Danny* constituted "one of the most powerful critiques [of media images of PWAs] that exists to date." Crimp, *Melancholia and Moralism*, 100.

58 Yang's use of performance in exhibiting his photographs also draws from the strong tradition of the monologue in contemporary performance art. See Cavenett, "William Yang, *Sadness*, between the Lines."

59 Musser, *Emergence of Cinema*, 15.

60 In fact, in many countries the lecturer (particularly the *benshi* in Japan) remained an important structural element of screen practice long after motion pictures had been developed. See Burch, *To the Distant Observer*.

61 Using recent historical scholarship to undermine Burch's binarism, Tom Gunning argues that the functions of the film lecturer in both the West and in Japan were far more complex than Burch suggests. Researchers have discovered a wide range of practices that seemed to have operated between Burch's two poles, combining elements from both. See Gunning, "Scene of Speaking."

62 *Sadness* won an award from the Australian Film Institute for its sound design.

63 See Watney, *Imagine Hope*, 216–27.

64 Like Nan Goldin, Yang uses only first names in his accompanying commentary, which contributes to the effect of intimacy in the work.

65 Shaun de Waal argues that the most plausible etymology for the South African slang term *moffie* is a Dutch term for hermaphrodite, *mofrodiet*. He also indicates how its recent affirmative resignification by gay men and transvestites parallels the transformations in the use of *queer* in the United States and Britain. See de Waal, "Etymological Note," xiii.

66 The debate over including lesbian and gay rights in the new South African constitution dramatically increased public discourse on homosexuality in South Africa during the early 1990s, despite a relatively weak and fragmented gay liberation movement still emerging from decades of apartheid suppression. See Croucher, "South Africa's Democratization."

67 Willemse was profiled in a feature on people living with HIV/AIDS published in the *Sunday Times*, and he delivered a public service announcement on HIV/AIDS discrimination for Cape Town radio.

68 Jack Lewis, e-mail to author, 25 July 2003.

69 See Chetty, "Drag at Madame Costello's."

70 Maynard Swanson notes that "medical officials and other public authorities in South Africa at the turn of the century were imbued with the imagery of infectious disease as a societal metaphor, and . . . this metaphor powerfully interacted with British and South African racial attitudes to influence the policies and shape the institutions of segregation . . . a major strand in the creation of urban apartheid." Quoted in Lund, "Healing the Nation," 93.

71 Wolf and Taylor, "On Fandom and Smalltown Boys," 658.

72 Wojnarowicz's Arthur Rimbaud in New York series has also been explicitly reworked by another young queer artist, Emily Roysdon, whose photo series Untitled (David Wojnarowicz Project) (2001) restages the original photographs using her own body and Wojnarowicz's face as the mask. See Carlomusto and Roysdon, "Radiant Spaces."

73 Hartman, Longest Shadow, 8.

74 Hirsch, "Surviving Images," 9.

75 Cvetkovich, Archive of Feelings, 7.

2. The Embodied Immediacy of Direct Action

1 While protesters at NBC were arrested before they could get near the news set, others at PBS successfully chained themselves to the desks on the MacNeil/Lehrer News Hour, disrupting the show for a considerable time as studio security worked to cut them loose.

2 Treichler, How to Have Theory in an Epidemic, 141.

3 Although ACT UP/New York became the principal locus for the intersection between direct action politics and AIDS video activism, radical activist groups elsewhere, such as Toronto's AIDS Action Now, also stimulated activist media in a similar vein, including through such works as John Greyson's The World Is Sick (sic) (1989) and The Pink Pimpernel (1989).

4 Rockville Is Burning was largely distributed informally through activist networks and shown in gay bars and clubs in New York.

5 Stam, "Television News and Its Spectator," 365. In his analysis of television journalism more generally, Bill Nichols discusses the spatial dynamics of such discursive authority: "Frontality of face, eyes, and trunk is the favored bodily position for commentators. . . . This commonly lends a heightened awareness not of the constructedness of an imaginary world or even the constructedness of a particular representation of the historical world, but of the authority, expository agency itself: this is the world according to Barbara Walters, Robin Leach, Oprah Winfrey, Arsenio Hall, or Ted Koppel, and the institutions for which they stand." Nichols, Representing Reality, 130.

6 Morse, "Television News Personality and Credibility," 62.

7 Over the past two decades in the United States, news anchors on the major networks and the cable news channels, such as CNN's Anderson Cooper, have,

however, increasingly moved out of the studio for their news reports, especially during times of national and international crisis. But the increased competition for television news and the enhanced capabilities of satellite technology that led to these changes have, on the other hand, also produced a revived fetishism for the studio, as can be seen in Wolf Blitzer's CNN show *The Situation Room*. The early television news coverage of AIDS during the 1980s nevertheless remained rooted in conventional studio-bound news anchoring and round-table discussions.

8 John Greyson wittily lampooned such conventions in *The World Is Sick (sic)*, in which Andrea Austin-Sibley, a pompous news correspondent (played in frumpy drag by David Roche) reports on the Fifth International Conference on AIDS in Montreal from several stand-up positions in the convention center. Constantly interrupted and irritated by off-screen activist chanting, Austin-Sibley shows a blatant preference for interviewing medical researchers and pharmaceutical executives rather than activists. She is subsequently kidnapped by AIDS activists, who force her to listen to their arguments and observe their activities. On being released at the end of the video, she dryly admits a degree of self-transformation: "I'm free to go now? Maybe it's the Patty Hearst syndrome, but I'm beginning to see your point. Is there a demonstration in the lobby?" She picks up an activist placard and starts chanting "AIDS Action Now!" The camp irony of drag here undermines the stand-up convention as a spatial mechanism of objectivity in news media.

9 Colby and Cook, "Epidemics and Agendas," 220. My account of the early U.S. television coverage of AIDS draws principally from this study.

10 Watney, "Spectacle of AIDS," 86.

11 See Meyer, "Rock Hudson's Body." Meyer borrows the analytical framework of the body/antibody of AIDS representation from Timothy Landers's influential essay, "Bodies and Anti-bodies."

12 For an analysis of this diversification of AIDS representation on U.S. television in the 1990s, see Treichler, *How to Have Theory in an Epidemic*, 140–48.

13 Wright, "AIDS, the Status Quo, and the Elite Media."

14 For a brief survey of how queer experimental film and video have taken up the issue of mainstream AIDS representation, see my article, "Resistant Corpus," which includes analysis of both Hammer's and Huff's video.

15 In her social history of emotion in ACT UP, Deborah B. Gould contends that the *Bowers vs. Hardwick* decision, while not specifically about AIDS, did prove to be a vital, anger-validating trigger for radicalizing gay men and lesbians, since it confirmed their exclusion from protection by the state. See Gould, "Passionate Political Processes," 167.

16 This is the self-definition that ACT UP groups used in a number of different contexts: to open their weekly meetings, to provide a description for media interviews and reportage, and to convey on posters and flyers.

17 See Román, *Acts of Intervention*, 1–43.

18 Gamson, "Silence, Death, and the Invisible Enemy," 356.

19 In her oral history of lesbians involved in ACT UP, Ann Cvetkovich illuminates the complexity of their various commitments to the group. See Cvetkovich, *Archive of Feelings*, chap. 5.

20 For a comprehensive account of the first three years of ACT UP and its visual strategies, see Crimp with Rolston, AIDS *Demo Graphics*.

21 Many artists and media makers in ACT UP had come through the influential Independent Study Program at the Whitney Museum of American Art, which put an emphasis on contemporary critical theory.

22 The original Testing the Limits collective consisted of Gregg Bordowitz, Jean Carlomusto, Sandra Elgear, Robyn Hutt, Hilery Joy Kipnis, and David Meieran. The founding members of DIVA TV were Robert Beck, Gregg Bordowitz, Jean Carlomusto, Rob Kurilla, Ray Navarro, Costa Pappas, George Plagianos, Catherine Saalfield, and Ellen Spiro. James Wentzy joined DIVA TV in 1990 shortly before it ceased to function as a collective due to activist burnout and the deaths of Pappas and Navarro. Wentzy subsequently continued the work of DIVA TV single-handedly and broadcast its tapes on AIDS *Community Television*, a weekly cable access show that he established in 1993. Alexandra Juhasz provides a detailed history of AIDS video activism in AIDS TV, 44–73.

23 Catherine Saalfield describes the particular dynamics of this working process in her essay, "On the Make: Activist Video Collectives."

24 Bordowitz recalls, "When David Meieran and I first showed up in ACT UP, young kids with the most unprofessional equipment, we couldn't get anyone's attention. They treated us like hobbyists. . . . When *Testing the Limits* was shown (in ACT UP) and then on television, people all of a sudden realized that these were serious young people, who were actually going to accomplish what they said they were going to do. . . . Larry Kramer is in *Testing the Limits* in a side shot, because Larry Kramer would not give us an interview. He did not think we were important enough to give us an interview to. So I had to stand next to an ABC reporter and point my camera at Larry Kramer while he was giving an interview to the local news." Gregg Bordowitz, interview with the author, New York City, 24 March 2001.

25 Bordowitz, "Picture a Coalition," 187.

26 Juhasz, AIDS TV, 32–44.

27 For a history of guerilla television and its influence on contemporary video activism, see Boyle, *Subject to Change*.

28 Bordowitz, interview, New York City, 24 March 2001.

29 Corner, *Art of Record*, 128–32. Corner cites Connie Field's *The Life and Times of Rosie the Riveter* (1980) as a quintessential example of this strategy.

30 Bordowitz, "Picture a Coalition," 195; emphasis original.

31 Zimmermann, *States of Emergency*, 98.

32 Unlike later digital video cameras, the analog video cameras used by AIDS activists in this period required their operators to look through the viewfinder when shooting hand-held.

33 See Patton, *Inventing AIDS*, 77–120; and Watney, *Practices of Freedom*, 103–20.

34 For an analysis of the use of space by Queer Nation (and a brief mention of ACT UP as its progenitor), see Berlant and Freeman, "Queer Nationality."

35 Gaines, "Political Mimesis."

36 Regarding the affinity group's name, Douglas Crimp and Adam Rolston note, "The group adopted the movie star's name as a camp gesture, and each time someone asked what it meant, CHER became an acronym for whatever could be concocted on the spot, anything from "Commie Homos Engaged in Revolution" to "Cathy Has Extra Rollers." Crimp with Rolston, *AIDS Demo Graphics*, 20.

37 "No More Business as Usual" was in fact the theme of ACT UP's very first action when it demonstrated on Wall Street on 24 March 1987. See Crimp with Rolston, *AIDS Demo Graphics*, 27–29.

38 Nichols, *Representing Reality*, 3.

39 Quoted in Crimp with Rolston, *AIDS Demo Graphics*, 138.

40 Of course, in no way were all the activists Catholics, but a large enough number of them were raised in the faith for it to become a major issue in ACT UP meetings.

41 Hilferty chose the "Dies Irae" ("Day of Wrath"), a liturgical hymn from the medieval Latin mass, for specific reasons: "The medieval trope is dynamically appropriated by Berlioz in symphonic form for the nightmare section of his programmatic symphony—I also use 'day of wrath' to refer to the justifiable anger gays have against the church." Robert Hilferty, e-mail to author, 13 April 2008.

42 For example, Larry Kramer defines the Catholic Church as "arrogant, sterile, retrograde, and blind," while a female activist comments, "It's the fundamentalist extreme wing of the Catholic Church which is in power right now. I'm no longer a practicing Catholic."

43 This form of counterwitnessing, which records hateful or oppressive speech for the purposes of mobilizing those very groups that the speech targets, has been widely used in lesbian and gay media activism against antigay political initiatives, including state and local referenda. *Sacred Lies, Civil Truths* (Catherine Saalfield and Cyrille Phipps, 1993), the most widely circulated lesbian and gay video during the infamous Colorado and Oregon initiatives in 1992, devotes its whole first section to such a counterwitnessing of the hatred espoused by the Religious Right. Cindy Patton argues that such show-and-tell strategies used by both sides of these political battles demonstrate the shifting dynamics of postmodern governmentality, which prioritize strategies around representation as depicting over ones that concentrate on representation as speaking for. See Patton, "Tremble, Hetero Swine!"

44 PBS statement quoted in Saalfield, "*Tongues Untied.*"

45 See Mookas, "Culture in Contest"; and Bullert, *Public Television*, 123–45.

46 Knee, "Feeling of Power," 97–98.

47 For an account of the collective's movement toward institutionalization, see Juhasz, *AIDS TV*, 60–64.

48 Patton, *Inventing* AIDS, 51.

49 Ben-Levi, *"Voices from the Front,"* 114.

50 Crimp, *Melancholia and Moralism*, 265, 267; emphasis original. Interestingly, ACT UP/Philadelphia, one of the vanguards of the current global AIDS activist movement, chose to screen *Voices from the Front* as a fundraiser to celebrate its twentieth anniversary in January 2008.

51 See Crimp, *Melancholia and Moralism*, 169–93; and Epstein, "AIDS Activism," 179–84.

52 Benjamin Shepard and Ronald Hayduk trace the lines of continuity and development between ACT UP and this new global coalition of social movements in their anthology *From* ACT UP *to the* WTO.

53 See Nogueira, "Birth and Promise."

54 It is this logic of activist convergence that differentiates *Pills, Profits, Protest* from *Pandemic:Facing* AIDS (Rory Kennedy, 2002) and *A Closer Walk* (Robert Bilheimer, 2003), two far more conventional (and better funded) documentaries about the global AIDS crisis that compete with *Pills, Profits, Protest* in the institutional market for educational documentaries. For an analysis of these two documentaries, see my essay, "Face of AIDS."

55 Catherine Saalfield notes that even after Testing the Limits had become institutionalized, it continued to share its extensive archive with other video collectives. Saalfield, "On the Make," 31. However, Jean Carlomusto, one of the collective's founding members, recalls a less sanguine situation, in which struggles developed over how to address the question of who owned the rights to the archive of the original collective after it had disbanded. See Carlomusto, "ACT UP Oral History Project," 14.

56 Jim Hubbard, e-mail to author, 23 August 2007. The New York Public Library collection also contains a number of videos documenting the memorial services for deceased activists.

57 Robert Garcia's memorial tape is archived with his collected papers held by the Human Sexuality Collection of Cornell University Library (series VIII, V-110).

58 Saalfield, "On the Make," 33.

59 Whereas memorial tapes circulated between the spaces of activism and mourning, the political funerals of Jon Greenberg, Mark Lowe, Tim Bailey, and Aldyn McKean, which ACT UP staged between 1993 and 1994, fused these spaces by bringing the memorial service into the street. James Wentzy recorded them for broadcast on AIDS *Community Television*.

60 Hilderbrand, "Retroactivism," 308.

61 The sociologist Deborah Gould has stressed the significance of affective dynamics, particularly in the relationships between women and gay men, for the fracturing of ACT UP during this time: "Scholars and activists alike tend to focus on the substance of a movement's conflicts, neglecting the emotional undercurrents that play a part in structuring the content, character, and effects of such conflicts. With the phrase emotional undercurrent I mean to point to the way the

feelings operating in a movement's internal conflicts are often unarticulated, unacknowledged, and submerged, but nevertheless have a force and direction to them, an insistence, affecting participants themselves as well as things like the content, shape, tone, texture, velocity and intensity of the conflicts. In this case, often unstated and unrecognized feelings of betrayal, non-recognition, resentment, mistrust, and anger were at the heart of ACT UP's internal conflicts." Gould, "Solidarity and Its Fracturing in ACT UP," 10. Ann Cvetkovich also takes up this issue in *Archive of Feelings*, 197–201.

3. Resisting Confession in Autobiographical Video

1 Dovey, *Freakshow*.

2 Muñoz, *Disidentifications*, 143–60.

3 The most widely known works of AIDS autobiography in literary form include Reinaldo Arenas's *Before Night Falls* (1993), Michael Callen's *Surviving AIDS* (1990), Cyril Collard's *Savage Nights* (1989), David Feinberg's *Eighty-Sixed* (1988) and *Queer and Loathing: Rants and Raves of a Raging AIDS Clone* (1994), Gary Fisher's *Gary in Your Pocket* (1996), Hervé Guibert's *To the Friend Who Did Not Save My Life* (1990), Derek Jarman's *Modern Nature* (1992), Eric Michael's *Unbecoming* (1997), Paul Monette's *Borrowed Time* (1988) and *The Last Watch of the Night* (1994), and David Wojnarowicz's *Close to the Knives: A Memoir of Disintegration* (1991). The works by Arenas, Collard, and Wojnarowicz were adapted into narrative feature films.

4 As its title might suggest, Guibert's video diary provoked concern at TF1, the French public television network, about its possibly sensationalist treatment of such culturally sensitive material, causing its broadcast in January 1992 to be postponed by over a week. For an account of the debate around the program, see Boulé, "The Postponing of *La Pudeur ou l'Impudeur*."

5 Dovey, *Freakshow*, 55–77. *Rubber Queen*, the video diary of the dancer and performance artist Adam Gale, was broadcast in regular installments on local cable access television in Washington, D.C. The Vancouver physician Peter Jepson-Young taped over one hundred video diary entries about his experience as a gay man with AIDS for a local television news program from 1990 until his death in 1992. The British television producer David Paperny later edited down the individual segments into a one-hour television documentary entitled *The Broadcast Tapes of Dr. Peter*, which was subsequently shown on the BBC in the United Kingdom and on HBO in the United States.

6 Gilmore, *Limits of Autobiography*, 2.

7 See Anderson, *Autobiography*, 1–17.

8 Sturrock, *Language of Autobiography*, 4.

9 Lejeune, "Autobiographical Contract," 193.

10 See Miller, "Representing Others"; Friedman, "Women's Autobiographical Selves"; and Mason, "Other Voice."

11 Friedman, "Women's Autobiographical Selves," 42.

12 Chambers, *Facing It*, 5–6.

13 For example, Jarman's *Modern Nature* and Fisher's *Gary in Your Pocket* are presented as diaries, whereas Feinberg's *Queer and Loathing* and Monette's *The Last Watch of the Night* are books of autobiographical essays.

14 Tougaw, "Testimony and the Subjects of AIDS Memoirs," 235.

15 It was Friedman who decided to use the footage from *Blackstar*. Joslin had originally wanted to use other forms of found footage in the project, such as clips from TV medical shows and Rutger Hauer's death scene in *Blade Runner*. This particular appropriation of popular culture resonates strongly with Mike Hoolboom's films, especially *Positiv* (1997), which I discuss at the beginning of chapter 5.

16 Seckinger and Jakobsen, "Love, Death, and Videotape," 152.

17 See Corner, *Art of the Record*, 1–8.

18 *Silverlake Life* problematizes the issue of medium specificity in a number of different ways. First, as a filmmaker, Friedman, like his mentor, reworks the "immediacy" and "coverage" of the video footage through the sensibility of the film medium, which Catherine Russell argues is characterized by the "structure of secondary revision." Unlike videomaking, filmmaking necessitates a temporal and spatial deferral in its production of an image. What is "captured" in the camera must be processed and screened in another time and space. Russell notes that "in the cinema, self-representation always involves a splitting of the self, a production of another self, another body, another camera, another time, another place. Video threatens to collapse the temporal difference of filmic memory . . . because of its 'coverage,' its capacity as an instrument of surveillance." Russell, *Experimental Ethnography*, 313. Second, *Silverlake Life* was, like *Fast Trip, Long Drop*, shot on video and subsequently transferred to film for festival and theatrical distribution as a means to supplement its primary distribution through public television broadcasting.

19 Renov, *Subject of Documentary*, 216–29.

20 See also Russell, *Experimental Ethnography*, 275–314; and Lionnet, *Autobiographical Voices*.

21 Nichols, *Blurred Boundaries*.

22 Mary Louise Pratt quoted in Russell, *Experimental Ethnography*, 277.

23 Renov, *Subject of Documentary*, 141.

24 Bruzzi, *New Documentary*, 154.

25 Thomas Waugh argues that the performative complexity and sophistication of lesbian and gay liberation–era documentaries, such as *Blackstar*, have long been overlooked. See Waugh, "Walking on Tippy Toes."

26 Although the shot of the television monitor might suggest that there was a second camera present in the room, the coproducer Jane Weiner revealed to me that the shot was taken at a later point during postproduction. Without it, Weiner noted, the scene would have been spatially confusing to the viewer. Knowing that it was a "cheat shot" does not lessen the power of the scene's self-reflexivity. Jane Weiner, personal communication, 29 April 2004.

27 Phelan, *Mourning Sex*, 173.

28 Sobchack, "Inscribing Ethical Space," 287.

29 Ehrenstein. "AIDS, Death, and Videotape."

30 The DVD release of *Silverlake Life* on its tenth anniversary in 2003 includes among its special features an epilogue produced by Parvez Sharma, in which the videographer Elaine Mayes and the filmmaker Peter Friedman discuss the two questions most commonly asked of them: What happened to Mark and how did the documentary get made after both deaths? The epilogue includes footage that Mayes shot of Massi shortly before his death, when his whole body was covered by painful KS lesions.

31 Warren, "Film."

32 "Love, AIDS and Videotape."

33 Friedman quoted in Graham, "A Matter of Life and Death."

34 Bullert, *Public Television*, 32.

35 Aufderheide, "Electronic Public Space," 35.

36 Aufderheide, "Vernacular Video," 47.

37 P.O.V. has since fully exploited Internet resources to develop a sophisticated and highly impressive structure for interactivity among its audience members, including a Web site with downloadable video responses and electronic bulletin boards dedicated to each individual program. See the site, www.pbs.org/pov.

38 The executive director of P.O.V., Ellen Schneider, provided me with access to both the video letters produced for "Talk Back" and the archive of letters received by P.O.V. The letter book contained just under fifty letters. Many more letters and responses were received by the local PBS affiliates that broadcast the program and were thus not consequently archived at the production offices for P.O.V. in New York City.

39 Renov, *Subject of Documentary*, 104–19.

40 Barthes, *Roland Barthes*, 177.

41 In this chapter, when I use quotation marks around Bordowitz's name, I am referring to the protagonist presented in the video as "Gregg Bordowitz." His name without quotation marks hence refers to the videomaker who has produced the video's discourse.

42 Bordowitz has commented, "*Fast Trip* is television. I watch television, I've always watched television, I think about the language and idioms of television." Meyer, "Art of Living," 90.

43 Renov, *Subject of Documentary*, 106.

44 Kun, "Archaeologies of Identity." Alisa Lebow notes the ambivalent tension between the video's exploration of Bordowitz's Jewish and queer identities, which she argues is a common characteristic of autobiographical documentaries made by gay and lesbian Jews. See Lebow, *First Person Jewish*, chap. 4.

45 See Harrington, "Some Transitions."

46 See Caruth and Keenan, "'AIDS Crisis Is Not Over,'" 256.

47 See Saalfield, "Positive Propaganda."

48 Meyer, "Art of Living," 89.

49 Juhasz, AIDS TV, 240.

50 The subgenres mentioned include at least six of the nine initial subgenres of alternative AIDS media that John Greyson first identified in his article "Strategic Compromises."

51 Bordowitz, AIDS Crisis Is Ridiculous, 251. Much of the testimony in Fast Trip, Long Drop can also be found in Bordowitz's essay "Dense Moments," in which there are far fewer formal attempts to disturb the autobiographical self. Originally published in 1994, "Dense Moments" is reprinted in The AIDS Crisis Is Ridiculous, 113–40. In her analysis of the video, Alisa Lebow reads a fractured performance of multiple selves by Bordowitz, not simply the bifurcated subject invoked by the videomaker himself. Yet I would argue that the multiply fractured subjectivity that Lebow identifies is less the performance of numerous distinct personae than the fracturing dynamic of the ambiguous movement between "Bordowitz" and Allesman. See Lebow, First Person Jewish, 141–48.

52 Bordowitz, AIDS Crisis Is Ridiculous, 43–67.

53 Charles Ludlam, "Manifesto: Ridiculous Theater; Scourge of Human Folly," reprinted in Bordowitz, AIDS Crisis Is Ridiculous, 44.

54 Lebow, First Person Jewish, 143. Alisa Lebow draws her discussion of the "conscious pariah" from Hannah Arendt's seminal work, The Origins of Totalitarianism (New York: Harcourt Brace, 1951), 56–68.

55 Crimp, Melancholia and Moralism, 265.

56 For example, Cyril Collard's Savage Nights (1993).

57 Chris, "Documents and Counter-documents," 8.

58 Jean Carlomusto's Shatzi Is Dying is the videomaker's complex autobiographical meditation on mortality, memory, and queer relationality in light of AIDS activist burnout. As she and her lover, Jane Rosett, witness the attenuated process of dying for their beloved Doberman, Shatzi, they reflect on the nature of experiencing loss and mortality, something that has profoundly shaped their lives over the past two decades. For an excellent analysis of the video, see Cvetkovich, Archive of Feelings, 262–67. Richard Fung's Sea in the Blood is a moving and poetic video essay that reflects on the experience of living in the shadow of illness by paralleling Fung's two most intimate relationships: that with his sister Nan, who died of thalassemia (literally, "sea in the blood") in 1977, and that with his lover Tim, who has been seropositive since 1980. Through a parallax structure that recalls William Yang's Sadness, Fung subtly traces the ways in which these two experiences of living intimately with another's illness have mutually informed one another. For an insightful reading of Sea in the Blood in relation to Fung's earlier AIDS videos, see Waugh, Romance of Transgression, 312–15.

59 Juhasz, "Artist's Statement."

60 Juhasz, "Video Remains," 319.

61 Bordowitz, AIDS Crisis Is Ridiculous, 270.

62 For an analysis of Pandemic, see my essay "Face of AIDS."

63 Crimp and Bordowitz, "A Noun and a Verb," 35.

64 Bordowitz, AIDS Crisis Is Ridiculous, 278.

4. *The Testimonial Space of Song*

1 Nero, "Diva Traffic and Male Bonding in Film," 48. Whereas Charles Nero takes issue with the ideological construction of race in this pedagogic encounter, Ross Chambers affirms the value of the operatic "visitation" that Andy brings to Joe, engendering a "brotherly love that implies some possibility of identification between himself and the homosexual, AIDS-infected other, Andy." Chambers, "Visitations," 44.

2 Farmer, "Fabulous Sublimity of Gay Diva Worship," 177; and Allen, "Homosexuality and Narrative," 625.

3 Felman and Laub, *Testimony*, 268–83.

4 In line with the concerns of the other chapters and my own disciplinary expertise, this chapter analyzes the discursive rather than the musicological aspects of song.

5 Waugh, *Romance of Transgression*, 291–92.

6 Greyson, "Figments."

7 Greyson, "Pils Slip," 52.

8 Cohan, *Incongruous Entertainment*, 18; emphasis original.

9 Patricia Wald provides the most comprehensive account of how Patient Zero emerged as a key figure in the dominant media representation of AIDS in *Contagious*, 213–63.

10 Greyson derives this tag line from a cover of *California Magazine* following the release of Shilts's book in 1987. The *New York Post* ran a similar headline on 6 October 1987: "The Man Who Gave Us AIDS."

11 Waugh further contends that the film's carefully organized arrangement of diverse styles of song numbers, including three reprises, ultimately worked to frame it for many critics as more of a homage to the classical integrated musical than a self-reflexive appropriation. Waugh, *Romance of Transgression*, 296.

12 Greyson's commitment to memorializing Dugas was already clear in a piece he wrote in 1989, "Requiem for Gaetan," portions of which were subsequently incorporated in "Liberace's Music Helped Cure Me," published in Greyson, *Urinal*, 252–71.

13 To avoid confusion, I will refer to the operatic character as "Zackie" and reserve the name Achmat for the historical person on whom the character is based (and who also appears in the opera in documentary video clips).

14 Achmat was given the Desmond Tutu Leadership Award (2003), named "Politician of the Decade" by the South African newspaper the *Financial Mail*, and named one of thirty-six "modern heroes" from around the world by *Time* magazine (2003). He and TAC also received the Jonathan Mann Award for Global Health and Human Rights in 2003.

15 Booth, *Experience of Songs*, 15; emphasis original.

16 Kostenbaum, *Queen's Throat*, 42.

17 Even integrated film musicals (which contain song numbers with elements or

events that propel the narrative forward) create a differentiated space during their performance, but to a lesser degree than nonintegrated film musicals.

18 Yet Jane Feuer argues that such a shift to direct address should not be taken as a modernist, distanciating quality of the Hollywood film musical since it ultimately works with other aspects of the self-reflexive musical to reinscribe the myth of entertainment. See Feuer, *Hollywood Musical*.

19 I am indebted to Steven Cohan for this insight.

20 Although contemporary installation art comprises a highly diverse set of aesthetic practices and historical influences, the experience of the viewer/visitor arguably remains the central preoccupation of the form. See Bishop, *Installation Art*.

21 Michel Foucault's genealogical method aims to break up the grand chains of historical continuity, to historicize that which has been deemed immutable or transcendent. Genealogy historicizes its object of study by focusing on the material conditions of discourse, on the disciplinary technologies within institutions that utilize knowledge as a function of modern power. See Foucault, *Discipline and Punish*.

22 Shilts, *And the Band Played On*, xxiii.

23 Greyson initiated his critique of Shilts's discourse in 1990 with a scathing and hilarious parody, "Realism Traps the Homosexual: A Documentary Novel About AIDS in America," in which a computer virus called Volodya fosters an online romance between Shilts and the gay novelist David Leavitt (whose *The Lost Language of Cranes* was a bestseller at the same time as *And the Band Played On*) and then proceeds to switch their writing styles, highlighting the hackneyed modes of realism and superannuated narrative tropes employed by each of these celebrated gay writers. The text was published in *Urinal*, 224–51.

24 Roland Barthes quoted in Crimp, *Melancholia and Moralism*, 53.

25 Shilts, *And the Band Played On*, xxiii.

26 Quoted in Fettner and Check, *Truth About AIDS*, 86.

27 Crimp, *Melancholia and Moralism*, 124.

28 See Levi, *Drowned and the Saved*. *Zero Patience* invokes the trope of the drowned in the Hall of Contagion's homoerotic mural of nameless naked sailors drowning after their ships were burned by the Dutch during the plague.

29 Except for AIDS, the proper nouns remained lowercase in the opening title shot.

30 Greyson and Schellenberg modeled the film's song on the musical idioms of late 1980s queer pop music, namely, on the B-52's, 10000 Maniacs, the Pet Shop Boys, and Erasure. See Greyson, "Pils Slip," 52. In its appropriation of the MGM musicals style, this number precisely duplicates a remarkable underwater shot from *Bathing Beauty* (George Sidney, 1944) in which Esther Williams swims directly into the camera. For an analysis of the camp dynamics of the water ballet finale of *Bathing Beauty*, see Cohan, *Incongruous Entertainment*, 41–45.

31 Todorov, *Poetics of Prose*, 73.

32 Zipes, afterword, 587.

33 Said, *Orientalism*, 195.

34 For a discussion of the diorama as a cinematic precursor, see Schwartz, "Cinematic Spectatorship before the Apparatus."

35 The diorama is the visual technology that according to Donna Haraway, functioned in the American Museum of Natural History to visualize the racial imaginary of imperialism and the emergent eugenics movement. Haraway describes the imaginary sustained by the diorama halls of the museum in the following way: "Western 'man' may begin again the first journey, the first birth from within the sanctuary of nature. . . . A hope is implicit in every architectural detail: in immediate vision of the origin, perhaps the future can be fixed. By saving the beginnings, the end can be achieved and the present can be transcended." Haraway, *Primate Visions*, 26.

36 Waugh usefully reads *Zero Patience* through Richard Dyer's theorization of the utopian desires that structure musical numbers. See Waugh, *Romance of Transgression*, 290–99.

37 Steven Cohan notes that "as a musical moves back and forth between the diegetic realism of story and extradiegetic awareness of the star's performance in numbers, the oscillation between indirect and direct address heightens the audience's sense of not observing the star play a character so much as witnessing her or his own authenticity, charisma, and talent without the mediation of fictional narrative or cinematic technology." Cohan, *Hollywood Musicals*, 13.

38 While the performative aspects of Miss HIV as a drag queen tend to forestall a sexist representation of disease, Greyson's use of female performers to depict all the smaller viruses is rather more ideologically problematic.

39 Waugh provides an extensive and highly incisive analysis of "Positive." See Waugh, *Romance of Transgression*, 297–99.

40 John Greyson interviewed in Cohen, "By Any Genre Necessary," 70; emphasis added.

41 Martin Rubin argues that it is this spatial disjunction that defines the spectacular form of the backstage musical: "The film must work to establish a space (or a series of homologous spaces) that are, to a certain extent, self-enclosed and independent of the surrounding narrative. This renders the space accessible to spectacular expansions and distortions that can be clearly in excess of the narrative without necessarily disrupting it. The main requirement is that this space be a special or bracketed space, adjoining the primary space of the narrative but not completely subordinated to it. The strong demarcation of the space of the numbers as distinct from that of the offstage narrative is an essential ingredient of Berkeleyesque cinema." Rubin, *Showstoppers*, 36.

42 Edison's kinetoscope marked a distinct appropriation for entertainment of a technology originally developed for scientific use (Étienne-Jules Marey's celluloid filmstrip).

43 For an analysis of the Royal Ontario Museum controversy, see Butler, *Contested*

Representations; and for discussion of the MoMA controversy, see Crimp, *Melancholia and Moralism*, 83–107.

44 Bennett, *Birth of the Modern Museum*, 79.

45 Having the diorama figures modeled by the same actors playing the contemporary characters Mary and George (Dianne Heatherington and Richardo Keens-Douglas) acts as another self-conscious device to indicate the historicity of AIDS representation.

46 This image also became one of the original film posters.

47 For a fuller account of these struggles, see Robins, "Long Live Zackie, Long Live"; and Hoad, "Thabo Mbeki's AIDS Blues."

48 Powers, "AIDS Rebel."

49 Achmat, "My Childhood as an Adult Molester," 325–41.

50 Mark Gevisser analyzes the constitutional protection for sexual orientation and its broader ramifications in South African society in his article, "Mandela's Stepchildren."

51 Posel, "Getting the Nation Talking About Sex," 15.

52 Schoonakker, "AIDS Warrior"; Power, "AIDS Rebel"; Carroll, "Good Man in Africa"; and Rosenberg, "In South Africa."

53 The documentary also includes several reenacted "flashbacks" of scenes from "My Childhood as an Adult Molester." In their sexual frankness, these confessional moments both refuse an easily consumable media hero and expose the intersection of race and sexuality in Achmat's queer childhood.

54 Greyson and Wall, *Fig Trees*, 18. *Fig Trees* has not been the only work of queer AIDS media to "video-ize" opera in a gallery context. The artist Simon Leung and the composer Michael Webster collaborated on *Proposal for "The Side of a Mountain,"* a four-channel video/architectural installation mounted at the Santa Monica Museum of Art in 2002. The side of the mountain refers to Griffith Park in Los Angeles, which serves as the location for this short experimental opera exploring the intersubjective relations of the queer public sex that takes place in the park. Like Greyson, Leung was influenced by Kostenbaum's queer understanding of the operatic voice: "Wayne Kostenbaum once said that the operatic voice is the sound of 'unadulterated rage,' which I interpret to mean a deep, larger-than-life emotion that can neither be contained nor adequately expressed through speech. . . . The operatic voice comes from a fragility of a mortal body and at the same time sounds superhuman, like a force of nature—it can at once be beautiful and terrifying." Leung, *Simon Leung*, 19. The libretto focuses on an anonymous sexual encounter between an older man (the baritone) and a younger man (the tenor) that is persistently interrupted by the calls of another man (the countertenor) calling out for his lost dog. The younger man hears the dog being attacked by a pack of coyotes (instrumental voices), but he hesitates calling out in assistance for fear of being caught by the police patrolling the park. In the midst of a sexual tryst that is both intensified by the ferocious sounds of the coyotes and disturbed by the desperate calls of the dog owner, both men mourn the loss of gay sexual

culture before AIDS, as the older man reminisces about a past sexual encounter and the younger man fantasizes about a future denied him. The affective complexity of opera provided Leung with a highly suitable form to explore the intricate layers of loss and denial haunting gay men in the post-AIDS era.

55 In addition to sharing the book's wit and irreverent affection for opera, *Fig Trees* also explicitly incorporates several of Kostenbaum's ideas and historical references.

56 See Linda Hutcheon and Michael Hutcheon's analysis of opera's tubercular heroine in their book *Opera*, 29–59.

57 The words excerpted for the libretto were highlighted in yellow in the full text hanging on the wall.

58 Greyson and Wall, *Fig Trees*, 19.

59 The title of the scene also hints at the questionable expediency of Stein and Thomson's search for new subjects.

60 The train motif also facilitates a thematic connection to a later scene, "Sushi Train."

61 The Latin lines translate as follows: "We enter the circle after dark . . . and are consumed by fire."

62 Waugh, *Romance of Transgression*, 302.

63 Greyson and Wall, *Fig Trees*, 21.

64 Greyson, "Figments," 21. As a U.S. AIDS activist with access to antiretrovirals, Bordowitz also invoked the safari trope in *Habit* to self-consciously acknowledge the ideological dynamics at play in his attendance of the Thirteenth International AIDS Conference in Durban, South Africa.

65 Quoted in Waugh, *Romance of Transgression*, 303–4.

66 Greyson, "Figments," 12.

67 A condensed installation of *Fig Trees* was mounted at the Scotiabank Dance Centre by Vancouver New Music in December 2007 as part of the city's World AIDS Day programming.

68 Greyson, "Pils Slips," 52.

69 I cannot discuss the feature film version in any greater detail since I have not been able to see it before this book goes to press.

5. Gay Cinephilia

1 Hoolboom also seizes clips from *L'age d'or* (The Golden Age) (Luis Buñuel, 1930); *Natural Born Killers* (Oliver Stone, 1994); *City of Lost Children* (Marco Caro and Jean-Pierre Jeunet, 1993); *Rumblefish* (Francis Ford Coppola, 1983); *Heavenly Creatures* (Peter Jackson, 1994); *A Matter of Life and Death* (Michael Powell and Emeric Pressburger, 1946); and Michael Jackson's music video for the song "Leave Me Alone" (1989).

2 See Creekmur and Doty, introduction, 1–11.

3 The engagement by gay experimental filmmakers with the affective dimensions

of the AIDS crisis was not without controversy, as Tom Kalin has revealed in talking about his widely screened and influential experimental short *They Are Lost to Vision Altogether* (1988). Feeling the pressure of AIDS cultural activism to make directly political work, he recut the ten-minute video in 1989 to make it more didactic and less elegiac. In retrospect, Kalin admits to preferring the original version to the thirteen-minute 1989 version that is in distribution. See Greyson, "Scoping Boys," 47.

4 Williams, *Marxism and Literature*, 132.

5 Williams's term seems particularly appropriate in this context, since he argued that such structures of feeling were often first made visible in art and literature: "The ideas of a structure of feeling can be specifically related to the evidence of forms and conventions—semantic figures—which, in art and literature, are often among the first indications that such a structure is forming" (133).

6 Odets, *In the Shadow of the Epidemic*, 14–15.

7 Although earlier works of queer AIDS media, such as Jerry Tartaglia's *A.I.D.S.C.R.E.A.M.* (1988) and *Ecce Homo* (1989), have appropriated images from pre-AIDS gay porn, recent works have pursued a more extensive exploration of the gay porn culture of the 1970s and early 1980s. These range from Joseph Lovett's conventional but revealing documentary *Gay Sex in the 70s* (2005) to William E. Jones's experimental opus, *v.o.* (2006), which illuminates the haunting erotic landscapes of the era by splicing together interstitial moments from classic gay porn and appropriated dialogue from international art cinema.

8 K.I.P. resonates with a comment made by Douglas Crimp in "Mourning and Militancy," when he describes the response of a young gay man to an early 1970s film shown at the Gay and Lesbian Experimental Film Festival in New York: "The young man was very excited about what seemed to me a pretty ordinary sex scene in the film, but then he said, 'I'd give anything to know what cum tastes like, somebody else's that is.' That broke my heart for two reasons: for him because he didn't know, for me because I do." Crimp, *Melancholia and Moralism*, 139. In the late 1980s, HIV prevention campaigns in New York and other U.S. cities—unlike in Canada and Europe—encouraged gay men to use condoms for oral sex. In his AIDS activist video *The Pink Pimpernel* (1989), John Greyson wittily incorporated this prevention debate into one of the safer-sex scenes that appropriated canonical queer films. Greyson presents "Safer Blow Job by Andy Warhol" in a New York and a Toronto version, with the former depicting oral sex with a condom and the latter without. The scene concludes with the intertitle: "Debate ensues between the two porn stars about different safer sex guidelines from different cities."

9 Odets, *In the Shadow of the Epidemic*, 72.

10 Jarman used the term to describe his filmmaking technique for *Angelic Conversation* (1985), for which he used a Nizo Super-8 camera that permits shooting at variable speeds. Shooting at a fast speed and projecting at a slow speed thus enables an attenuated duration of the frame, like a series of slides: "The single frame makes for extreme attention, a concentration that is voyeuristic. Time seems

suspended. The slightest movement is amplified. This is the reason I call it 'a cinema of small gestures.'" Jarman, *Last of England*, 146.

11 While the appropriative dynamic in cinephilia would suggest calling it "queer cinephilia," I have chosen *gay cinephilia* to emphasize its historical significance for postwar gay identity formation.

12 My analysis of gay male cultural production here resonates with the conclusions drawn by Joy Van Fuqua's study of two lesbian videomakers' use of their own star obsessions with Elizabeth Taylor and Anna Magnani in bearing witness to AIDS. Van Fuqua argues that videos by Jean Carlomusto (*L Is for the Way You Look* [1991] and *To Each Her Own* [1994]) and Joan Braderman (*Joan Does Dynasty* [1986] and *Joan Sees Stars* [1993]) appropriate the "raw material of popular culture" to "document the presumably private practices of AIDS mourning." See Van Fuqua, *Tell the Story*, 88–122.

13 See, for instance, Mayne, *Cinema and Spectatorship*, 157–72; Doty, *Making Things Perfectly Queer*; White, *UnInvited*; Harris, *Rise and Fall of Gay Culture*; and Farmer, *Spectacular Passions*.

14 Mayne, *Cinema and Spectatorship*, 166.

15 Farmer, *Spectacular Passions*, 27.

16 Harris, *Rise and Fall of Gay Culture*, 15.

17 See Arthur, "Lost and Found."

18 La Valley, "Great Escape," 29.

19 Farmer, *Spectacular Passions*, 28. In developing his notion of "gay cinematic capital," Brett Farmer adapts Sarah Thornton's concept of "subcultural capital," which he defines as "the extensive and often highly developed systems of tastes, knowledges, and competences developed and used by subcultures as marks of distinction and group affiliation" (Farmer, *Spectacular Passions*, 27).

20 For a history of cinephilia's impact on classical film theory, see Keathley, *Cinephilia and History*.

21 Willemen, *Looks and Frictions*, 227; emphasis added.

22 Sontag, "Decay of Cinema," 60.

23 Cardinal, "Pausing over Peripheral Detail," 124.

24 Willemen, *Looks and Frictions*, 237; emphasis added.

25 Both the impressionist discourse on *photogénie* and contemporary cinephilia entail a rich imbrication of spectatorship, criticism, and filmmaking practice. *Photogénie* emerged in the film culture of the French *ciné-clubs*, forerunners to the film festival, which provided a space in which the dynamics of all three practices came together.

26 Willemen, *Looks and Frictions*, 126.

27 For the analysis of found-footage filmmaking as a practice of postmodern resignification, see Wees, *Recycled Images*; and Bonet, *Desmontaje*.

28 Anbian, "Phelan Filmmaking Award-Winners Interviewed," 17–18.

29 Ahlgren, "Personal Story Decoded in Bits of Old Footage."

30 Kalin, "Identity Crisis," 29.

31 In the context of HIV prevention and psychotherapy, this return of traumatic experience has been formulated in discussions of the role that self-esteem plays in seroconversion rates among gay men. See Odets, *In the Shadow of the Epidemic.*

32 See Kalin, "Identity Crisis"; and Haynes, "A Gay Kind of Film," 3. Kalin further observes that "during both the screenings of *The Place Between Our Bodies* that I attended an AZT beeper happened to go off in the audience, a signal not only to a person with AIDS to take medication but also a sign of just how long ago 1975 seems" (30).

33 Michael Renov uses the term *attenuated indexicality* to describe the specific semiotic and material qualities of photographic images that have been repeatedly reproduced. He discussed the concept during his response to Marianne Hirsch's and Leo Spitzer's lecture "'There Never Was a Camp Here!': Retracing Images, Re-placing History," presented at the Center for Culture, Media, and History at New York University, 15 February 2002.

34 Jacobson, "Matthias Müller," 47; translation mine.

35 This is not the only time that *Aus der Ferne* appropriates a classic German film. Arnold Fanck's *Bergfilme* (mountain films) provide shots for the avalanche imagery, which sets off the expression of crisis at the film's beginning.

36 The zoetrope was an optical toy and cinematic precursor invented in the 1830s, but not patented until 1867. It consisted of a thin, slot-pierced metal drum that revolved about its axis by turning horizontally on a pivot. Multiple images of a figure in various stages of movement lined the inside of the drum, so that the viewer could gain the illusion of perpetual motion when she or he looked through the slots as the zoetrope spun.

37 Alternatively, Gabriele Jutz reads the zoetrope and the film's pervasive iconography of revolving movement as a metaphor for life. See Jutz, "Die Physis des Films."

38 In both its formal and thematic embrace of alchemy, *Aus der Ferne* bears distinct relations to the Super-8 films of Derek Jarman, a filmmaker who has undoubtedly influenced Müller.

39 Kuzniar, *Queer German Cinema*, 209.

40 Müller, "Mes films s'écartent de cette vision des choses," 306; translation mine.

41 See Sitney, *Visionary Film*, 30–31.

42 *Pensão Globo* incorporates three pieces of found footage: a solarized shot from a home movie in which Müller's mother is nursing him as a baby; shots of a doctor holding up an X-ray; and a shot of a young man taking a written exam (seen on a television screen). The two latter shots are both from *The Incredible Shrinking Man* (Jack Arnold, 1957).

43 Kuzniar also reads the seductive stranger as a doppelgänger: "The lead character follows his apparition down the streets, perhaps in desire, perhaps longing for death. The two are never shown together in the same frame; instead the editing cuts back and forth between them, suggesting that this angel of death is a hallucination of the dying man (we only hear one set of footsteps)." Kuzniar, *Queer German Cinema*, 210.

44 Kuzniar, *Queer German Cinema*, 211. Alternatively, Peter Tscherkassky suggests that this technique constitutes an allusion to the classical Hollywood conventions for depicting ghosts in which "characters' deaths have been represented by showing their souls leaving their bodies but maintaining the same physical aspects." See Tscherkassky, "Poet of Images," 173.

45 Curiously, Technicolor has of course demonstrated a far greater resistance to chromatic deterioration than other postwar film stocks, such as Kodachrome.

46 Truffaut, *Films in My Life*, 149.

47 Hoberman, *Vulgar Modernism*, 248.

48 Elsaesser, "Tales of Sound and Fury," 53.

49 Mary Beth Haralovich notes of Sirk's use of color: "While the realist narrative space provides 'normal' sources for all the colors, *All That Heaven Allows* also uses the ability of color to function as an emphasis in itself: as spectacle, as excess, and as potentially distractive of the primacy of narration." Haralovich, "*All That Heaven Allows*," 70–71.

50 Müller, "Mes films s'écartent de cette vision des choses," 306.

51 Jacobson, "Matthias Müller," 45; translation mine.

52 Fassbinder, "Imitation of Life," 89.

53 Müller has stated that "I feel very close to melodrama. . . . It is very important to me that my films produce a great emotional effect." Müller, "Mes films s'écartent de cette vision des choses," 306; translation mine.

54 See Dyer, *Heavenly Bodies*, 141–94; and La Valley, "Great Escape," 33.

55 Farmer, *Spectacular Passions*, 176.

56 Philippe Ariès notes, "Beginning in the eighteenth century, the *memento mori* that had previously been objects of piety became mourning lockets. Their purpose was not so much to help prepare the wearer for death, but to perpetuate the memory of the deceased." Ariès, *Images of Man and Death*, 243–47. *Memento Mori* is dedicated to Greg Robbins and David Feinberg.

57 Dickinson, *Complete Poems of Emily Dickinson*, 489.

58 Chin, "Super-8 and the Aesthetics of Intimacy."

59 Zimmermann, *Reel Families*, 154. Matthias Müller speaks of his embrace of Super-8 as a redemption of an ideologically circumscribed format: "First of all it was an old, home-movie, amateur gauge for fathers whose reactionary films all looked alike in a permanent repetition of themes: family, holidays, Christmas. We had to free Super-8 from the cliché that it could only be used for individual memory." Hoolboom, "Old Children and AIDS," 90.

60 John Belton notes: "Even though CinemaScope remained associated with classical narrative films, it introduced a level of visual spectacle that often threatened to overwhelm the narrative. This threat could be contained only by a shift in terms of the kinds of films that were made—a shift to historical spectacle—which functioned to naturalize pictorial spectacle." Belton, *Widescreen Cinema*, 194.

61 Belton notes the specific tension between realism and spectacle in the exploitation of these film technologies: "The 'greater realism' produced by the new

technology was understood, it would seem, as a kind of excess, which was in turn packaged as spectacle." Belton, *Widescreen Cinema*, 195.

62 For a cogent account of such memorializing practices, see Watney, *Imagine Hope*, 163–68.

63 James notes: "The underground's opposition to Hollywood was accompanied by dialogues with it, which make clear that while the underground may have been inspired and stylistically nourished by extra-industrial priorities, by other art forms, and preeminently by social developments, the most significant determinant upon it was Hollywood itself." See James, *Allegories of Cinema*, 141.

64 Following James's revisionist lead, Juan A. Suárez argues that the underground films of Anger, Smith, and Warhol must be understood in the context of their use of mass culture and their engagement with gay cultural practices. See Suárez, *Bike Boys*.

65 Arthur, "Lost and Found," 17.

6. The Corporeal Implication of Witnessing

1 Lombardo, "Cruellement bleu," 133.

2 Experimental cinema has a long tradition of "cameraless" filmmaking, most notably the work of Stan Brakhage, Len Lye, Oskar Fischinger, and Man Ray. Digital film technology now has also made this kind of film production prevalent in mainstream cinema.

3 Wees, *Light Moving in Time*, 54; emphasis added.

4 Smith, "Blue and the Outer Limits," 19.

5 Darke, "*Blue*," 41. Darke thus connects *Blue* to structuralist filmmaking like Hollis Frampton's *Hapax Legomena II: Poetic Justice* (1972), in which filmed pages of a rudimentary script displace the responsibility of visualization from the filmmaker onto the viewer.

6 Walter Ruttmann's twelve-minute sound montage over a black screen combines the sounds, speech fragments, and silence of a Berlin weekend during the Weimar period.

7 See Petley, "Lost Continent."

8 See Driscoll, "Rose Revived"; Iles, "Derek Jarman"; and O'Pray, "New Romanticism."

9 Kenneth Anger's wordless "magick" films were an important early cinematic influence on Jarman during his years at the Slade School of Art. See Peake, *Derek Jarman*, 112.

10 Quoted in Watson, "Archaeology of Soul," 47.

11 Quotes taken from Watson, "Archaeology of Soul," 47; and Sexton, "St. Derek."

12 Macdonald, "Gay Champion Dies."

13 Watney, "Derek Jarman," 119.

14 See Peake, *Derek Jarman*, 415.

15 Watney labelled him a "Queer William Morris of the '90s," who also belonged to

"the England of the Elizabethan philosopher/astrologer John Dee, of the 17th-century diarist and antiquarian John Evelyn and the mystic and medical man Sir Thomas Browne, and of the metaphysical poets—John Donne, George Herbert, Henry Vaughan." Watney, "Derek Jarman," 85.

16 Quoted in Calhoun, "Genius of Derek Jarman," 14.

17 Andrew Moor argues that this and other similar paintings constitute an intertextual antimony to *Blue*: "Blue and red, spirit and matter, segregated into different media: the gap between these regimes is seemingly unbreachable in Jarman's final output." Moor, "Spirit and Matter," 64. Yet Moor's dichotomization between the film and the paintings neglects both the complexity of affect in *Blue* and the visceral experience it produces for its viewers.

18 Quoted in Brown, "Dying Wishes."

19 Jarman's innovative garden at Dungeness arguably broadened his appeal in Britain more than any other aspect of his work. Isaac Julien notes that the garden now attracts over 250,000 visitors each year. Julien, "Derek Jarman," 29.

20 Barber, "Derek Jarman."

21 On Jarman's canonization, see Peake, *Derek Jarman*, 484–85.

22 Peake suggests the 1974 Klein exhibit at the Tate Gallery as the probable catalyst. See Peake, *Derek Jarman*, 196.

23 Quoted in Stich, *Yves Klein*, 77.

24 Blue has also historically been the most tangible color in an economic sense due to the rarity and expense of premodern blue pigments like lapis lazuli. Since their use in commissioned artwork constituted an act of conspicuous consumption, these pigments came to function as materialist fetishes, as much abstract as representational. Jarman imaginatively engages with this history of lapis lazuli in the spoken script of *Blue*. For an extensive material history of the color blue, see Pastoureau, *Blue*.

25 In his deobjectifying use of blue, Klein ironically appropriated a color long-prized not only for its economic value but also for its symbolic significance in Western art. Since the late Middle Ages, blue has been associated with the melancholy of the Virgin Mary. See Pastoureau, *Blue*, 49–84.

26 Stich, *Yves Klein*, 78.

27 Quoted in Peake, *Derek Jarman*, 398.

28 After a second performance in London, the event traveled without Jarman to Bari, Ghent, Rome, Berlin, and Tokyo to generate the kind of cultural interest that would facilitate the eventual funding of the film.

29 As the two most expensive materials available to the artist in the late Middle Ages and the Renaissance, lapis lazuli and gold leaf were frequently combined in commissioned works of art.

30 The film script omits the initial four pages of the chapter "Into the Blue" from Jarman's *Chroma* (103–6), which present a parataxis of blue associations, ranging from the "black blue sadness in Geertgen's *Nativity at Night*" to "the blues of Japan. The work clothes, the blue of the roofs of its houses." This opening sec-

tion of the chapter also includes the only mention of Klein: "The great master of blue—the French painter Yves Klein. No other painter is commanded by blue, though Cézanne painted more blues than most" (104).

31 Jarman shared Klein's intense passion for alchemy, which is present in many of his films. Tony Peake traces the origins of Jarman's early interest in alchemy to his research on sixteenth-century alchemists that he carried out as a set designer for Ken Russell's *The Devils* (1971). See Peake, *Derek Jarman*, 190–92.

32 This was perhaps a sly homage on Jarman's part to Klein's famous postcard invitations to a double show he put on at the Iris Clert and Collette Allendy galleries in 1957. Although Klein painted over all the stamps with International Klein Blue, the French postal system franked and processed all the postcards.

33 Del Re, "Blue CD-Rom," 45.

34 Metz, *Imaginary Signifier*, 43.

35 Schwenger, "Derek Jarman," 421.

36 Although the history of experimental cinema has produced key champions of sound, including Dziga Vertov, Hollis Frampton, and Michael Snow, it has been largely dominated until quite recently by filmmakers dedicated to what Melissa Ragona dubs "the phenomenal purity of visual experience." Ragona, "Hidden Noise," 98.

37 Chion, *Voice in Cinema*, 3.

38 Although it is grounded in the consideration of narrative cinema, Chion's theorization of film sound remains pertinent for analyzing experimental film, since the history of the latter cannot be understood outside its dialectical relationship to narrative film, which, as the dominant mode of cinema, has historically shaped the habits and assumptions of film spectatorship.

39 Chion uses the example of Fritz Lang's Dr. Mabuse in *Das Testament des Dr. Mabuse/ The Testament of Dr. Mabuse* (1932), who is the voice of an absent yet omniscient body, ultimately revealed to be no more than a microphone behind a screen. In this way, Mabuse is literally a metaphor for cinema. See Chion, *Voice in Cinema*, 17–29.

40 Ricco, *Logic of the Lure*, 47.

41 I am indebted to Tina Lee for this insight. The blue screen in fact masks a more fundamental and unsettling sign of lack: electronic noise, with its snowy image and monotonous buzz.

42 Chion, *Voice in Cinema*, 51; emphasis original.

43 *Live Blue Roma (The Archaeology of Sound)*, Mute Records, 1995.

44 Chion, *Voice in Cinema*, 53.

45 See Spector, *Felix Gonzalez-Torres*, 139–78.

46 Smith, "Blue and the Outer Limits," 19.

47 In this sense, watching *Blue* mirrors the experience of encountering one of James Turrell's light installations. See Richard, "James Turrell."

48 Marks, *Skin of the Film*, 162.

49 Marks explains the concept of "intercultural cinema" in the following terms: "'Intercultural' means that a work is not the property of one culture, but medi-

ates in at least two directions. It accounts for the encounter between different cultural organisations of knowledge, which is one of the sources of intercultural cinema's synthesis of new forms of expression and new kinds of knowledge." Marks, *Skin of the Film*, 7.

50 Schwenger, "Derek Jarman," 420.

51 Marks discusses synesthesia as another significant dynamic in intercultural cinema. See Marks, *Skin of the Film*, 213.

52 I have transcribed these words from film since the published film script omits the whispered refrain of names from this section.

53 The trope of "walking out of life" recurs several times in the script.

54 Clive Myer, e-mail to author, 23 February 2008. Myer lived at the time in a remote part of Wales that had no television reception.

55 Several queer artists also turned to a conceptually oriented visual iconoclasm in their moving image installations about AIDS. Jonathan Horowitz's video installation *Countdown* (1995) challenges the sentimental pedagogy of Jonathan Demme's *Philadelphia* by blocking virtually the entire image track of the original film with white mattes imprinted with transparent ascending numbers. Horowitz's decision to determine the pace of the numerical toll by tying it to the cuts in Demme's film not only urges viewers to consider what this particular text *cuts* out but also foregrounds the limitations and problems of turning to statistical information to communicate the magnitude of AIDS. Despite its rhetorical force, the use of a numerical toll necessarily involves a systematic abstraction and objectification of bodies and lives that merely become information.

Focusing its visual iconoclasm on words rather than numbers, Yann Beauvais's video installation *Tu, sempre* (You, always) (2001) elaborates on AIDS as an epidemic of signification by spatializing it. The installation involves streams of AIDS discourses, including autobiographical, activist, and scientific texts, which are projected onto a screen that rotates in a gallery space. Since one side of this rotating screen is a mirror, these streams are refracted around the gallery space. Visitors are caught in the apparatus, not only surrounded by the incessant flow of AIDS discourse but also subject to its very projection on their bodies.

56 The installation was also exhibited in a group show at the Andrea Rosen Gallery in New York from 11 July to 11 August 1995.

57 Jonathan Kahana, e-mail to author, 28 February 2008. For the theatrical premiere of the film in December 1993, the producer James McKay had requested that the Walker "play the sound a fair bit louder than you would on a dialogue film. Loud but not painfully so." Letter to Bruce Jenkins, 1 December 1993, Walker Art Center Archive.

58 These technical details are taken from Murphy's instructions, which have been archived by the Walker.

59 Moviegoers can also walk out of the theater before the screening has ended, but doing so constitutes more of a deliberate act of resistance to the work than does exiting a gallery installation after only a short period.

60 Billed as "a national day of mourning and action in response to the AIDS crisis,"

the Day without Art was launched in 1989 by the recently formed arts organization Visual AIDS. Over eight hundred institutions in the United States participated in the first year. Programming ranged from the temporary closure of institutions and the removal of artworks to the exhibition of art about AIDS and the organization of HIV/AIDS education events. Visual AIDS changed the name to Day with(out) Art in 1997, "to highlight the proactive programming of art projects by artists living with HIV/AIDS, and art about AIDS, that was taking place across the country. It had become clear that active interventions within the annual program were far more effective than actions to negate or reduce the programs of cultural centers." Day with(out) Art, www.thebody.com/visualaids/dwa (accessed 3 March 2008). For a critique of Day without Art, see Crimp, *Melancholia and Moralism*, 166–68.

61 Jessica Weiss, "Campus Artwork Cloaked in Black," *Michigan Daily*, 2 December 1999.

62 Julien, "Derek Jarman," 29.

63 Swinton, "Letter to an Angel."

64 Brooke, "*Blue*," 85.

Afterword

1 See Jenkins, *Convergence Culture*, 1–24. Jenkins's analysis of this new "participatory culture" (3) acknowledges that any understanding of its potential for political and cultural resistance must be understood in relation to the attempts by new media businesses to "harness" the commercial power of such "collective intelligence" (20).

2 Green and Jenkins, "Moral Economy of Web 2.0."

3 The roots of such media piracy can be traced to the work of certain independent documentary videomakers in the 1990s, whom Patricia Zimmermann has named "Pirates of the New World Image Orders." See Zimmermann, *States of Emergency*, 154–97.

4 See Gregory, "Transnational Storytelling," 199–201.

5 The DIVA TV netcasts are available at www.actupny.org/divatv/netcasts/index.html. Bob Huff's videos are available on YouTube at youtube.com/user/bobinevu (both accessed 28 April 2008).

6 See Cvetkovich, *Archive of Feelings*, 162; and Hilderbrand, "Retroactivism," 310. Alisa Lebow also mentions it in Alexandra Juhasz's video *Video Remains*.

7 Quoted in Schmelling, "Documenting Social Change."

8 For an elaboration of her critique of such narratives, see Schulman, *Stagestruck*.

9 Sarah Schulman, interview with author, 17 August 2005. All subsequent Schulman quotations are taken from this interview, unless otherwise indicated.

10 ACT UP Oral History Project, home page of project Web site. www.actuporalhistory.org/index1.html (accessed 28 April 2008).

11 Bethany Winkler, e-mail to Dudley Saunders, 15 August 2005.

12 As of August 2008, there were one hundred completed interviews and seventy-seven available on the Web site. Schulman notes that funding continues to be intermittent and that support has come from lesbians (working at major foundations) rather than from gay men (e-mail to author, 28 August 2008).

13 Sarah Schulman, e-mail to author, 28 August 2008.

14 Jim Hubbard, e-mail to author, 17 August 2005.

15 Manovich, *Language of New Media*, 218.

16 After its institutional move to a permanent home at the University of Southern California (USC) in 2006, the organization changed its full name from the Survivors of the Shoah Visual History Foundation to the USC Shoah Foundation Institute for Visual History and Education.

17 See Carlson, "Index of Horror."

18 Drawing on his experience using the full online archive at the University of Southern California, Noah Shenker has noted the risks of distraction in its interface: "The fact that multiple cognitive tasks converge around the use of the database screen raises the issue of how the archive positions sustained viewing of testimony. In my experience with both individual and classroom uses of the database, the close proximity of viewing and search options has posed a hindrance to allowing survivor stories to unfold as they were originally recorded." Shenker, "Searching for Memory," 9. The redesign of the public Web site in 2007 included changes to the interface of the "Online Testimony Viewer" that permitted the user to shift to full-screen mode when viewing the talking head testimonies, which could mitigate distraction, but it was still an option that the user would have to initiate.

19 For a comparison of the witnessing dynamics between the Fortunoff archive and the Shoah Foundation, see Stier, *Committed to Memory*, 93–109.

20 As an example, Schulman cites the discovery that abortion remained the only non-AIDS specific issue that never created division within the group, unlike gay rights, which generated sufficient disagreement within ACT UP to necessitate the formation of a new group, Queer Nation.

21 Ultra Red was formed in 1994 by two ACT UP members, Dont Rhine and Marco Larsen. Originally based in Los Angeles, the collective now has members across North America and Europe and develops sound art practices with a wide range of social movements.

22 Ultra Red, "Time for the Dead."

23 Freire, *Pedagogy of Freedom*, 105.

24 Ultra Red, artist's talk, Art Gallery of Ontario, Toronto, 16 August 2006, available as podcast at www.artmatters.ca/blog/uploads/sounds/mp3/ultra-red1.mp3 (accessed 10 March 2008).

25 The performances have taken place at the Baltimore Museum of Art, the Hammer Museum of Art in Los Angeles, the Banff Centre for the Arts, the Andy Warhol Museum of Art in Pittsburgh, Concordia University in Montreal, Southern Illinois University in Carbondale, the Art Gallery of Ontario in Toronto, and the

Sixteenth International AIDS Conference in Toronto. Ultra Red's Web site (www
.ultrared.org) contains details of the procedures for each performance.

26 Robert Semper, e-mail to the author, 12 March 2008.

27 The minutes are available at www.ultrared.org/publicrecord/archive (accessed 10
March 2008).

28 Robert Semper, e-mail to the author, 12 March 2008.

□

Bibliography

Aaron, Michele. *New Queer Cinema: A Critical Reader*. Edinburgh: University of Edinburgh Press, 2004.

Achmat, Zackie. "My Childhood as an Adult Molester: A Salt River Moffie." In *Defiant Desire: Gay and Lesbian Lives in South Africa*, ed. Mark Gevisser and Edwin Cameron, 325–41. Johannesburg: Ravan Press, 1994.

ACT UP Oral History Project (Web site), www.actuporalhistory.org/index1.html.

Agamben, Giorgio. *Remnants of Auschwitz: The Witness and the Archive*. Trans. Daniel Heller-Roazen. New York: Zone, 1999.

Ahlgren, Calvin. "Personal Story Decoded in Bits of Old Footage." *San Francisco Chronicle*, 25 June 1989.

Allen, Dennis. "Homosexuality and Narrative." "Sexuality and Narrative," ed. Judith Roof, special issue, *Modern Fiction Studies* 41, nos. 3–4 (1995): 609–34.

Anbian, Robert. "Phelan Filmmaking Award-Winners Interviewed." *Release Print* (December/January 1988–89): 7, 9, 17–18.

Anderson, Linda. *Autobiography*. New York: Routledge, 2001.

Ariès, Philippe. *Images of Man and Death*. Trans. Janet Lloyd. Cambridge: Harvard University Press, 1985.

Arroyo, José. "Death, Desire, and Identity: The Political Unconscious of 'New Queer Cinema.'" In *Activating Theory: Lesbian, Gay, and Bisexual Politics*, ed. Joseph Bristow and Angela R. Wilson, 70–96. London: Lawrence and Wishart, 1993.

Arthur, Paul. "Lost and Found: American Avant-Garde Film in the Eighties." In *A Passage Illuminated: The American Avant-Garde Film, 1980–1990*, ed. Nelly Voorhuis, 15–29. Amsterdam: Stichting Mecano, 1991.

———. "No Longer Absolute: Portraiture in American Avant-Garde and Documentary Films of the Sixties." In *Rites of Realism: Essays on Corporeal Cinema*, ed. Ivone Margulies, 93–118. Durham: Duke University Press, 2003.

Atkins, Robert. "The Unfashionability of AIDS." *Artery: The AIDS—Arts Forum*, 2000, artistswithaids.org/artery/symposium/symposium_motion.html (accessed 6 November 2007).

Aufderheide, Patricia. "Electronic Public Space." *Progressive*, July 1997, 34–35.

———. "Vernacular Video." *Columbia Journalism Review*, January–February 1995, 46–48.

Barber, Lynn. "Derek Jarman: The Lynn Barber Interview." *Independent on Sunday*, 18 August 1991.

Barthes, Roland. *Roland Barthes by Roland Barthes*. Trans. Richard Howard. London: Macmillan, 1977.

Bazin, André. *What Is Cinema?* 2 vols. Ed. and trans. Hugh Gray. Berkeley: University of California Press, 1967.

Belton, John. *Widescreen Cinema*. Cambridge: Harvard University Press, 1992.

Ben-Levi, Jack. "*Voices from the Front*." *Felix* 1, no. 3 (1993): 113–16.

Bennett, Tony. *The Birth of the Modern Museum: History, Theory, Politics*. London: Routledge, 1995.

Berlant, Lauren, and Elizabeth Freeman. "Queer Nationality." In *Fear of a Queer Planet: Queer Politics and Social Theory*, ed. Michael Warner, 193–229. Minneapolis: University of Minnesota Press, 1994.

Bishop, Claire. *Installation Art: A Critical History*. New York: Routledge, 2005.

Bonet, Eugeni, ed. *Desmontaje: Film, vídeo/apropriación, reciclaje*. Valencia: Institut Valencià d'Art Modern, 1993.

Booth, Mark W. *The Experience of Songs*. New Haven: Yale University Press, 1981.

Bordowitz, Gregg. *The AIDS Crisis Is Ridiculous and Other Writings, 1986–2003*. Cambridge: MIT Press, 2004.

———. "Guest List for a Cocktail Party." *Camerawork* 25, no. 1 (1998): 4–9.

———. "Picture a Coalition." *AIDS Cultural Analysis/Cultural Activism*, ed. Douglas Crimp, 183–96. Cambridge: MIT Press, 1988.

Boulé, Jean-Pierre. "The Postponing of *La Pudeur ou l'Impudeur*: Modesty or Hypocrisy on the Part of French Television?" *French Cultural Studies* 3, no. 9 (1992): 289–304.

Bowen, Peter. "Not in Your Local Listings: Aids Videos and Their Public(s)." *Public Art Issues*, spring 1992, n.p.

Boyle, Deirdre. *Subject to Change: Guerilla Television Revisited*. New York: Oxford University Press, 1997.

Brooke, Michael. "Blue." *Sight and Sound*, October 2007, 85.

Brown, Mick. "The Dying Wishes of Derek Jarman." *Daily Telegraph*, 16 August 1993.

Bruzzi, Stella. *New Documentary: A Critical Introduction*. London: Routledge, 2000.

Bullert, B. J. *Public Television: Politics and the Battle over Documentary Film*. New Brunswick: Rutgers University Press, 1997.

Burch, Noël. *To the Distant Observer: Form and Meaning in the Japanese Cinema*. Berkeley: University of California Press, 1979.

Burke, Peter. *Eyewitnessing: The Uses of Images as Historical Evidence*. Ithaca: Cornell University Press, 2001.

Butler, Judith. "Critically Queer." *GLQ: A Journal of Lesbian and Gay Studies* 1, no. 1 (1993): 17–32.

Butler, Shelley Ruth. *Contested Representations: Revisiting "Into the Heart of Africa."* Amsterdam: Gordon and Breach, 1999.

Calhoun, Dave. "The Genius of Derek Jarman." *Time Out London*, 6 February 2008, 14.

Cardinal, Roger. "Pausing over Peripheral Detail." *Framework*, nos. 30–31 (1986): 112–33.

Carlomusto, Jean. "ACT UP Oral History Project," interview no. 15, 19 December 2002. www.actuporalhistory.org/interviews/images/carlomusto.pdf (accessed 31 January 2009).

Carlomusto, Jean, and Emily Roysdon. "Radiant Spaces: An Introduction to Emily Roysdon's Photograph Series *Untitled*." *GLQ: A Journal of Lesbian and Gay Studies* 10, no. 4 (2004): 671–79.

Carlson, Scott. "An Index of Horror." *Chronicle of Higher Education*, 15 June 2007, 32.

Caruth, Cathy, ed. *Trauma: Explorations in Memory*. Baltimore: Johns Hopkins University Press, 1995.

Caruth, Cathy, and Thomas Keenan, "'The AIDS Crisis Is Not Over': A Conversation with Gregg Bordowitz, Douglas Crimp, and Laura Pinsky." In *Trauma: Explorations in Memory*, ed. Caruth, 256–71. Baltimore: Johns Hopkins University Press, 1995.

Cavenett, Wendy. "William Yang, *Sadness*, between the Lines." *iMagazine*, online publication, www.thei.aust.com/isite/btl/btlinyang.html (accessed 8 February 2004).

Chamberlain, Joy, et al. "'Filling the Lack in Everybody Is Quite Hard Work, Really . . .': A Roundtable Discussion." In *Queer Looks: Perspectives on Lesbian and Gay Film and Video*, ed. Martha Gever, John Greyson, and Pratibha Parmar, 41–60. New York: Routledge, 1993.

Chambers, Ross. *Facing It: AIDS Diaries and the Death of the Author*. Ann Arbor: University of Michigan Press, 1998.

———. "Visitations: Operatic Quotation in Three AIDS Films," *UTS Review* 2, no. 2 (1996): 24–67.

Chapnick, Howard. *Truth Needs No Ally: Inside Photojournalism*. Columbia: University of Missouri Press, 1994.

Chetty, Dhianaraj. "A Drag at Madame Costello's: Cape Moffie Life and the Popular Press in the 1950s and 1960s." In *Defiant Desire: Gay and Lesbian Lives in South Africa*, ed. Mark Gewisser and Edwin Cameron, 115–27. New York: Routledge, 1995.

Chin, Daryl. "Super-8 and the Aesthetics of Intimacy." *Jump Cut*, no. 37 (1992): 78–81.

Chion, Michel. *The Voice in Cinema*. Ed. and trans. Claudia Gorbman. New York: Columbia University Press, 1999.

Chris, Cynthia. "Documents and Counter-documents: AIDS Activist Video at the Crossroads," *Afterimage*, November 1994, 6–8.

Coady, C. A. J. *Testimony: A Philosophical Study*. Oxford: Oxford University Press, 1992.

Cohan, Steven, ed. *Hollywood Musicals: The Film Reader*. New York: Routledge, 2002.

———. *Incongruous Entertainment: Camp, Cultural Value, and the MGM Musical*. Durham: Duke University Press, 2005.

Cohen, Cathy J. *The Boundaries of Blackness: AIDS and the Breakdown of Black Politics.* Chicago: University of Chicago Press, 1999.

Cohen, Lisa. "By Any Genre Necessary." *Village Voice,* 5 April 1994, 70.

Colby, David C., and Timothy E. Cook. "Epidemics and Agendas: The Politics of Nightly News Coverage of AIDS." *Journal of Health Politics, Policy and Law* 16, no. 2 (1991): 215–49.

Corner, John. *The Art of Record: A Critical Introduction to Documentary.* Manchester: Manchester University Press, 1996.

Creekmur, Corey K., and Alexander Doty. Introduction to *Out in Culture: Gay, Lesbian, and Queer Essays on Popular Culture,* ed. Creekmur and Doty, 1–11. Durham: Duke University Press, 1995.

Crimp, Douglas, ed. *AIDS: Cultural Analysis, Cultural Activism.* Cambridge: MIT Press, 1988.

———. *Melancholia and Moralism: Essays on AIDS and Queer Politics.* Cambridge: MIT Press, 2002.

———. "Mourning and Militancy," *October,* no. 51 (1989): 3–18.

Crimp, Douglas, with Adam Rolston. *AIDS Demo Graphics.* Seattle: Bay Press, 1990.

Crimp, Douglas, and Gregg Bordowitz. "A Noun and a Verb." In *Drive: The AIDS Crisis Is Still Beginning,* 29–38. Chicago: WhiteWalls, 2002.

Croucher, Sheila. "South Africa's Democratization and the Politics of Gay Liberation." *Journal of Southern African Studies* 28, no. 2 (2002): 315–30.

Cvetkovich, Ann. *An Archive of Feelings: Trauma, Sexuality, and Lesbian Public Cultures.* Durham: Duke University Press, 2003.

———. "Video, AIDS, and Activism." *Afterimage,* September 1991, 8–11.

Dangerous Bedfellows, eds. *Policing Public Sex: Queer Politics and the Future of AIDS Activism.* Boston: South End Press, 1996.

Danzig, Alex. "Acting Up: Independent Video and the AIDS Crisis." *Afterimage,* May 1989, 5–7.

Darke, Chris. "Blue." *Sight and Sound,* October 1993, 41.

De Waal, Shaun. "Etymological Note: On 'Moffie.'" *Defiant Desire: Gay and Lesbian Lives in South Africa,* ed. Mark Gewisser and Edwin Cameron, xiii. New York: Routledge, 1995.

Deitcher, David. "What Does Silence Equal Now?" In *Art Matters: How the Culture Wars Changed America,* ed. Philip Yenawine, Marianne Weems, and Brian Wallis, 95–125. New York: New York University Press, 1999.

Del Re, Gianmarco. "Blue CD-Rom." *Flash Art* 29, no. 190 (October 1996): 45.

Denizet-Lewis, Benoit. "Double Lives on the Down Low." *New York Times Magazine,* 3 August 2003, 28–33, 48, 52–53.

Derek Jarman: Brutal Beauty. London: Koenig, 2008. Published in conjunction with the exhibition "Derek Jarman: Brutal Beauty" shown at the Serpentine Gallery, London, 23 February–13 April 2008, and curated by Isaac Julien.

Dickinson, Emily. *The Complete Poems of Emily Dickinson.* Ed. Thomas H. Johnson. Boston: Little, Brown, 1960.

Doty, Alexander. *Making Things Perfectly Queer: Interpreting Mass Culture.* Minneapolis: University of Minnesota Press, 1993.

Dovey, Jon. *Freakshow: First Person Media and Factual Television.* London: Pluto, 2000.

Dowsett, Gary, and David McInnes. "Gay Community, AIDS Agencies, and the HIV Epidemic in Adelaide: Theorising 'Post-AIDS.'" *Social Alternatives* 15, no. 4 (1996): 29–32.

Driscoll, Lawrence. "'The Rose Revived': Derek Jarman and the British Tradition." In *By Angels Driven: The Films of Derek Jarman,* ed. Chris Lippard, 65–83. Trowbridge, U.K.: Flicks Books, 1996.

Du Bois, W. E. B. *The Souls of Black Folk.* Chicago: A. C. McClurg, 1903.

Dyer, Richard. *Heavenly Bodies: Film Stars and Society.* New York: St. Martin's Press, 1986.

Egan, Susanna. "Encounters in Camera: Autobiography as Interaction." *Modern Fiction Studies* 40, no. 3 (1994): 593–618.

Ehrenstein, David. "AIDS, Death, and Videotape." *Los Angeles Times,* 14 March 1993.

Elsaesser, Thomas. "Tales of Sound and Fury: Observations on the Family Melodrama." *Home Is Where the Heart Is: Studies in Melodrama and the Woman's Film,* ed. Christine Gledhill, 43–69. London: British Film Institute, 1987.

Epstein, Steven. "AIDS Activism and State Policies in the United States." In *No Name Fever: AIDS in the Age of Globalization,* ed. Maj-Lis Follér and Håkan Thörn, 167–91. Lund: Studentlitteratur, 2005.

Farmer, Brett. "The Fabulous Sublimity of Gay Diva Worship," *Camera Obscura,* no. 65 (2005): 165–99.

———. *Spectacular Passions: Cinema, Fantasy, Gay Male Spectatorships.* Durham: Duke University Press, 2000.

Fassbinder, Rainer Werner. "Imitation of Life: On the Films of Douglas Sirk." *The Anarchy of the Imagination: Interviews, Essays, Notes,* 77–89. Trans. Krishna Winston. Baltimore: Johns Hopkins University Press, 1992.

Felman, Shoshana, and Dori Laub. *Testimony: Crises of Witnessing in Literature, Psychoanalysis, and History.* New York: Routledge, 1992.

Feneley, Stephen. "William Yang and the Art of Society." Australian Broadcasting Corporation (Web site), 1998, www.abc.net.au/arts/visual/stories/s424388.htm (accessed 28 January 2009).

Fettner, Ann Giudici, and William A. Check. *The Truth about AIDS: Evolution of an Epidemic.* New York: Henry Holt, 1984.

Feuer, Jane. *The Hollywood Musical.* 2nd edition. Bloomington: Indiana University Press, 1993.

Foucault, Michel. *The Archaeology of Knowledge.* Trans. A. M. Sheridan Smith. New York: Pantheon, 1972.

———. *Discipline and Punish: The Birth of the Prison.* Trans. Alan Sheridan. New York: Pantheon, 1978,

———. "Politics and the Study of Discourse." In *The Foucault Effect: Studies in Governmentality; With Two Lectures by and an Interview with Michel Foucault,* ed.

Graham Burchell, Colin Gordon, and Peter Miller, 53–72. London: Harvester Wheatsheaf, 1991.

Freeman, Gregory A. "In Search of Death." *Rolling Stone*, 6 February 2003, 44–48.

Freire, Paulo. *Pedagogy of Freedom: Ethics, Democracy, and Civic Courage*. Trans. Patrick Clarke. Lanham, Md.: Rowan and Littlefield, 1998.

Friedman, Susan Stanford. "Women's Autobiographical Selves: Theory and Practice." In *The Private Self: Theory and Practice of Women's Autobiographical Writings*, ed. Shari Benstock, 34–62. Chapel Hill: University of North Carolina Press, 1988.

Fung, Richard. "Shortcomings: Questions about Pornography as Pedagogy." In *Queer Looks: Perspectives on Lesbian and Gay Film and Video*, ed. Martha Gever, John Greyson, and Pratibha Parmar, 355–67. New York: Routledge, 1993.

Fuss, Diana, ed. *Inside/Out: Lesbian Theories, Gay Theories*. New York: Routledge, 1991.

Gaines, Jane M. "Political Mimesis." In *Collecting Visible Evidence*, ed. Gaines and Michael Renov, 84–102. Minneapolis: University of Minnesota Press, 1999.

Gamson, Josh. "Silence, Death, and the Invisible Enemy: AIDS Activism and Social Movement 'Newness.'" *Social Problems* 36, no. 4 (1989): 351–67.

Gever, Martha. "Pictures of Sickness: Stuart Marshall's *Bright Eyes*." In *AIDS Cultural Analysis/Cultural Activism*, ed. Douglas Crimp, 109–26. Cambridge: MIT Press, 1988.

Gever, Martha, John Greyson, and Pratibha Parmar, eds. *Queer Looks: Perspectives on Lesbian and Gay Film and Video*. New York: Routledge, 1993.

Gevisser, Mark. "Mandela's Stepchildren: Homosexual Identity in Post-Apartheid South Africa." In *Different Rainbows*, ed. Peter Drucker, 111–36. London: Gay Men's Press, 2000.

Gilmore, Leigh. *The Limits of Autobiography: Trauma and Testimony*. Ithaca: Cornell University Press, 2001.

Goldin, Nan, ed. *Witnesses: Against Our Vanishing*. New York: Artists Space, 1989.

Gott, Ted, ed. *Don't Leave Me This Way: Art in the Age of AIDS*. Canberra: National Gallery of Australia, 1994.

Gould, Deborah B. "Passionate Political Processes: Bringing Emotions Back into the Study of Social Movements." In *Rethinking Social Movements: Structure, Meaning, and Emotion*, ed. Jeff Goodwin and James M. Jasper, 155–75. Lanham, Md.: Rowman and Littlefield, 2004.

———. "Solidarity and Its Fracturing in ACT UP." *AREA Chicago: Art, Research, Education, Activism*, no. 3 (2006): 10–13.

Graham, Trey. "A Matter of Life and Death." *Washington Blade*, 11 June 1993.

Green, Jesse. "When Political Art Mattered." *New York Times Magazine*, 7 December 2003, 68–74.

Green, Joshua, and Henry Jenkins. "The Moral Economy of Web 2.0." Online paper, 18 March 2008, www.henryjenkins.org/2008/03/the_moral_economy_of_web_20_pa.html.

Gregory, Sam. "Transnational Storytelling: Human Rights, WITNESS, and Video Advocacy." *American Anthropologist* 108, no. 1 (2006): 195–204.

Greyson, John. "Figments; or, The Queen's Sore Throat." Paper presented at Concordia University, Montreal, 19 January 2006.

———. "Pils Slip." *Vertigo* 2, no. 9 (2005): 52–53.

———. "Scoping Boys: Tom Kalin, Andy Fabo, and Mike Hoolboom in Conversation." *MIX* 23, no. 1 (1997): 42–47.

———. "Strategic Compromises: AIDS and Alternative Video Practices." In *Reimaging America: The Arts of Social Change*, ed. Mark O'Brien and Craig Little, 60–74. Philadelphia: New Society Publishers, 1990.

———. *Urinal and Other Stories*. Toronto: ArtMetropole/Power Plant, 1993.

Greyson, John, and David Wall. *Fig Trees*. Oakville, Ontario: Oakville Galleries, 2003.

Grindon, Leger. "Q & A: Poetics of the Documentary Film Interview." *Velvet Light Trap*, no. 60 (2007): 4–12.

Grover, Jan Zita, ed. *AIDS: The Artists' Response*. Columbus: Ohio State University, 1989.

———. "Visible Lesions: Images of the PWA in America." In *Fluid Exchanges: Artists and Critics in the AIDS Crisis*, ed. James Miller, 23–43. Toronto: University of Toronto Press, 1992.

Guerin, Frances, and Roger Hallas, eds. *The Image and the Witness: Trauma, Memory, and Visual Culture*. London: Wallflower Press, 2007.

Gunning, Tom. "The Scene of Speaking: Two Decades of Discovering the Film Lecturer." *Iris*, no. 27 (1999): 67–79.

Haaken, Janice. "The Recovery of Memory, Fantasy, and Desire: Feminist Approaches to Sexual Abuse and Psychic Trauma." *Signs: Journal of Women in Culture and Society* 21, no. 4 (1996): 1069–94.

Hallas, Roger. "'The Face of AIDS': Commodity Compassion and the Global Pandemic." In *What Democracy Looks Like: A New Critical Realism for a Post-Seattle World*, ed. Amy Schrager Lang and Cecelia Tichi, 88–101. New Brunswick: Rutgers University Press, 2006.

———. "The Resistant Corpus: Queer Experimental Film and Video and the AIDS Pandemic." *Millennium Film Journal* 41 (2003): 53–60.

Halperin, David M. *What Do Gay Men Want?: An Essay on Sex, Risk, and Subjectivity*. Ann Arbor: University of Michigan Press, 2007.

Haralovich, Mary Beth. "All That Heaven Allows: Color, Narrative Space, and Melodrama." In *Close Viewings: An Anthology of New Film Criticism*, ed. Peter Lehman, 57–72. Tallahassee: Florida State University Press, 1990.

Haraway, Donna. *Primate Visions: Gender, Race, and Nature in the World of Modern Science*. New York: Routledge, 1988.

Harper, Phillip Brian. "Eloquence and Epitaph: Black Nationalism and the Homophobic Impulse in Responses to the Death of Max Robinson." In *Fear of a Queer Planet: Queer Politics and Social Theory*, ed. Michael Warner, 239–63. Minneapolis: University of Minnesota Press, 1994.

Harrington, Mark. "Some Transitions in the History of AIDS Treatment Activism." In

Acting on AIDS: *Sex, Drugs, and Politics*, ed. Joshua Oppenheimer and Helena Reckitt, 273–86. London: Serpent's Tail, 1997.

Harris, Daniel. *The Rise and Fall of Gay Culture.* New York: Hyperion, 1997.

Hartman, Geoffrey. *The Longest Shadow: In the Aftermath of the Holocaust.* Bloomington: Indiana University Press, 1996.

Hawkins, Peter S. "Naming Names: The Art of Memory and the NAMES Project AIDS Quilt." *Critical Inquiry* 19, no. 4 (1993): 752–79.

Haynes, Todd. "A Gay Kind of Film." *Afterimage*, December 1988, 3.

Hemphill, Essex, ed. *Brother to Brother: New Writings by Black Gay Men.* Boston: Alyson, 1991.

Hilderbrand, Lucas. "Retroactivism." GLQ: *A Journal of Lesbian and Gay Studies* 12, no. 2 (2006): 303–17.

Hirsch, Marianne. "Surviving Images: Holocaust Photographs and the Work of Post-memory." *Yale Journal of Criticism* 14, no. 1 (2001): 5–37.

Hoad, Neville. "Thabo Mbeki's AIDS Blues: The Intellectual, the Archive, and the Pandemic." *Public Culture* 17, no. 1 (2005): 101–28.

Hoberman, J. *Vulgar Modernism: Writing on Movies and Other Media.* Philadelphia: Temple University Press, 1991.

Hoolboom, Mike. "Old Children and AIDS: An Interview with Matthias Müller." *Independent Eye* 11, nos. 2–3 (1990): 89–98.

Hubbard, Jim. "A Report on the Archiving of Film and Video Work by Makers with AIDS," report prepared for Media Network, 1996, www.actupny.org/diva/Archive.html (accessed 6 November 2007).

Hutcheon, Linda, and Michael Hutcheon. *Opera: Desire, Disease, Death.* Lincoln: University of Nebraska Press, 1996.

Iles, Chrissie. "Derek Jarman." In *Derek Jarman: Brutal Beauty*, 64–77. London: Koenig, 2008.

Jacobson, Alexandra. "Matthias Müller, der Maximalist." *Pioniere, Tüftler, Illusionen: Kino in Bielefeld*, ed. Frank Bell, 37–48. Bielefeld: Westfalen Verlag, 1995.

James, David. *Allegories of Cinema: American Film in the Sixties.* Princeton: Princeton University Press, 1988.

Jarman, Derek. *Chroma: A Book of Color.* Woodstock: Overlook Press, 1995.

——. *The Last of England.* London: Constable, 1987.

Jay, Martin. *Downcast Eyes: The Denigration of Vision in Twentieth-Century French Thought.* Berkeley: University of California Press, 1993.

Jenkins, Henry. *Convergence Culture: Where Old and New Media Collide.* New York: New York University Press, 2006.

Juhasz, Alexandra. AIDS TV: *Identity, Community, and Alternative Video.* Durham: Duke University Press, 1995.

——. "Artist's Statement." Press packet for *Video Remains*, 2005, pzacad.pitzer.edu/~ajuhasz/video_remains/cast_crew_statement.html (accessed 30 March 2008).

——. "Interview with Jim Hubbard and Sarah Schulman." *Corpus* 4, no. 1 (2006): 80–87.

———. "Video Remains: Nostalgia, Technology, and Queer Archive Activism." *GLQ: A Journal of Lesbian and Gay Studies* 12, no. 2 (2006): 319–28.

Julien, Isaac. "Derek Jarman (1942–1994): Brutal Beauty." In *Derek Jarman: Brutal Beauty*, 28–31. London: Koenig, 2008.

Jutz, Gabriele. "Die Physis des Films: Techniken der Körperrepräsentation in der Filmavantgarde." In *Unter die Haut: Signaturen des Selbst im Kino der Körper*, ed. Jürgen Felix, 351–64. St Augustin, Germany: Gardez! Verlag, 1998.

Kalin, Tom. "Flesh Histories." In *A Leap in the Dark: AIDS, Art, and Contemporary Politics*, ed. Allan Klusacek and Ken Morrison, 120–35. Montreal: Véhicule Press, 1992.

———. "Identity Crisis: The Lesbian and Gay Experimental Film Festival." *Independent Film and Video Monthly*, January–February 1989, 29.

Keathley, Christian. *Cinephilia and History; or, The Wind in the Trees*. Bloomington: Indiana University Press, 2006.

Kleinhans, Chuck, and Julia Lesage. "Listening to the Heartbeat: Interview with Marlon Riggs." *Jump Cut*, no. 36 (1991): 119–26.

Knee, Adam. "The Feeling of Power: AIDS Activism on/through Video." *Minnesota Review*, no. 40 (1993): 94–101.

Kostenbaum, Wayne. *The Queen's Throat: Opera, Homosexuality, and the Mystery of Desire*. New York: Poseidon Press, 1993.

Kotz, Liz. "Aesthetics of 'Intimacy.'" In *The Passionate Camera: Photography and the Bodies of Desire*, ed. Deborah Bright, 204–15. London: Routledge, 1998.

Kramer, Larry. *Reports from the Holocaust: The Making of an AIDS Activist*. New York: St. Martin's Press, 1999.

Kun, Josh. "Archaeologies of Identity: An Interview with Gregg Bordowitz." N.d. www.tattoojew.com/gregg.html (accessed 15 March 2001).

Kuzniar, Alice A. *The Queer German Cinema*. Stanford: Stanford University Press, 2000.

Landers, Timothy. "Bodies and Anti-bodies: A Crisis in Representation." *Independent Film and Video Monthly*, January–February 1988, 18–24.

Lane, Jim. *The Autobiographical Documentary in America*. Madison: University of Wisconsin Press, 2002.

La Valley, Al. "The Great Escape." *American Film* 10, no. 6 (1985): 28–31.

Lawrence, Amy. "Staring the Camera Down: Direct Address and Women's Voices." In *Embodied Voices: Representing Female Vocality in Western Culture*, ed. Leslie C. Dunn and Nancy A. Jones, 166–78. Cambridge: Cambridge University Press, 1994.

Lebow, Alisa. *First Person Jewish*. Minneapolis: University of Minnesota Press, 2008.

Lejeune, Philippe. "The Autobiographical Contract." In *French Literary Theory Today*, ed. Tzvetan Todorov, 192–222. Cambridge: Cambridge University Press, 1982.

Lesage, Julia. "The Political Aesthetics of the Feminist Documentary Film." *Quarterly Review of Film Studies* 3, no. 4 (1978): 507–23.

Leung, Simon. *Simon Leung: Proposal for The Side of the Mountain: An Opera by Michael Webster and Simon Leung*. Santa Monica: Santa Monica Museum of Art, 2002.

Levi, Primo. *The Drowned and the Saved*. Trans. Raymond Rosenthal. New York: Random House, 1989.

Levin, David Michael. *The Philosopher's Gaze: Modernity in the Shadows of the Enlightenment.* Berkeley: University of California Press, 1999.

Levinas, Emmanuel. "Ethics as First Philosophy." In *The Levinas Reader*, ed. Sean Hand, 75–87. London: Blackwell, 1989.

———. *Totality and Infinity: An Essay on Exteriority.* Trans. Alphonso Lingis. The Hague: Nijhoff, 1979.

Lionnet, Françoise. *Autobiographical Voices: Race, Gender, Self-Portraiture.* Ithaca: Cornell University Press, 1989.

Loftus, Elizabeth. *Eyewitness Testimony.* Cambridge: Harvard University Press, 1979.

Lombardo, Patrizio. "Cruellement bleu." *Critical Quarterly* 36, no. 1 (1994): 131–33.

Long, Thomas L. *AIDS and American Apocalypticism: The Cultural Semiotics of an Epidemic.* Albany: State University of New York Press, 2005.

"Love, AIDS, and Videotape." *On Air Magazine*, June 1993.

Lund, Giuliana. "'Healing the Nation': Medicolonial Discourse and the State of Emergency from Apartheid to Truth and Reconciliation." *Cultural Critique*, no. 54 (2003): 88–119.

Macdonald, Marianne, and Stephen Ward. "Gay Champion Dies on Eve of New Age." *Independent* (London), 21 February 1994.

Manovich, Lev. *The Language of New Media.* Cambridge: MIT Press, 2001.

Marks, Laura U. *The Skin of the Film: Intercultural Cinema, Embodiment, and the Senses.* Durham: Duke University Press, 2000.

———. *Touch: Sensuous Theory and Multisensory Media.* Minneapolis: University of Minnesota Press, 2002.

Marshall, Stuart. "The Contemporary Political Use of Gay History: The Third Reich." In *How Do I Look?: Queer Film and Video*, ed. Bad Object-Choices, 65–89. Seattle: Bay Press, 1991.

———. "Picturing Deviancy." In *Ecstatic Antibodies: Resisting the AIDS Mythology*, ed. Tessa Boffin and Sunil Gupta, 19–36. London: Rivers Oram Press, 1993.

Mason, Mary G. "The Other Voice: Autobiographies of Women Writers." In *Autobiography: Essays Theoretical and Critical*, ed. James Olney, 207–35. Princeton: Princeton University Press, 1980.

Mayne, Judith. *Cinema and Spectatorship.* London: Routledge, 1993.

McBride, Dwight A. *Impossible Witnesses: Truth, Abolitionism, and Slave Testimony.* New York: New York University Press, 2001.

McGovern, Thomas. *Bearing Witness (to AIDS).* New York: Visual AIDS/A.R.T. Press, 1999.

Metz, Christian. *The Imaginary Signifier: Psychoanalysis and the Cinema*, trans. Celia Britton, Annwyl Williams, Ben Brewster, and Alfred Guzzetti. Bloomington: Indiana University Press, 1982.

Meyer, James. "Art of Living: James Meyer Talks with Gregg Bordowitz." *Artforum* June 1995, 89–90, 128.

Meyer, Richard. *Outlaw Representation: Censorship and Homosexuality in Twentieth Century American Art.* Oxford: Oxford University Press, 2002.

————."Rock Hudson's Body." In *Inside/Out: Lesbian Theories, Gay Theories*, ed. Diana Fuss, 259–88. New York: Routledge, 1991.

Miller, Nancy K. "Representing Others: Gender and Subjects of Autobiography." *differences* 6, no. 1 (1994): 1–27.

Monk, Lorraine. *Photographs That Changed the World: The Camera as Witness, The Photograph as Evidence*. New York: Doubleday, 1999.

Mookas, Ioannis. "Culture in Contest: Public TV, Queer Expression, and the Radical Right," *Afterimage*, April 1992, 8–9.

Moor, Andrew. "Spirit and Matter: Romantic Mythologies in the Films of Derek Jarman." In *Territories of Desire: Challenging the Boundaries of Contemporary Queer Culture*, ed. David Alderson and Linda Anderson, 49–67. Manchester: Manchester University Press, 2000.

Morse, Margaret, "Talk, Talk, Talk: The Space of Discourse on Television." *Screen* 26, no. 2 (1985): 2–15.

————. "The Television News Personality and Credibility." In *Studies in Entertainment: Critical Approaches to Mass Culture*, ed. Tania Modleski, 55–79. Bloomington: Indiana University Press, 1986.

Müller, Matthias. "Mes films s'écartent de cette vision des choses." In *Scratch Book, 1983/1998*, ed. Yann Beauvais and Jean-Damien Collin, 302–7. Paris: Light Cone, 1999.

Muñoz, José Esteban. *Disidentifications: Queers of Color and the Performance of Politics*. Minneapolis: University of Minnesota Press, 1999.

Musser, Charles. *The Emergence of Cinema: The American Screen to 1907*. New York: Charles Schribner's Sons, 1990.

Nero, Charles I. "Diva Traffic and Male Bonding in Film: Teaching Opera, Learning Gender, Race, and Nation." *Camera Obscura* 56 (2004): 47–73.

Nichols, Bill. *Blurred Boundaries: Questions of Meaning in Contemporary Culture*. Bloomington: Indiana University Press, 1994.

————. *Representing Reality: Issues and Concepts in Documentary*. Bloomington: Indiana University Press, 1991.

Nogueira, Ana. "The Birth and Promise of the Indymedia Revolution." *From ACT UP to the WTO: Urban Protest and Community Building in the Era of Globalization*, ed. Benjamin Shepard and Ronald Hayduck, 290–97. New York: Verso, 1990.

Odets, Walt. *In the Shadow of the Epidemic: Being HIV-Negative in the Age of AIDS*. Durham: Duke University Press, 1995.

O'Pray, Michael. "'New Romanticism' and the British Avant Garde Film in the Early 1980s." In *The British Cinema Book*, 2nd edition, ed. Robert Murphy, 256–62. London: British Film Institute, 2001.

Orgeron, Devin, and Marsha Orgeron. "Megatronic Memories: Errol Morris and the Politics of Witnessing." In *The Image and the Witness: Trauma, Memory, and Visual Culture*, ed. Frances Guerin and Roger Hallas, 238–52. London: Wallflower Press, 2007.

Osborne, Thomas. "The Ordinariness of the Archive." *History of the Human Sciences* 12, no. 2 (1999): 51–64.

Parker, Andrew, and Eve Kosofsky Sedgwick, eds. *Performativity and Performance.* New York: Routledge, 1995.

Pastoureau, Michel. *Blue: The History of a Color.* Trans. Markus I. Cruse. Princeton: Princeton University Press, 2001.

Patten, Mary. "The Thrill Is Gone: An ACT UP Post-mortem (Confessions of a Former AIDS Activist)." In *The Passionate Camera: Photography and Bodies of Desire,* ed. Deborah Bright, 385–406. New York: Routledge, 1998.

Patton, Cindy. *Inventing AIDS.* New York: Routledge, 1990.

———. "Reconfiguring Social Space." In *Social Postmodernism: Beyond Identity Politics,* ed. Linda J. Nicholson and Steven Seidman, 216–49. Cambridge: Cambridge University Press, 1996.

———. "Safe Sex and the Pornographic Vernacular." *How Do I Look?: Queer Film and Video,* ed. Bad Object-Choics. Seattle: Bay Press, 1991.

———. "Tremble, Hetero Swine!" In *Fear of a Queer Planet: Queer Politics and Social Theory,* ed. Michael Warner, 143–77. Minneapolis: University of Minnesota Press, 1994.

Peake, Tony. *Derek Jarman.* London: Little, Brown, 1999.

Petley, Julian. "The Lost Continent." In *All Our Yesterdays: Ninety Years of British Cinema,* ed. Charles Barr, 98–119. London: British Film Institute, 1986.

Phelan, Peggy. *Mourning Sex: Performing Public Memories.* New York: Routledge, 1997.

Posel, Deborah. "'Getting the Nation Talking About Sex': Reflections on the Politics of Sexuality and 'Nation-Building' in Post-Apartheid South Africa." Paper presented for the On the Subject of Sex seminar series, Wits Institute for Social and Economic Research, University of Witwatersrand, 25 February 2002.

Powers, Samantha. "The AIDS Rebel." *New Yorker,* 19 May 2003, 54–67.

Ragona, Melissa. "Hidden Noise: Strategies of Sound Montage in the Films of Hollis Frampton." *October,* no. 109 (2004): 96–118.

Reid, Roddey. "UnSafe at Any Distance: Todd Haynes' Visual Culture of Health and Risk." *Film Quarterly* 51, no. 3 (1998): 32–43.

Renov, Michael. *The Subject of Documentary.* Minneapolis: University of Minnesota Press, 2004.

Rhodes, John David. "Allegory, Mise-en-Scène, AIDS: Interpreting *Safe*." In *The Cinema of Todd Haynes: All That Heaven Allows,* ed. James Morrison, 68–78. London: Wallflower Press, 2007.

Ricco, John Paul. *The Logic of the Lure.* Chicago: University of Chicago Press, 2002.

Rich, B. Ruby. "New Queer Cinema." *Sight and Sound,* September 1992, 30–34.

Richard, Frances. "James Turrell and the Nonvicarious Sublime." In *On the Sublime: Mark Rothko, Yves Klein, and James Turrell,* 85–107. Berlin: Deutsche Guggenheim, 2001.

Robins, Steven. "'Long Live Zackie, Long Live': AIDS, Activism, Science, and Citizenship After Apartheid." *Journal of Southern African Studies* 30, no. 3 (2004): 651–72.

Rofes, Eric. *Dry Bones Breathe: Gay Men Creating Post-AIDS Identities and Cultures.* New York: Hayworth Press, 1998.

Román, David. *Acts of Intervention: Performance, Gay Culture, and AIDS.* Bloomington: Indiana University Press, 1998.

————. "Not-About-AIDS." *GLQ: A Journal of Lesbian and Gay Studies* 6, no. 1 (2000): 1–28.

Rosenberg, Tina. "In South Africa, a Hero Measured by the Advance of a Deadly Disease." *New York Times*, 13 January 2003.

Rubin, Martin. *Showstoppers: Busby Berkeley and the Tradition of Spectacle*. New York: Columbia University Press, 1993.

Russell, Catherine. *Experimental Ethnography: The Work of Film in the Age of Video*. Durham: Duke University Press, 1999.

Saalfield, Catherine. "On the Make: Activist Video Collectives." *Queer Looks: Perspectives on Lesbian and Gay Film and Video*, ed. Martha Gever, John Greyson, and Pratibha Parmar, 21–37. New York: Routledge, 1993.

————. "Positive Propaganda: Jean Carlomusto and Gregg Bordowitz on AIDS Media." *Independent Film and Video Monthly*, December 1990, 19–21.

————. "*Tongues Untied*: Homophobia Hamstrings PBS." *Independent Film and Video Monthly*, October 1991, 4.

Saalfield, Catherine, and Ray Navarro. "Shocking Pink Praxis: Race and Gender on the ACT UP Frontlines." In *Inside/Out: Lesbian Theories, Gay Theories*, ed. Diana Fuss, 341–69. New York: Routledge, 1991.

Said, Edward. *Orientalism*. London: Peregrine, 1987.

Sanger, Kerran L. *"When the Spirit Says Sing!": The Role of Freedom Songs in the Civil Rights Movement*. New York: Garland, 1995.

Schmelling, Sarah. "Documenting Social Change: NIH Seminar Details History of ACT UP." *NIH Record*, 7 September 2007, 1, 8.

Schoonakker, Bonny. "AIDS Warrior Finds Love and Ends Drug Fast." *Sunday Times* (South Africa), 31 August 2003.

Schulman, Sarah. *Stagestruck: Theater, AIDS, and the Marketing of Gay America*. Durham: Duke University Press, 1998.

Schwartz, Vanessa R. "Cinematic Spectatorship Before the Apparatus: The Public Taste for Reality in Fin-de-Siècle Paris." In *Viewing Positions: Ways of Seeing Film*, ed. Linda Williams, 87–113. New Brunswick: Rutgers University Press, 1994.

Schwenger, Peter. "Derek Jarman and the Colour of the Mind's Eye." *University of Toronto Quarterly* 65, no. 2 (1996): 419–26.

Scott, Joan. "The Evidence of Experience." In *The Lesbian and Gay Studies Reader*, ed. Henry Abelove, Michèle Aina Barale, and David M. Halperin, 397–415. New York: Routledge, 1993.

Seckinger, Beverly, and Janet Jakobsen. "Love, Death, and Videotape: *Silverlake Life*." In *Between the Sheets, in the Streets: Queer, Lesbian, Gay Documentary*, ed. Chris Holmlund and Cynthia Fuchs, 144–57. Minneapolis: University of Minnesota Press, 1997.

Sedgwick, Eve Kosofsky. "Queer Performativity: Henry James's *The Art of The Novel*." *GLQ: A Journal of Lesbian and Gay Studies* 1, vol. 1 (1993): 1–16.

Sekula, Allan. "The Body and the Archive." *October* 39 (winter 1986): 3–64.

Sexton, David. "St. Derek of Dungeness." *Sunday Telegraph*, 21 April 1996.

Shattuc, Jane. *The Talking Cure: TV Talk Shows and Women.* New York: Routledge, 1997.

Shenker, Noah. "Searching for Memory: The Pedagogical and Narrative Possibilities of Holocaust Testimony in the Survivors of the Shoah Visual History Archive." Paper presented at the South Atlantic Modern Language Association, Roanoke, Virginia, 12–14 November 2004.

Shepard, Benjamin, and Ronald Hayduk, eds. *From ACT UP to the WTO: Urban Protest and Community Building in the Era of Globalization.* New York: Verso, 2002.

Shilts, Randy. *And the Band Played On: Politics, People, and the AIDS Epidemic.* New York: St. Martin's Press, 1987.

Sitney, P. Adams. *Visionary Film: The American Avant-Garde, 1943–1978.* 2nd edition. Oxford: Oxford University Press, 1979.

Smith, Paul Julian. "Blue and the Outer Limits." *Sight and Sound,* October 1993, 18–19.

Smyth, Cherry. "Queer Questions." *Sight and Sound,* September 1992, 35–36.

Sobchack, Vivian. "Inscribing Ethical Space: Ten Propositions on Death, Representation, and Documentary." *Quarterly Review of Film Studies* 9, no. 4 (1984): 283–300.

Solomon-Godeau, Abigail. "Inside/ Out." In *Public Information: Desire, Disaster, Document,* 49–61. San Francisco: San Francisco Museum of Modern Art, 1994.

Sontag, Susan. "The Decay of Cinema." *New York Times Magazine,* 25 February 1996, 60–61.

Specter, Michael. "Higher Risk." *New Yorker,* 23 May 2005, 38–45.

Spector, Nancy. *Felix Gonzalez-Torres.* New York: Guggenheim Museum, 1995.

Spencer, Jon Michael. *Protest and Praise: Sacred Music of Black Religion.* Minneapolis: Fortress Press, 1990.

Stam, Robert. "Television News and Its Spectator." In *Film and Theory: An Anthology,* ed. Stam and Toby Miller, 361–80. Malden, Mass.: Blackwell, 2000.

Stein, Arlene. "Whose Memories? Whose Victimhood?: Contests for the Holocaust Frame in Recent Social Movement Discourse." *Sociological Perspectives* 41, no. 3 (1998): 519–40.

Stich, Sidra. *Yves Klein.* Ostfildern, Germany: Cantz, 1994.

Stier, Oren Baruch. *Committed to Memory: Cultural Mediations of the Holocaust.* Amherst: University of Massachusetts Press, 2003.

Straayer, Chris, and Tom Waugh. "Queer Film and Video Festival Forum, Take One: Curators Speak Out." *GLQ: A Journal of Lesbian and Gay Studies* 11, no. 4 (2005): 579–603.

Sturken, Marita. *Tangled Memories: The Vietnam War, the AIDS Epidemic, and the Politics of Remembering.* Berkeley: University of California Press, 1997.

Sturrock, John. *The Language of Autobiography: Studies in the First Person Singular.* Cambridge: Cambridge University Press, 1993.

Suárez, Juan A. *Bike Boys, Drag Queens, and Superstars: Avant-Garde, Mass Culture, and Gay Identities in the 1960s Underground Cinema.* Bloomington: Indiana University Press, 1996.

Sullivan, Andrew. "When Plagues End: Notes on the Twilight of an Epidemic." *New York Times Magazine,* 10 November 1996, 52–62, 76–77, 84.

Swinton, Tilda. "Letter to an Angel." *Guardian*, 12 August 2002.

Tagg, John. *The Burden of Representation: Essays on Photographies and Histories*. Amherst: University of Massachusetts Press, 1988.

Todorov, Tzvetan. *The Poetics of Prose*. Trans. Richard Howard. Ithaca: Cornell University Press, 1977.

Tomso, Gregory. "Bug Chasing, Barebacking, and the Risks of Care." *Literature and Medicine* 23, no. 1 (2004): 88–111.

Tougaw, Jason. "Testimony and the Subjects of AIDS Memoirs." *a/b: Auto/Biography Studies* 13, no. 2 (1998): 235–56.

Treicher, Paula. *How to Have Theory in an Epidemic: Cultural Chronicles of AIDS*. Durham: Duke University Press, 1999.

Trites, Allison. *The New Testament Concept of Witness*. Cambridge: Cambridge University Press, 1977.

Tropiano, Stephen. *The Prime Time Closet: A History of Gays and Lesbians on TV*. New York: Applause, 2002.

Truffaut, François. *The Films in My Life*. Trans. Leonard Mayhew. New York: Simon and Schuster, 1978.

Tscherkassky, Peter. "A Poet of Images." In *Trenta-Sesto Mostra Internazionale del Nuovo Cinema*, 167–86. Milan: Castoro, 2000.

Ultra Red. "Time for the Dead to Have a Word with the Living: The AIDS Uncanny." *Journal of Aesthetics and Protest* 1, no. 4 (2005): 82–94.

Van Fuqua, Joy. "Tell the Story: AIDS in Popular Culture." PhD diss., University of Pittsburgh, 1997.

Wainberg, Milton L., Andrew J. Kolodny, and Jack Drescher, eds. *Crystal Meth and Men Who Have Sex with Men: What Mental Health Care Professionals Need to Know*. New York: Haworth Medical Press, 2006.

Wald, Patricia. *Contagious: Cultures, Carriers, and the Outbreak Narrative*. Durham: Duke University Press, 2008.

Walker, Janet. *Trauma Cinema: Documenting Incest and the Holocaust*. Berkeley: University of California Press, 2005.

Warren, Steve. "Film: Silverlake Life." *Au Courant*, 17 May 1993.

Watney, Simon. "Art AIDS NYC." *Art and Text*, no. 38 (1991): 59–98.

———. "Derek Jarman, 1942–94: A Political Death." *Artforum*, May 1994, 84–85, 119, 125.

———. *Imagine Hope: AIDS and Gay Identity*. London: Routledge, 2000.

———. *Policing Desire: Pornography, AIDS, and the Media*. Minneapolis: University of Minnesota Press, 1987.

———. *Practices of Freedom: Selected Writings on HIV/AIDS*. Durham: Duke University Press, 1994.

———. "Representing AIDS." In *Ecstatic Antibodies: Resisting the AIDS Mythology*, ed. Tessa Boffin and Sunil Gupta, 165–92. London: Rivers Oram Press, 1990.

———. "The Spectacle of AIDS." In *AIDS Cultural Analysis/Cultural Activism*, ed. Douglas Crimp, 71–86. Cambridge: MIT Press, 1988.

Watson, Gray. "An Archaeology of Soul." In *Derek Jarman: A Portrait*, 33–48. London: Thames and Hudson, 1996.

Watson, Steven. *Prepare for Saints: Gertrude Stein, Virgil Thomson, and the Mainstreaming of American Modernism*. New York: Random House, 1999.

Waugh, Thomas. "Mike Hoolboom and the Second Generation of AIDS Films in Canada." In *North of Everything: English-Canadian Cinema Since 1980*, ed. William Beard and Jerry White, 416–29. Alberta: University of Alberta Press, 2002.

———. *The Romance of Transgression in Canada: Queering Sexualities, Nations, Cinemas*. Montreal: McGill-Queen's University Press, 2006.

———. "Walking on Tippy Toes: Lesbian and Gay Liberation Documentary of the Post-Stonewall Period, 1969–84." In *Between the Sheets, in the Streets: Queer, Lesbian, Gay Documentary*, ed. Chris Holmlund and Cynthia Fuchs, 107–24. Minneapolis: University of Minnesota Press, 1997.

Wees, William. *Light Moving in Time: Studies in the Visual Aesthetics of Avant-Garde Film*. Berkeley: University of California Press, 1992.

———. *Recycled Images: The Art and Politics of Found Footage Films*. New York: Anthology Film Archives, 1993.

Weiss, Jessica. "Campus Artwork Cloaked in Black." *Michigan Daily*, 2 December 1999.

White, Ian. "Stuart Marshall." *Lux Online*, www.luxonline.org.uk/artists/stuart_marshall/essay(1).html (accessed 7 November 2007).

White, Patricia. *UnInvited: Classical Hollywood Cinema and Lesbian Representability*. Bloomington: Indiana University Press, 1999.

Willemen, Paul. *Looks and Frictions: Essays in Cultural Studies and Film Theory*. London: British Film Institute, 1994.

Williams, Raymond. *Marxism and Literature*. Oxford: Oxford University Press, 1977.

Winston, Brian. *Claiming the Real: The Documentary Film Revisited*. London: British Film Institute, 1995.

Wolf, Matt, and Marvin J. Taylor. "On Fandom and Smalltown Boys." *GLQ: A Journal of Lesbian and Gay Studies* 10, no. 4 (2004): 657–70.

Woods, Donald. "Prescription." In *Brother to Brother: New Writings by Black Gay Men*, ed. Essex Hemphill, 162–64. Boston: Alyson, 1991.

Wright, Kevin B. "AIDS, the Status Quo, and the Elite Media: An Analysis of the Guest Lists of *The MacNeil/Lehrer News Hour* and *Nightline*." In *Power in the Blood: A Handbook on AIDS, Politics, and Communication*, ed. William N. Elwood, 281–92. Mahwah, N.J.: Lawrence Erlbaum, 1999.

Zimmermann, Patricia R. *Reel Families: A Social History of Amateur Film*. Bloomington: Indiana University Press, 1995.

———. *States of Emergency: Documentaries, Wars, Democracies*. Minneapolis: University of Minnesota Press, 2000.

Zipes, Jack. Afterword to *Arabian Nights: The Marvels and Wonders of the Thousand and One Nights*, ed. Zipes, 584–91. New York: Signet, 1991.

□

Index

Roger Hallas is an assistant professor of English
at Syracuse University. He is the coeditor of *The Image
and the Witness: Trauma, Memory, and Visual Culture*.

□

Library of Congress
Cataloging-in-Publication Data
Hallas, Roger, 1970–
Reframing bodies : AIDS, bearing witness, and
the queer moving image / Roger Hallas.
p. cm.
Includes bibliographical references and index.
ISBN 978-0-8223-4583-1 (cloth : alk. paper)
ISBN 978-0-8223-4601-2 (pbk. : alk. paper)
1. Homosexuality in motion pictures.
2. Gay motion picture producers and directors.
3. AIDS (Disease) in motion pictures. I. Title.
PN1995.9.H55H35 2009
791.43′6352664—dc22
2009013113